I0875110

Noninvasive Ventilation Technologies and Healthcare for Geriatric Patients

César Fonseca
Universidade de Évora, Portugal

Manuel José Lopes
Universidade de Évora, Portugal

David Mendes
Universidade de Évora, Portugal

Jose Garcia-Alonso
University of Extremadura, Spain

Felismina Mendes
Universidade de Évora, Portugal

A volume in the Advances in Medical Diagnosis, Treatment, and Care (AMDTC) Book Series

IGI Global
PUBLISHER of TIMELY KNOWLEDGE

Published in the United States of America by
IGI Global
Medical Information Science Reference (an imprint of IGI Global)
701 E. Chocolate Avenue
Hershey PA, USA 17033
Tel: 717-533-8845
Fax: 717-533-8661
E-mail: cust@igi-global.com
Web site: http://www.igi-global.com

Copyright © 2020 by IGI Global. All rights reserved. No part of this publication may be reproduced, stored or distributed in any form or by any means, electronic or mechanical, including photocopying, without written permission from the publisher.
Product or company names used in this set are for identification purposes only. Inclusion of the names of the products or companies does not indicate a claim of ownership by IGI Global of the trademark or registered trademark.

Library of Congress Cataloging-in-Publication Data

Names: Fonseca, César, 1973- editor. | Lopes, Manuel Jose, editor. | Mendes, David, 1966- editor. | Garcia-Alonso, José, editor. | Mendes, Felismina R. P., editor.
Title: Noninvasive ventilation technologies and healthcare for geriatric patients / César Fonseca, Manuel Lopes, David Mendes, José García-Alonso, Felismina Mendes, editors.
Description: Hershey, PA : Medical Information Science Reference (an imprint of IGI Global), [2020] | Includes bibliographical references and index. | Summary: "This book explores noninvasive ventilation technologies and healthcare for geriatric patients"-- Provided by publisher.
Identifiers: LCCN 2019057182 (print) | LCCN 2019057183 (ebook) | ISBN 9781799835318 (hardcover) | ISBN 9781799835325 (ebook)
Subjects: MESH: Noninvasive Ventilation | Aged
Classification: LCC RA575.5 (print) | LCC RA575.5 (ebook) | NLM WF 145 | DDC 363.739/20846--dc23
LC record available at https://lccn.loc.gov/2019057182
LC ebook record available at https://lccn.loc.gov/2019057183

This book is published in the IGI Global book series Advances in Medical Diagnosis, Treatment, and Care (AMDTC) (ISSN: 2475-6628; eISSN: 2475-6636)

British Cataloguing in Publication Data
A Cataloguing in Publication record for this book is available from the British Library.

All work contributed to this book is new, previously-unpublished material.
The views expressed in this book are those of the authors, but not necessarily of the publisher.

For electronic access to this publication, please contact: eresources@igi-global.com.

Advances in Medical Diagnosis, Treatment, and Care (AMDTC) Book Series

ISSN:2475-6628
EISSN:2475-6636

MISSION

Advancements in medicine have prolonged the life expectancy of individuals all over the world. Once life-threatening conditions have become significantly easier to treat and even cure in many cases. Continued research in the medical field will further improve the quality of life, longevity, and wellbeing of individuals.

The **Advances in Medical Diagnosis, Treatment, and Care (AMDTC)** book series seeks to highlight publications on innovative treatment methodologies, diagnosis tools and techniques, and best practices for patient care. Comprised of comprehensive resources aimed to assist professionals in the medical field apply the latest innovations in the identification and management of medical conditions as well as patient care and interaction, the books within the AMDTC series are relevant to the research and practical needs of medical practitioners, researchers, students, and hospital administrators.

COVERAGE

- Medical Testing
- Patient-Centered Care
- Disease Prevention
- Medical Procedures
- Cancer Treatment
- Diagnostic Medicine
- Alternative Medicine
- Chronic Conditions
- Experimental Medicine
- Critical Care

IGI Global is currently accepting manuscripts for publication within this series. To submit a proposal for a volume in this series, please contact our Acquisition Editors at Acquisitions@igi-global.com or visit: http://www.igi-global.com/publish/.

The Advances in Medical Diagnosis, Treatment, and Care (AMDTC) Book Series (ISSN 2475-6628) is published by IGI Global, 701 E. Chocolate Avenue, Hershey, PA 17033-1240, USA, www.igi-global.com. This series is composed of titles available for purchase individually; each title is edited to be contextually exclusive from any other title within the series. For pricing and ordering information please visit http://www.igi-global.com/book-series/advances-medical-diagnosis-treatment-care/129618. Postmaster: Send all address changes to above address. Copyright © 2020 IGI Global. All rights, including translation in other languages reserved by the publisher. No part of this series may be reproduced or used in any form or by any means – graphics, electronic, or mechanical, including photocopying, recording, taping, or information and retrieval systems – without written permission from the publisher, except for non commercial, educational use, including classroom teaching purposes. The views expressed in this series are those of the authors, but not necessarily of IGI Global.

Titles in this Series

For a list of additional titles in this series, please visit:
http://www.igi-global.com/book-series/advances-medical-diagnosis-treatment-care/129618

Biopsychosocial Perspectives and Practices for Addressing Communicable and Non-Communicable Diseases
Simon George Taukeni (University of Namibia, Namibia)
Medical Information Science Reference • © 2020 • 368pp • H/C (ISBN: 9781799821397) • US $265.00

Oncological and Endoscopical Dilemmas in Modern Gynecological Clinical Practice
Konstantinos Dinas (Aristotle University of Thessaloniki, Greece) Stamatios Petousis (Aristotle University of Thessaloniki, Greece) Matthias Kalder (Philipps-University Marburg, Germany) and George Mavromatidis (Aristotle University of Thessaloniki, Greece)
Medical Information Science Reference • © 2020 • 300pp • H/C (ISBN: 9781799842132) • US $345.00

Role of Nutrition in Providing Pro-/Anti-Inflammatory Balance Emerging Research and Opportunities
Uğur Günşen (Bandırma Onyedi Eylül University, Turkey) and Ramazan Mert Atan (Bandırma Onyedi Eylül University, Turkey)
Medical Information Science Reference • © 2020 • 214pp • H/C (ISBN: 9781799835943) • US $235.00

Handbook of Research on Prenatal, Postnatal, and Early Childhood Development
Neriman Aral (Ankara University, Turkey)
Medical Information Science Reference • © 2020 • 470pp • H/C (ISBN: 9781799829522) • US $365.00

Ethnomedicinal Plant Use and Practice in Traditional Medicine
Akash (Gurukul Kangri University, India) Navneet (Gurukul Kangri University, India) and B.S. Bhandari (Garhwal University, India)
Medical Information Science Reference • © 2020 • 380pp • H/C (ISBN: 9781799813200) • US $295.00

For an entire list of titles in this series, please visit:
http://www.igi-global.com/book-series/advances-medical-diagnosis-treatment-care/129618

IGI Global
PUBLISHER of TIMELY KNOWLEDGE

701 East Chocolate Avenue, Hershey, PA 17033, USA
Tel: 717-533-8845 x100 • Fax: 717-533-8661
E-Mail: cust@igi-global.com • www.igi-global.com

Table of Contents

Detailed Table of Contents

Respiratory failure decreases a person's quality of life. Noninvasive ventilation therapy plays a key role in the stabilization of respiratory disease, which translates into evident gains for the patient. The objective of this chapter is to describe the gains and application of NIV and associated respiratory rehabilitation in patients with respiratory failure and the role of rehabilitation nursing. Seven articles were collected from the scientific databases, including only articles made in the last 10 years. The importance of NIV in the stabilization of respiratory disease is consensual. Respiratory rehabilitation is essential for improving respiratory functionality and should be performed during and after crisis. NIV is a therapy with recognized advantages in the control of respiratory failure: it's safe, effective, comfortable for the patient, and applicable to a wide range of events and chronic conditions. Respiratory rehabilitation reduces symptoms, improving quality of life. The rehabilitation nurse has an important role in success.

Non-invasive ventilation is, nowadays, a well received, successful therapeutic strategy for the treatment of different varieties of respiratory failure. Associated to respiratory rehabilitation and exercise training, NVI brings numerous advantages to the person, namely in the control of symptoms, in the quality of life, in the reduction of the perception of dyspnea, in the increase of the tolerance to the activity, and in the decrease in the use of health services. The intervention of the specialist nurse in rehabilitation nursing is essential in order to maximize health gains. However, the bibliography that supports these gains with the intervention of the EEER needs greater investment in the research area.

The objective of this chapter is to analyze articles on the adaptation of the elderly to NIV. The methodology is integrative literature review, using the PICO methodology. After analyzing the content covered, the authors found that there are common factors regarding the adaptation of elderly users to NIV. COPD users are the main users of NIV. This technique promotes an improvement in the quality of life. The introduction of NIV in the user's daily life requires behavioral and lifestyle changes involving health professionals, the user, and caregivers. The choice of the type of ventilator and interfaces is important, in issues such as late assessment of the user's condition and the influence of external factors in adapting to NIV, such as the use of drugs. The adaptation of the elderly user to NIV is influenced by socio-demographic, pathological, anatomical, and associated factors.

The use of invasive mechanical ventilatory support has been increasingly used in the treatment of respiratory insufficiency, since it replaces the respiratory work while reversing the pathological processes that led to its necessity, allowing the recovery of respiratory function. The critical patient's ventilatory weaning requires a rigorous assessment by qualified professionals to reduce complications and the eventual need for (re) intubation, referring to the design and implementation of rehabilitation nursing programs. The nurse specialist in rehabilitation nursing intervenes in an early, autonomous, and differentiated way, avoiding complications and incapacities, promoting effective ventilatory weaning. This integrative review of the literature made evident the gains obtained in the critical patient undergoing invasive mechanical ventilation and included in an early rehabilitation program, revealing significant impact for both the patient and the hospital institution.

The objective of this chapter is to identify the latest evidence on the elderly critical patient with chronic obstructive pulmonary disease. Nine articles were analysed. The effectiveness of NIV has been demonstrated in cases of elderly critically ill patients with acute COPD. Evidence has been shown to decrease hospital stay and mortality, although long-term survival has been shown to be short. The prediction of NIV failure is multifactorial, including very old age, comorbidities, low analytical values of albumin, simplified severity index II, pH < 7.3 of arterial blood, PaCO2

This chapter is a literary review based on the experience of patients with ambulatory oxygen therapy treatment that analysed the way in which this treatment influences patients from an occupational point of view. The relationship of these pathologies and treatments with mental health, especially with depression, anxiety, and stress, is also addressed, with an interest in the treatment of possible functional limitations from the intervention of the discipline of occupational therapy. Oxygen therapy allows patients to continue in their performance contexts, although it can generate new limitations and deficiencies derived from episodes of anxiety and mood disorders, causing greater occupational disfunction. A function-dysfunction process that can be approached from occupational therapy with the aim of minimizing the impact both physical and psychological, enhancing the autonomy and independence of these patients.

The use of non-invasive ventilation (NIV) has markedly increased over the last decades, and NIV has now become an important alternative to invasive ventilation and has gained popularity particularly as treatment option for patients with obstructive sleep apnea, chronic obstructive pulmonary disease (COPD), and acute respiratory failure. The most prominent forms of NIV are noninvasive positive pressure ventilation (NPPV) and the recently introduced high-flow nasal cannula (HFNC) therapy. Many patients who received NIV may also benefit from the administration of pharmaceutical aerosols, typically bronchodilators, which are best delivered without interrupting respiratory support. For example, nowadays, the use of NIV is considered the standard of care for some forms of acute respiratory failure such as COPD exacerbation and acute cardiogenic pulmonary edema. Patients with COPD exacerbation also benefit from inhaled bronchodilator therapy.

Preface

Population aging, the indoor and outdoor exposition to particulates, and harmful agents contribute to the increase of chronic respiratory diseases with a social and economically global impact. The Non-Invasive Ventilation (NIV) is now-a-days a therapeutic resource to which we can associate health gains, but also quality of life and functionality, but these concepts will only make sense if the care processes using NIV are centered on people and their contexts.

The assistance process is an interactive process to which NIV is a part of and, based on this assumption, the objectives laid are not limited to reducing ventilatory effort or improving respiratory parameters. Adherence to therapy, as addressed in this work, provides health professionals with resources and strategies that support care in standards of good practice, but simultaneously challenges the questioning and construction of knowledge. Current data document that in patients with COPD who initiate NIV at home, non-adherence to treatment is close to 10%. Non-adherence is a multifactorial process of which health literacy, the relationship with professionals, and increasing age or self-efficacy are highlighted.

The NIV depends in the increasing technologies that effectively combine method and equipment safety with a user-friendly interface. The relationship between the patient and the equipment is mediated with a device which assesses problems such as loss of effectiveness, discomfort, and integumentary changes. For the authors, the physical relationship between the patient and the equipment is not only a necessary condition for health gains, but also an element that increases self-care. The patient's ability to safely handle the interface combines professional action in teaching and training, with the requirement for safe, compatible and comfortable masks. A care process centered on self-care is seen as a foundation for therapeutic adherence.

The work takes the reader through a sequence of chapters that present NIV in different care contexts, ranging from home care, to patients with COPD, neuromuscular diseases and sleep apnea, to highly complex hospital care such as the treatment of respiratory failure or ventilatory weaning. The specifics of each context are presented in a perspective centered on the patient and the care needs that, associated with NIV, contribute to the objectives of improving the quality of life and functionality.

Respiratory rehabilitation emerges as an area of knowledge with the competence to correct or mitigate respiratory signs and symptoms, thus contributing to optimize the therapeutic results of NIV. Muscle fatigue, asynergies in ventilatory dynamics and airway cleaning are focuses of attention that require continuous monitoring and follow-up and are presented from the perspective of the professionals' skills, and also in the measures for training the patient in effort management and control techniques symptoms. Rehabilitation, understandably centered on the functions of ventilation and breathing, is part of the care process for patients with NIV, but assumes broader objectives such as self-care and participation activities.

Musculoskeletal changes, associated with aging, lead to increased ventilatory work with a consequent reduction in lung capacity and, when associated with immobility or the condition of chronic respiratory disease or neuromuscular disease, create a complex context that has to be included in the diagnostic evaluation, to be the target of specific interventions and results evaluation. Self-care and participation activities require voluntary action and effort aimed at a certain purpose, such a goal must be achieved through the training of specific techniques that associate the lowest energy outflow with maximum efficiency and are reconciled with the implemented ventilatory assistance. Maintaining or recovering musculoskeletal function, is part of the care process and studies show results that need to be strengthened in the sense of evidence regarding the benefits of physical exercise in patients with NIV.

This work would not be complete without reserving a space for deep reflection on non-professional caregivers. Among the health results from NIV, the transition from patients from the hospital to the home, stands out with the consequent adaptation of the family's functions to this condition. Intervention plans, that include teaching, training, communication and monitoring strategies aimed at caregivers, respond to continuity of care and are themselves monitored for safety and results. It is also in the transition from the assistance level, that partnerships in care are made concrete by discussing and sharing the objectives, when jointly defining outcome indicators and analyzing difficulties or obstacles with a view to mitigating them. To be a partner is to participate effectively in the care plan for patients with NIV. Professionals are responsible for using instruments to assess family and non-professional caregivers, in order to monitor resources, their use, and results. The care plan directed to care is therefore dynamic, supported by evidence of good practices and assessed on accountability for the safety of all participants.

The trajectory of care that the authors present constitutes an evidence base that, due to its relevance and innovative perspective, places the reader in a condition of excellence to reflect, analyze, and act on the different contexts where NIV is a therapeutic resource that is not without risks or complications.

Section 1

Promotion of Self-Care and Respiratory Rehabilitation

Chapter 1
Respiratory Rehabilitation Gains in People With Respiratory Insufficiency Submitted to Noninvasive Ventilation:
Systematic Review of Literature

Marco António Polido Jacinto
São Bernardo's Hospital, Portugal

Cheila Reis
São Bernardo's Hospital, Portugal

Tânia Leite
Beatriz Angelo's Hospital, Portugal

César Fonseca
https://orcid.org/0000-0001-6975-612X
Universidade de Évora, Portugal

ABSTRACT

Respiratory failure decreases a person's quality of life. Noninvasive ventilation therapy plays a key role in the stabilization of respiratory disease, which translates into evident gains for the patient. The objective of this chapter is to describe the gains and application of NIV and associated respiratory rehabilitation in patients with respiratory failure and the role of rehabilitation nursing. Seven articles were

DOI: 10.4018/978-1-7998-3531-8.ch001

Copyright © 2020, IGI Global. Copying or distributing in print or electronic forms without written permission of IGI Global is prohibited.

collected from the scientific databases, including only articles made in the last 10 years. The importance of NIV in the stabilization of respiratory disease is consensual. Respiratory rehabilitation is essential for improving respiratory functionality and should be performed during and after crisis. NIV is a therapy with recognized advantages in the control of respiratory failure: it's safe, effective, comfortable for the patient, and applicable to a wide range of events and chronic conditions. Respiratory rehabilitation reduces symptoms, improving quality of life. The rehabilitation nurse has an important role in success.

INTRODUCTION

Respiratory failure consists of the inability of the respiratory system to properly perform blood oxygenation and consequent elimination of carbon dioxide (Ceriana & Nava, 2006). It is associated with chronic respiratory disease or with acute events and affects the activity and quality of life of the person (Ceriana & Nava, 2006; Shu, Mandal and Hart, 2013).

Currently, respiratory failure accounts for 19.3% of hospitalizations in Portugal and 11.8% of deaths (excluding death because of respiratory failure due to lung cancer) (OE, 2018). Thus, it becomes pertinent to approach respiratory failure in a broad perspective, considering gains to the individual (Roque *et al.*, 2014). Noninvasive ventilation (NIV) can be used as treatment intended to correct gas exchange through the application of positive airway pressure (Roque *et al.*, 2014).

NIV can be used in invasive ventilation weaning, thus avoiding muscle fatigue and postextubation respiratory failure, as well as in the context of respiratory failure, whether acute or chronic (Cordeiro & Menoita, 2012; Shu *et al.*, 2013).

The use of resources for noninvasive ventilation dates from the beginning of the nineteenth century, wherein the first ventilators used negative pressure during inspiration by placing the surface of the thorax under subatmospheric pressures (Cordeiro & Menoita2012, OE 2018). It was advantageous to use it in individuals with muscle weakness during the polio epidemic; however, it was expensive and could not be transported, compromising an individual's independence (Cordeiro & Menoita, 2012; OE, 2018).

In the 1940s and 1950s, the NIV technique was developed using positive pressure; however, during the Second World War and in the 1960s and 1970s, it was abandoned due to the development of ventilators and tracheal tubes (Cordeiro & Menoita, 2012). In the 1980s, interest in NIV was resumed for the treatment of acute and chronic respiratory failure, and it was considered the first-line therapy in several acute respiratory diseases (Cordeiro & Menoita, 2012; Faverio *et al.*, 2018).

Currently, NIV is used to manage respiratory changes in both the acute and community phases because it decreases respiratory work, promotes the resting of respiratory muscles, and improves gas exchange (Dyer *et al.*, 2018; Suh *et al.*, 2013).

This therapy can be used in situations of acute or chronic respiratory disease. In the acute phase, it shows benefit in terms of CO_2 retention in individuals with Chronic Obstructive Pulmonary Disease (COPD), pulmonary tuberculosis status, neuromuscular diseases, and anomalies in the thoracic wall (mainly after thoracoplasty and kyphoscoliosis) (Dyer *et al.*, 2018; Suh *et al.*, 2013).

It is also frequently used because it is an asset in situations of acute pulmonary edema or when extubation support is needed[2]. NIV is also indicated in individuals with chronic health conditions or respiratory diseases requiring ventilatory support at home, as in cases of obesity syndrome and chronic symptomatic hypoventilation during sleep (Cordeiro & Menoita, 2012; Dyer *et al.*, 2018).

However, there are contraindications for NIV adaptation, such as cardiorespiratory arrest, coma, severe encephalopathy, severe gastrointestinal bleeding, severe hemodynamic instability, facial surgery or trauma, upper airway obstruction, inability to protect the upper airways and/or high risk of aspiration, excessive secretions in the airways with inability to eliminate them and recent abdominal surgery (Cordeiro & Menoita, 2012).

Among these contraindications, only cardiorespiratory arrest, upper airway obstruction and facial deformities/facial trauma/facial surgery that prevent interface adjustments are considered absolute contraindications for the initiation of NIV (OE, 2018). If NIV is not effective, as in situations of person/ventilator asynchrony, interface intolerance, absence of ventilatory improvement or abundant secretion, invasive mechanical ventilation (IMV) should be used (Cordeiro & Menoita, 2012).

NIV has many advantages for the restoration of gas exchange and respiratory function. Because it avoids the need for orotracheal intubation, it can be performed intermittently and allows speech and swallowing, maintains ventilation with an adapted ventilatory mode, adequate air humidification and heating, and physiological cough and provides easier weaning (Cordeiro & Menoita, 2012; Menadue *et al.*, 2014).

The main advantage is the reduction of the morbidity and mortality rates; however, close monitoring is important because the correction of gas exchange disturbances is performed more slowly and problems related to interfaces, leakage and difficulty accessing the lower airways (in individuals with bronchial hypersecretion) (Cordeiro & Menoita, 2012; Shu *et al.*, 2013) sometimes exist.

Rehabilitation Nurse (RN) play a key role in the implementation, adherence and success of NIV because they can teach the patient about therapy so that the patient will be prepared, choose the appropriate material, verify compliance with the necessary oxygen support, monitor the ventilatory mode considering the hemodynamic status of the affected person, and educate and inform the family and peers about the therapy so that the individual can obtain the greatest benefit from it (Cordeiro & Menoita, 2012).

NSRNs also play a key role in the functional respiratory re-education program (FRR) because it seems to improve exercise tolerance, decrease dyspnea and ensure airway permeability (Cordeiro & Menoita, 2012; Shu *et al.* 2013). FRR should be applied considering the pathology that led to the need for ventilation, as well as the person's tolerance (Cordeiro & Menoita, 2012).

During NIV, FRR aims to promote the person's participation in the program, promote synchronization and adaptation to the interface and ventilator, improve the ventilation/perfusion ratio, maintain airway permeability through secretion mobilization, and prevent/correct positioning (Cordeiro & Menoita, 2012; Shu. *et al.,* 2013). The participation of the person and family involvement in this therapy are essential to its success, and part of NSRN's role is to explain the purpose of NIV and, thus, reduce anxiety and increase confidence in treatment (Cordeiro & Menoita, 2012).

NSRNs should also assist in positioning the patient, performing functional respiratory re-education exercises and optimizing airway clearance through the thinning and elimination of secretions (Cordeiro & Menoita, 2012). Additionally, NSRNs play an important role in preventing and excluding NIV complications such as ventilatory maladaptation, skin ulceration, retention of secretions, decreased SpO_2 or interface intolerance (Cordeiro & Menoita, 2012; Dyer *et al.,* 2018).

NIV presents a notable contribution; however, rehabilitation nursing specialists must apply NIV at the appropriate level for respiratory rehabilitation to have a beneficial effect on the prognosis of the disease, lower the number of exacerbations and lower mortality (OE, 2018).

Thus, the present systematic review of the literature is presented to evaluate the role of rehabilitation, more particularly NSRNs, in the care of persons under NIV.

METHODOLOGY

As a guideline of the systematic review of the literature, the following was elaborated according to the PICO methodology: "What are the gains of respiratory rehabilitation in the person with respiratory failure under NIV?".

After choosing the theme and goal to be reached, the EBSCO platform was searched, and all available databases were selected: *CINAHL Complete; MEDLINE Complete*; *Nursing & Allied Health Collection: Comprehensive; Cochrane Central Register of Controlled Trials; Cochrane Database of Systematic Reviews; Cochrane Methodology Register; Library, Information Science & Technology Abstracts;* and

MedicLatina. The databases Plus (full text), MEDLINE (full text) and B-on were also used from October to November 2018.

The discriminators that were used to start the selection of the articles were verified and validated through the Health Sciences Descriptors (DeCS) platform. Their combination in English was used to increase the spectrum of results, and the discriminators were "*Rehabilitation*", "*Rehabilitation Nursing*", "*Respiratory Insufficiency*", "*Respiratory*", "*Non-Invasive Ventilation*", "*Pulmonary*" and "*Quality of Life*". The search was performed using the boolean operators "*AND*" and "*OR*" and the truncation system with "*".

This review included articles from January 1, 2008, to November 2018, all quantitative or qualitative, whether primary or secondary, to increase the spectrum of literature already produced on the theme. The exclusion criteria included studies that were not indexed in electronic databases, duplicated articles, articles that were not available in full text and articles that were not published in English.

The search carried out in the databases using the interconnection between the various discriminators led to 1,215 articles. However, after applying the inclusion criteria, namely, the time when the article was published and search delimiters, 138 articles were obtained. After reading all the titles, 44 articles were selected, and their abstracts were subsequently read. Thereafter, 34 articles were excluded. Of the 10 articles selected, after their full reading, 7 articles that met the inclusion criteria were selected.

In preparing the review, we considered that, for the surveyed studies to be included in the review, they had to be identified with more than 50% of the items contained in the respective inclusion frameworks of the Joanna Briggs Institute (JBI)

In all our studies, the methodological quality was evaluated through the "FAME" framework of JBI, and we used the same assumption above—that is, for the studies to present a strong methodological quality, they would have to present more than 50% of positive responses in the applied frameworks. Finally, the level of scientific evidence was evaluated, considering the type of study included, using as a guide the frameworks of scientific evidence of efficacy, prognosis and significance of 2014 from JBI. The selected articles are outlined in Table 1.

RESULTS AND DISCUSSION OF RESULTS

After the analysis of the mentioned articles, it is possible to perceive that NIV plays an important role with respect to respiratory failure; according to Faverio *et al.* (2018), when NIV is initiated in the acute phase, it is associated with a higher survival rate in an initial period of 30 days because it promotes better tissue oxygenation.

Table 1. Article selection

	Title of Article	**Study Type - Level of Evidence**
1	Non-invasive ventilation during exercise training for people with chronic obstructive pulmonar disease (review) – Menadue, et al (2014)	1.a
2	Non-invasive ventilation (NIV) as na aid to rehabilitation in acute respiratory disease - Dyer, et al (2011)	3.a
3	Management of acute respiratory failure in interstitial lung diseases: overview and clinical insights - Faverio, et al (2018)	2.a
4	Introducing the national COPD resources and outcomes Project – Stone, et al (2009)	4.d
5	Does the addition of non-invasive ventilation during pulmonary rehabilitation in patients with chronic obstructive pulmonary disease augment patient outcome in exercise tolerance? A literature review - Corner & Garrod (2009)	1.b
6	Audit of acute exacerbations of chronic obstructive pulmonary disease at Waitemata District Health Board, New Zealand - Johnson, et al (2013)	3.b
7	Admission prevention in COPD: non-pharmacological management - Suh, et al (2013)	4.a

According to Dyer *et al.* (2011), going against what was mentioned in the study by Menadue *et al.* (2014), NIV can significantly increase cardiorespiratory fitness and exercise tolerance in individuals with acute exacerbations of chronic respiratory diseases by reducing desaturation during exercise and is a practical, safe and well-tolerated resource. Menadue *et al.* (2014) also point out that NIV may have benefits in terms of increased lower limb work and tolerance to higher intensity exercise, with a reduction in serum lactate in the bloodstream.

Suh *et al.* (2013) reinforce that NIV is well established regarding the treatment of acute hypercapnia, particularly in individuals affected by COPD, and that it reduces hospitalization time and mortality. The same author also mentions that NIV increases the ventilatory response at rest and during exercise compared with room air respiration, resulting in higher volumes and higher expiratory capacity (particularly in severe or very severe patients), corroborating the study by Corner and Garrod (2009) and reducing the sensation of dyspnea.

Contudo Faverio *et al.* (2018) state that, in cases of mild respiratory failure (not necessarily in COPD), NIV may fail as a treatment; yet, the test of the application of this therapy facilitates the recognition of its response, which may lead to better results in the short term.

Suh *et al.* (2013) emphasize that the use of NIV at home was shown to be very beneficial and has significantly reduced the number of recurrent hospitalizations due to acute COPD. However, the same authors also state that the evidence is not yet consistent in this regard and that there is still some disagreement among authors. Some evidence also suggests that NIV improves maximal cardiorespiratory fitness and endurance, but these data are not consistent for other exercise measures and require further investigation according to the study by Menadue *et al.* (2014).

Dyer *et al.* (2011) also state that the selection of cases in which NIV may be used should be judicious because there are cases in which interventions with NIV-assisted exercises involve short-term care, individuals may present clinical fragility or comorbidities, or they may even refuse this therapeutic measure.

According to Corner and Garrod (2009), concerns about NIV and failure in the application of NIV may be directly related to poor adaptation to the chosen interface; according to the authors, nasal interface is the best tolerated interface and the pressure ventilation mode is the most advised. According to the same study, therapy is suggested during exercise; however, this may be impractical and time consuming; thus, the authors refer to the importance of cost-benefit calculation (Corner & Garrod, 2009).

Johnson *et al.* (2013) are in agreement with the other authors, such as Stone *et al.* (2009) and Suh *et al.* (2009), and highlight the importance of information and continuous training of professionals, as well as advocates, regarding the existence of weaning protocols for NIV and education of individuals undergoing this therapy. Johnson *et al.* (2013) further state that follow-up and complementary treatment are essential, as well as the use of spirometry and arterial blood gas tests during therapy.

To complement the treatment of respiratory failure using NIV, Suh *et al.* (2013) state that there are respiratory rehabilitation programs, which are multidisciplinary interventions with evidence-based nutritional follow up aimed at reducing symptoms, optimizing the functional status, increasing individual participation, and reducing health costs through stabilization or reversal of disease manifestations.

Menadue *et al.* (2014) corroborate Suh *et al.* (2013) and mentions that physical training is an important component and aims to increase the physical capacity, improving the relationship between the load and capacity of the respiratory muscles. According to the same authors, this reduces effort-related dyspnea because gas changes affect muscle function, and hypoxemia is associated with muscle weakness and proteolysis, whereas hypercapnia aggravates muscle fatigue and diaphragm endurance (Menadue *et al.*, 2014; Suh *et al., 2013).*

Several authors point to the growing evidence on the usefulness of respiratory rehabilitation in the prevention of exacerbations and in the initial recovery period after exacerbation, with teaching about future warning signs (Johnson *et al.*, 2013; Menadue *et al.*, 2014; Stone *et al.,* 2009; Suh *et al.*, 2013).

Regarding respiratory rehabilitation in individuals with stable COPD, the studies are not consistent; according to Stone *et al.* (2009), the availability of financed rehabilitation programs that are included in health units with multidisciplinary teams is crucial.

CONCLUSION

NIV has several applications and may have benefits in acute or chronic respiratory failure, in health institutions or at home (Suh et al, 2013). NIV reduces muscular effort, increases cardiorespiratory fitness and reduces dyspnea associated with pathology (Dyer *et al.,* 2018; Faverio *et al*., 2018; Menadue *et al*., 2014; Suh *et al.,* 2013). It should be used as early as possible in situations of severe respiratory failure (Faverio *et al*., 2018). However, although there are apparently no benefits in using NIV in mild pathologies, its use can help in the perception of its necessity or not.

By improving cardiorespiratory fitness and reducing exertion and dyspnea, NIV increases exercise tolerance and as such can be used during physical training (Dyer et al. al., 2018). However, the scientific evidence is inconsistent regarding other measures of exercise fitness, so its application during training should be better studied, including a greater range of precipitating pathologies (Stone et al. al., 2009).

Respiratory rehabilitation is beneficial in the treatment of respiratory failure, and rehabilitation should be integrated into multidisciplinary programs. These programs should be applied during hospitalization with follow-up at home; they are important for reducing symptoms, optimizing functional status, increasing social participation of the person and leading to increased quality of life (Dyer *et* al., 2018; Faverio *et al.,* 2018; Suh *et al*., 2013). Information transmitted to those affected is also important, which promotes health education and identification/control of warning signs for future crises.

Thus, NSRNs play a key role in assessing the person and applying and monitoring NIV, in conjunction with the multidisciplinary team. The application of NIV together with a multidisciplinary team is suggested in periods of exertion and physical training whenever appropriate (Dyer *et* al., 2018; Faverio *et al.,* 2018; Menadue *et* al., 2014; Suh *et al*., 2013). Likewise, it has a fundamental role with respect to functional respiratory rehabilitation and to educating and informing the affected person as well as his/her family and peers.

REFERENCES

Ceriana, P., & Nava, S. (2006). Hypoxic and hypercapnic respiratory failure. *European Respiratory Society Monograph, 36*, 1–15. doi:10.1183/1025448x.00036001

Cordeiro, M., & Menoita, E. (2012). *Manual de Boas Práticas na Reabilitação Respiratória – Conceitos, princípios e técnicas*. Lusociência.

Corner, E., & Garrod, R. (2009). Does the addition of noninvasive ventilation during pulmonary rehabilitation in patients with chronic obstructive pulmonary disease augment patient outcome in exercise tolerance? A literature review. *Fisiotherapy Research International, 15*(1), 5–15. doi:10.1002/pri.451 PMID:20033880

dos Enfermeiros, O. (2018). Guia Orientador de Boa Prática - Reabilitação Respiratória. Ordem dos Enfermeiros.

Dyer, F., Flude, L., & Bazari, F. (2018). Noninvasive ventilation (NIV) as an aid to rehabilitation in acute respiratory disease. *BioMedCentral Pulmonary Medicine, 11*(58). Advance online publication. doi:10.1186/1471-2466-11-58 PMID:22177338

Faverio, P., Giacomi, F., & Sardella, L. (2018). Management of acute respiratory failure in interstitial lung diseases: Overview and clinical insights. *BioMedCentral Pulmonary Medicine, 18*(70), 70. Advance online publication. doi:10.118612890-018-0643-3 PMID:29764401

Johnson, C., Connolly, M., & Clover, S. (2013). Audit of acute exacerbations of chronic obstructive pulmonary disease at Waitemata District Health Board, New Zealand. *The New Zealand Medical Journal, 126*(1378), 15–25. PMID:24045312

Menadue, C., Piper, A., Van 't Hul, A., & Wong, K. (2014). Non-invasive ventilation during exercise training for people with chronic obstructive pulmonary disease. *Cochrane Database of Systematic Reviews, 5*. Advance online publication. doi:10.1002/14651858.CD007714.pub2 PMID:24823712

Roque. (2014). Ventilação Não-Invasiva. Vital Aire: Centro Hospitalar Lisboa Norte.

Stone, R., Harrison, B., Lowe, D., Buckingham, R. J., Pursey, N. A., Hosker, H. S. R., Potter, J. M., & Roberts, C. M. (2009). Introducing the national COPD resources and outcomes project. *BioMedCentral Health Services Research., 9*(173), 173. Advance online publication. doi:10.1186/1472-6963-9-173 PMID:19778416

Suh, E., Mandal, S., & Hart, N. (2013). Admission prevention in COPD: Nonpharmacological management. *BioMedCentral Medicine, 11*(247). Advance online publication. doi:10.1186/1741-7015-11-247 PMID:24252219

Chapter 2
Rehabilitation Nursing Care for the Person in the Context of Non-Invasive Ventilation

Pedro Teixeira
Centro Hospitalar Lisboa Norte, Portugal

Monica Pinto
Centro Hospitalar Lisboa Norte, Portugal

Lucilia Alves
Centro Hospitalar Lisboa Norte, Portugal

Ana Filipa Henriques
Centro Hospitalar Lisboa Norte, Portugal

ABSTRACT

Non-invasive ventilation is, nowadays, a well received, successful therapeutic strategy for the treatment of different varieties of respiratory failure. Associated to respiratory rehabilitation and exercise training, NVI brings numerous advantages to the person, namely in the control of symptoms, in the quality of life, in the reduction of the perception of dyspnea, in the increase of the tolerance to the activity, and in the decrease in the use of health services. The intervention of the specialist nurse in rehabilitation nursing is essential in order to maximize health gains. However, the bibliography that supports these gains with the intervention of the EEER needs greater investment in the research area.

DOI: 10.4018/978-1-7998-3531-8.ch002

Copyright © 2020, IGI Global. Copying or distributing in print or electronic forms without written permission of IGI Global is prohibited.

INTRODUCTION

Non-Invasive Ventilation (NIV) is a method of ventilatory support applied to the upper airway, using an interface and without the presence of an invasive method, such as the endotracheal tube or the laryngeal mask (Keenan et al, 2011), partially or totally replacing the person's ventilatory function.

The use of NIV has as mains objectives to increase alveolar ventilation; correct and improve gas exchange in order to reverse/prevent respiratory failure; reduce signs/symptoms such as dyspnea and ventilatory work; decrease the mortality rate; avoid tracheal intubation and hospitalization time (Keenan et al., 2011).

NIV is indicated in cases of acute or chronic respiratory failure. In case of respiratory failure in which clinical degradation is foreseen, ventilatory support must be started early, requiring great availability and dedication from the professional, with frequent reassessments, especially in the initial phase (first 4 to 8 hours), and should not be delayed until it becomes an emerging measure (Ferreira, 2009). Gasometry helps in the decision to start ventilatory support; however the final decision must be based on clinical judgment (Windisch, 2010).

The main contraindications to the use of NIV are: cardiorespiratory arrest; hemodynamic instability; myocardial ischemia or arrhythmias, non-participation or agitation of the person; the inability to protect the airway; the high risk of aspiration; recent surgery and / or burns; active bleeding from the upper gastrointestinal tract; severe hypoxemia; severe encephalopathy; upper airway obstruction; facial trauma and inability to drain tracheobronchial secretions (Ferreira et al., 2009; Society of Critical Care Medicine, 2008). NIV has been considered an alternative to conventional mechanical ventilation in people with acute respiratory failure, as it is a safe and effective ventilation mode, more comfortable for the person, as the orotracheal intubation is avoided, the need for sedation is reduced and the appearance of lesions in the airway, thus decreasing the risk of infection associated with health care. It allows the person to maintain speech, swallowing and the defense mechanisms of the airways, allowing the elimination of secretions, in a physiological way because it allows it to be used intermittently. It also requires shorter hospital stay, lower cost, easier weaning, and causes less mortality (Conti et al., 2004; Felgueiras et al, 2006; Ferreira et al, 2009; Sousa & Duque, 2012). However, there may be some adverse effects such as nasal congestion, dryness of mucous membranes, erythema / pressure ulcers, conjunctivitis, leakage, gastric distension and aspiration pneumonia. (Ferreira et al, 2009).

Respiratory Rehabilitation (RR) is a global and multidisciplinary intervention program, aimed at symptomatic people with chronic respiratory disease, and often with reduced participation in their ADL (Daily Life Activity) in order to contribute to improving their ability to exercise, to reduce dyspnea, to improve quality of life, to reduce levels of depression and anxiety (Cordeiro & Menoita, 2012; General Directorate of Health, 2009; Global Obstructive Lung Disease, 2019).

RR may be decisive in the treatment of people whose respiratory symptoms are associated with a decrease in functional capacity and quality of life (Pamplona & Morais, 2007). It is indicated in obstructive diseases (COPD, Bronchial Asthma, Bronchiectasis and Cystic Fibrosis), in restrictive diseases (interstitial diseases, chest diseases and neuromuscular diseases) and other situations, such as pre- and postoperative lung transplantation, morbid obesity, sleep apnea and lung cancer (Canteiro, 2003; Order of Nurses, 2018; Pamplona & Morais, 2007).

The person with chronic respiratory disease often has physical and emotional limitations that condition active life, promoting inactivity and disease progression (McCarthy et al, 2015). As dyspnea increases, ADLs (such as walking) become more and more difficult. The evolution of the disease, results in reduced physical activity and, consequently, poor cardiovascular performance, muscle weakness and, in some cases, nutritional deficits. Associated with the lack of physical conditioning, anxiety and depression often appear, which further contribute to the restriction of normal physical activity, due to the fear of triggering dyspnea. RR programs play a role in complementing pharmacological treatment, increasing tolerance to effort, improving quality of life, reducing dyspnea and minimizing the impact of the disease on ADLs. (General Directorate of Health, 2009). Its success is due to the "… ability to positively influence systemic effects, namely physical deconditioning, psychosocial dysfunction and co-morbidities, particularly cardiovascular (General Directorate of Health, 2009, p. 2). Therefore, it is not possible to talk about RR without addressing functional respiratory re-education, exercise training, health education, psychosocial and behavioral intervention and nutritional intervention. (General Directorate of Health, 2009; Global Obstructive Lung Disease, 2019; Order of Nurses, 2018).

The nurse specialist in rehabilitation nursing (EEER), due to the privileged position he occupies in the multidisciplinary team, has a preventive, treatment and rehabilitation role, as far as respiratory disease is concerned. (Cordeiro & Menoita, 2012).

The main objectives and health gains that are intended when associating RR to the person submitted to NIV are those that relate to the control of symptoms, safety, quality of life and decreased use of health services. In this sense, RR interventions are focused on preventing or improving secretion retention; improve the ability to cough; reduce the perception of dyspnea; increase tolerance to physical activity (Ambrosino & Cigni, 2015; Hill & Holland, 2014; Keenan et al., 2011; Order of Nurses, 2018; Spruit et al., 2013); obtain measurable improvements in maximum oxygen volume (VO2) and exercise heart rate (HR); compensate for the intrinsic limitations to exercise; decrease the need for IV or tracheostomy; prolong life; reduce rates of hospitalization and readmission; increase the person/family's knowledge of the therapeutic regime; improve the life quality; allow greater comfort to the person (Aboussouan, 2009; Araújo et al, 2017; Bach e Martinez, 2011; Costa et al, 2010; Dyer, 2011; Hoo, 2003; Hill & Holland, 2014; Order of Nurses, 2018; Sousa & Duque, 2012; Tzeng e Bach, 2000), with the possibility of staying in a rehabilitation program in association with NIV at home (Sousa & Duque, 2012).

RR can be combined with NIV by reducing the work of the respiratory muscles with improved pulmonary function, minimizing dyspnea and, consequently, improving the ability to perform ADL with increased tolerance to effort (Araújo et al., 2017, Duiverman et al., 2011; Simonds, 2003).

The EEER should make an initial assessment with the collection of information from the person in need of RR care and under NIV. The assessment of the clinical situation must include the symptomatological assessment, using physical examination and complementary means of diagnosis, relevant to each case and context. (Heuer & Scanlan, 2013). The assessment of functional capacity, respiratory function, muscle function and quality of life, anxiety and depression should be taken into account. (DesJardins, Burton & Timothy, 2015; General Directorate of Health, 2009; Heuer, & Scanlan, 2013).

Scientific evidence recommends the use of systematic instruments for assessing the person in two moments: before and after the implementation of the RR program (American Association of Cardiovascular & Pulmonary Rehabilitation, 2011).

The main focuses of rehabilitation nursing intervention in the person with respiratory pathology in need of NIV are: Ventilation; Airway Cleaning / Expectorate and Activity Intolerance (Order of Nurses, 2016). As for ventilation, airway cleaning and expectoration, as examples of measurement instruments, the following are the Clinical COPD Questionnaire (Molen, 2003; Silva, 2012); London Chest Activity of Daily Living Scale (Garrod, 2000); Modified Borg scale - assessment of dyspnea (Borg, 1982); Modified Medical Research Council Dyspnea Scale (Kovelis, 2008) and St George's Respiratory Questionaire (Jones, 1991). Regarding the **activity intolerance** focus, in addition to the modified Borg scale, the 6-minute gait test (Dourado, 2011) and the 1-minute sit to stand test (Bohannon, 1995) or the Timed up and go Test (Podsiadlo, 1991). It is noteworthy that the person with respiratory pathology may present other focuses of intervention that lack other assessment tools such as the Barthel index (Mahoney, 1965) to assess BADL, the functional independence measurement scale - MIF (Granger et al., 1986) to assess functionality and the modified MRC scale (Florence et. al, 1984) to assess gains in muscle strength. There are also scales that assess the risk of falls and pressure ulcers, Morse (Costa-Dias et al., 2014) and Braden (Paranhos & Santos 1999), respectively.

The planning and execution of an RR program for the person in need of carrying out NIV maintains and enhances the existing capacities for functional independence and for the promotion of autonomy. The evidence points to a RR program which incorporates breathing exercises, and a progressive and early mobilization, becoming healthy for the person, with numerous benefits in functional, psychological and ventilatory terms, favoring ventilatory weaning. The RR program helps to prevent respiratory changes associated with immobility and to promote muscle strength. However, there is no consensus on the intensity, frequency and duration of interventions (Order of Nurses, 2018).

NIV has been used as an adjunctive therapy for rehabilitation in reconditioning the effort in people with respiratory pathology (eg, the bicycle, the treadmill and the resisted exercises) and in reducing respiratory work during the implementation of airway cleaning techniques, with improvement of pulmonary function and dyspnea, so the safety and effectiveness of the implementation of airway cleaning and effort reconditioning techniques is assumed during the implementation of NIV (Corner & Garrod, 2010; Moran, Bradley & Piper, 2013).

NIV as a therapeutic option can be considered a first-line therapeutic modality, due to the benefits it brings. Combined with RR, it produces beneficial effects, decreasing dyspnea, increasing symptom control and the ability to tolerate physical exercise (Sousa & Duque, 2012).

Therefore, it is essential to include in the RR programs the breathing techniques and exercises associated with rest and relaxation, **the airway cleaning techniques; energy management techniques** and **physical exercise** to ensure increased tolerance to activities.

Respiratory functional re-education (RFR) is based on a set of techniques for controlling breathing, positioning and movement. It acts on the mechanical component of breathing (external ventilation) in order to improve alveolar ventilation; reduce psychic and muscular tension; increase alveolar recruitment in order to improve pulmonary ventilation, gas exchange and oxygenation; mobilize and remove bronchial secretions, promoting airway cleaning and permeabilization; optimize the thoraco-abdominal movement pattern to decrease respiratory work; promote costal mobility and correct vicious positions; increase endurance, exercise capacity and independence in functionality, when associated with exercise training; increase understanding of the lung condition; and empower the person to manage their disease (Order of Nurses, 2018).

Muscle relaxation techniques and the teaching of resting positions reduce psychic tension, respiratory work and muscle overload. As a consequence, they reduce the sensation of dyspnea and promote better control of breathing, preparing the person for the rehabilitation process. Thoracic and scapular waist mobilization improves the inspiratory process, by improving the inspired volume and muscle efficiency with reduced dyspnea (Bott et al., 2009).

Postural correction is indicated in the person with respiratory pathology in order to prevent or correct postural defects, thoracic deformities and ventilatory asynergies.

The latter tend to appear due to the type of breathing, which is more superficial, costal and superior, so it is essential to implement breathing exercises such as breathing control, diaphragmatic and costal respiratory reeducation, exhalation with semi-closed lips and the adoption of positions that promote ventilatory optimization (Cordeiro & Menoita, 2012).

Breathing control is important for the relief and control of dyspnea, reducing the dynamic hyperinflation of the rib cage, thus improving gas exchange. It also increases the strength and resistance of the respiratory muscles and optimizes the breathing pattern (Gosselink et al., 2003, 2011).

Learning abdominal-diaphragmatic breathing is necessary for a more effective breathing process and consequent reduction of dyspnea (Bott et al., 2009; Hough, 2001). Exhalation with semi-closed lips promotes alveolar clearance and overcomes positive pressure maintained at the end of exhalation (Langer et al., 2009; Nici et al., 2006).

The effectiveness of airway cleaning techniques in RR programs is widely known and when used in conjunction with breathing exercises, it has similar effects on lung function. The active cycle of breathing, directed coughing, autogenic drainage and forced expiration are effective in addressing the person with respiratory disease under NIV, as well as external oscillation devices. With less evidence of efficacy, due to the small number of studies, techniques such as postural drainage, percussion, percussive intrapulmonary ventilation and positive expiratory pressure are found (Bott et al., 2009; Ides et al., 2011; Nici et al., 2006).

In order to avoid airway collapse during forced expiration in people who have a reduction in elastic lung retraction, the literature suggests performing PEEP or autogenic drainage (Holland & Button, 2006; Holland, Wadell & Spruit, 2013).

Energy management techniques are extremely important for people with dyspnea to perform ADLs, as they allow daily routines combining respiratory control through breathing with parted lips, spending less energy and reducing the feeling of tiredness and shortness of breath (Velloso et al., 2006). While the person is performing his tasks he must try to control his breathing so that the most tiring movement is performed simultaneously with the exhalation phase. For better energy management in ADLs, the person must learn to plan and establish priority tasks, carrying out the heaviest tasks at the time of the day when he feels with more energy using moments of rest. It should be noted that all tasks that can be performed sitting, should be avoided being done standing up (Velloso et al., 2006).

Physical exercise is now considered an essential pillar of RR. Exercise training increases maximum oxygen consumption, slows the anaerobic threshold, decreases heart rate for a given oxygen consumption, increases mitochondrial enzymatic capacity and increases the density of the muscle capillary network. In fact, physical exercise decreases the ventilatory requirements for a given task, as well as the reduction of dead space by increasing the tidal volume, decreasing the residual volume and the respiratory rate, thus contributing to a more effective ventilatory pattern with reduction of dyspnea of effort.

Education programs for physical exercise combine resistance training, aerobically, with strength training, anaerobic, generating important benefits in the treatment of peripheral muscle dysfunction in people with respiratory diseases and under NIV (Rabinovich et al., 2010; Spruit et al., 2013; Vilaró et al, 2008). Scientific evidence has been supporting the benefit of exercise training in people with COPD, but also with other pathologies such as asthma, cystic fibrosis, bronchiectasis, pulmonary fibrosis and lung cancer (ACSM, 2014).

A regular exercise program for most adults should include a variety of exercises in addition to activities performed as part of everyday life. It should include a warm-up phase (in order to avoid injuries - 5 to 10 min of aerobic activity of light to moderate intensity, so that the body adjusts to changes in physiological, biomechanical and bio-energetic needs); an exercise phase (preferably combining several types - at least 20 to 60 min of aerobic, resistance and neuro-motor activities); a resting phase, at least every 5 to 10 min of light to moderate cardiorespiratory activity allowing a gradual recovery of HR and blood pressure (TA) and the removal of metabolic end products; and a phase of flexibility (stretching) at least 10 min corresponding to a form of physical exercise in which the muscle is stretched or stretched in order to increase the range of motion, improving its elasticity and enabling more coordinated and efficient movements (Alencar et al., 2010; McHugh et al., 2010).

When prescribing physical exercise, some fundamental principles must be taken into account. Thus, according to ACSM (2014), it is based on the FITT-VP principle (frequency, intensity, duration, type / modality, volume and progression) (Garber et al., 2011). This principle, depending on the situations, may be related to a certain order of exercises to be performed, in order to allow rest and recovery of muscle groups. For example, in people with chronic pain and easy tiredness, the resistance test can be performed before the strength test and can be alternated between the upper and lower extremities (ACSM, 2014).

The **frequency** of exercise refers to the number of days per week dedicated to the exercise program, contributing to the improvement of physical and cardiorespiratory fitness. Aerobic exercise is recommended for 3 to 5 days a week for most adults, with a frequency that varies with the intensity of the exercise (Garber et al., 2011; Haskell et al., 2007; Nelson et al., 2007). In the case of a person with asthma, a minimum of 2 to 3 days a week is recommended (Lee, Simmonds & Jones, 2002; Mendes et al, 2011); Ram et al., 2005) and in the case of the person diagnosed with COPD 3 to 5 days a week (ACSM, 2014).

The **intensity** of the exercise in the person with chronic respiratory pathology should be well defined; however it is not always easy taking into account the state of health and other factors such as physical capacity, lifestyle and age. Therefore, an exercise intensity corresponding to between 40% and 85% of the oxygen uptake reserve (O2) (residual oxygen volume (vO2R) - difference between vO2 max and vO2 at rest, measured in the respiratory function tests, is recommended) or heart rate reserve (RFC) (difference between maximum HR and resting HR). There are some formulas available that calculate HR max. possible, being the most common "220-age" for its simplicity and ease of use, however it is not totally reliable as it can under or overestimate HR max measure (Gellish et al, 2007; Gulati et al, 2010; Tanaka, Monahan & Seals, 2001; Zhu, 2010). Aerobic exercise of moderate intensity (40% to 60% of HR reserve) to intense (60% to 90% of RFC) is recommended for most adults and aerobic exercise of light intensity (30 to 40% of RFC) moderate can be beneficial for people with changes in physical and cardiorespiratory fitness (ACSM, 2014).

The normal AT response to increasing dynamic exercise consists of a progressive increase in systolic blood pressure (BIT), and should be suspended if BAC values greater than 250 mmHg. Hypotension on exertion (SAD that does not increase or decrease [less than 10 mmHg]) can mean myocardial ischemia and / or left ventricular dysfunction. Diastolic blood pressure (DBT) greater than or equal to 110 mmHg, decrease in SBT greater than 10 mmHg during exercise with increasing work, the presence of significant ventricular arrhythmias with or without associated signs / symptoms, second or third heart block degrees, symptoms of exercise intolerance including angina, severe dyspnea (Borg scale assessment) and electrocardiographic changes suggestive of ischemia, should lead to interruption of exercise. People at rest with SAD greater than 180 mmHg and / or SAD greater than 110 mmHg should not start exercise training (Hare et al., 1999).

In people with respiratory disease, SpO2 should remain above 85%. The decrease of more than 5% in SpO2 during exercise is considered an abnormal response suggestive of exercise-induced hypoxemia (Balady et al, 2010). In these people, the intensity of aerobic exercise can be intense corresponding to 60 to 80% of the peak of the exercise tests or light corresponding to between 30 to 40%. The intensity should be adjusted according to the person's perception of dyspnea, so it should be below score 6 on the Borg scale. Light intensity training results in improvement in symptoms, quality of life and ADL performance. With vigorous intensity training, significant gains were demonstrated with a reduction in RR and HR (Nici et al, 2006)

Regarding Duration, most adults should perform 30 to 60 min per day of moderate intensity exercise, 20 to 60 min per day of vigorous intensity exercise or a combination of moderate and vigorous exercise per day to obtain volumes recommended exercise. This recommended amount of exercise can be accumulated in one continuous session or in sessions over 10 min over the course of a day. Shorter than recommended lengths may be beneficial for some individuals, particularly those who are in a weakened physical shape due to physical inactivity (ACSM, 2014), for example, people with respiratory pathology who, due to feeling dyspneic, do not have physical exercise routinely instituted. In the case of the person with moderate or severe COPD, the person may be able to exercise only at a specific intensity for a few minutes at the beginning of the training program. Intermittent exercise can also be used for the initial training sessions until the person tolerates the exercise at greater intensities and durations. With regard to the person with asthma, the recommended time is at least 20 to 30 min per day (Fanelli et al, 2007; Mendes et al, 2011; Ram et al, 2005; Turner et al, 2011).

Regarding the **type/modality** (for example aerobic exercises, strength training, endurance/endurance, flexibility or combined training), the rhythmic aerobic exercise of moderate intensity and involving large muscle groups requiring little specific skill for its performance is recommended to improve cardiorespiratory fitness. Other exercises that require greater skills to perform or higher levels of fitness are recommended only for individuals who have the ability to perform them (Garber et al, 2011).

Muscle strength training is the anaerobic component of exercise training programs and comprises "... the use of high intensity and short duration stimuli, more localized to small muscle groups ..." (Pamplona et al., 2007, p.103). Muscle strength training causes less dyspnea than resistance training, being a safe alternative for people with severe dyspnea (Spruit et al., 2013).

To strengthen the lower limbs, bicycles, mobilizations, open / closed kinetic chain exercises and gait training can be used. (Silva & Dourado, 2008). Respiratory muscle training should be included in exercise training programs as an adjunct to people with respiratory disease, as it has effects on strength and endurance without having effects on dyspnea or exercise capacity (Garcia et al, 2008; Spruit et al, 2013). In the case of people with COPD or asthma, the recommended modalities are walking, running and/or cycling. There is also, transcutaneous neuromuscular electrical stimulation of peripheral muscles that is well tolerated and increases the musculature of the lower limbs with gains in exercise capacity and in the reduction of dyspnea in people with stage 4 COPD. It is a technique that involves stimulation passive muscle contraction by electricity (Napolis et al, 2011; Vieira et al, 2014), being a safe procedure (Sillen et al, 2008).

Resistance is an exercise modality that requires repetitive physical activity over a period of time in order to modulate resistance (Ries et al, 2007). Thus, it increases the concentration of oxidative mitochondrial enzymes, allows muscle hypertrophy and the increase of type I oxidative fibers and the conversion of type II glycolytic fibers into type II oxidative fibers, increases the density of the muscle capillary network, enhancing oxygenation and thereby increasing performance in AVDF (Dourado et al, 2004; Rabinovich et al., 2010; Troosters et al, 2005).

The exercise **volume** corresponds to the product resulting from frequency, intensity and time (duration). For example, in the case of resistance exercises (oriented by series and repetitions), also recommended for the person with respiratory pathology, namely in COPD, each muscle group should be trained in a total of 2 to 4 series with 8 to 12 repetitions per series and with a 2 to 3 min rest interval between sets to improve neuromuscular conditioning (ACSM, 2009; Garber et al 2011; Peterson, Rhea&Alvar, 2005).

In order to outline which resistance to use in this type of exercise, the maximum resistance that the person can perform for a given movement in a repetition must be established, that is, if the person for elbow flexion reaches a maximum of 8 kg, then it should be used a resistance of approximately 5 to 6.5 kg of weight (60% to 80% of the maximum weight lifted in a repetition [1-RM]). For the elderly and infirm, at least a series of 10 to 15 repetitions of exercise against resistance of moderate intensity (60 to 70% 1-RM) is recommended. The greater the intensity or resistance, the less repetitions must be completed. Each set should be performed up to the point of muscle fatigue, but not insufficiency because exercising the muscles to this level increases the likelihood of injury or late muscle pain. If the objective is mainly to improve localized muscular endurance and not strength or increase in muscle mass, a greater number of repetitions, between 15 to 25 per set should be performed together with shorter rest intervals and less sets. This regimen requires less resistance intensity, generally not more than 50% of 1-RM. (ACSM, 2009; Garber et al., 2011; Peterson, Rhea & Alvar, 2005).

Progress in the exercise program depends on the person's health, fitness, training responses and the goals of the person's exercise program. Progress may consist of increasing any of the components of the FITT principle tolerated by the person. However, it must be progressive and adapted to minimize the risk of muscle cramps and injuries (Garber et al, 2011).

The progression of exercise training implies in most situations a progressive implementation of intensity. In people with COPD and under NIV it should not only be based on the maximum heart rate, due to the ventilatory limitation and the maximum effort normally present, but also on the perceived values of the effort or dyspnea (values of 5 and 6 in 10 of the Borg scale modified), as they allow the adjustment of the intensity during the exercise (Langer et al, 2009). t is usually prescribed 3 to 5 times a week, with high intensity (60% maximum muscle load), 20 to 60 minutes per session (Spruit et al, 2013). Take as examples of this training modality walking, running, cycling, rowing and swimming. However, in hospitalized patients, at an early stage, and always taking into account the Borg scale and hemodynamic status, progress can be guided. In an initial phase, mobilizations in the bed can be carried out, each time more intense until progressive lifting is possible, exercises in the sitting position, progressing to gait training combined with resistance exercises and later climbing and descending stairs. Interval training can be an option to increase the total volume or the average intensity of exercises performed during an exercise session. This consists of a modified form of resistance training in which alternating periods of discharge with low intensity or periods of exercise with pause times (Spruit et al., 2013).

HEALTH EDUCATION

In this area, one must highlight the importance of the educational context of the person with respiratory diseases, with the purpose to change behaviors, improve knowledge of chronic disease and learn how to life with it, namely with its limitations (General Directorate of Health, 2009).

The educational strategies must include knowledge about the disease, control of symptoms and prevention of complications; decrease of risk factors such as active smoking; the benefits of physical activities; breath control and energy management techniques; anxiety and stress management; bronchial hygiene; therapeutic management, mainly inhalation; respiratory assistant equipment (how to operate and maintenance); nutritional advisement (General Directorate of Health, 2005; General Directorate of Health, 2009; Global Initiative for Chronic Obstructive Lung Disease, 2019).

Smoking cessation is the intervention with the greatest capacity to influence the natural history of the person with respiratory pathology. Therefore, the evaluation of the long-term smoking cessation component, through a multicenter study indicates that, with effective resources and time, it will be achieved (Global Initiative for Chronic Obstructive Lung Disease, 2019).

Vaccination against influenza and pneumococcus is another example of intervention that should be facilitated for the person with a respiratory pathology, appearing to be more effective in the older sick person, with more serious diseases or with cardiac comorbidity (Rocha, 2017).

Optimization of inhalation therapy is essential and should be taken into account in order to enhance respiratory rehabilitation programs. In this way, there are gains in quality of life and tolerance, to activities obtained when complemented with programs, in which exercise training must also be introduced. (Global Initiative for Chronic Obstructive Lung Disease, 2019; Ries et al., 2008; Troosters et al., 2005)

CONCLUSION

NIV is, nowadays, a well received, successful therapeutic strategy for the treatment of different varieties of respiratory failure. This type of ventilation associated with RR brings numerous advantages for the person, namely in the control of symptoms, in the quality of life, in the reduction of the perception of dyspnea, in the increase of the tolerance to the activity and in the decrease in the use of health services. However, the bibliography that supports these gains with the intervention of the EEER needs greater investment in the research area. Therefore comes the need to carry out experimental studies of effectiveness that explore the intervention of the EEER concomitant to the execution of NIV as well as the exercise training in the person under NIV.

REFERENCES

Aboussouan, L. S. (2009). Mechanisms of exercise limitation and pulmonary rehabilitation for patients with neuromuscular disease. *Chronic Respiratory Disease*, *6*(4), 231–249. doi:10.1177/1479972309345927 PMID:19858353

Alencar, T. A. M. D., & Matias, K. F. D. S. (2010). Princípios fisiológicos do aquecimento e alongamento muscular na atividade esportiva. *Revista Brasileira de Medicina do Esporte*, *16*(3), 230–234. doi:10.1590/S1517-86922010000300015

Ambrosino, N., & Cigni, P. (2015). Non invasive ventilation as an additional tool for exercise training. *Multidisciplinary Respiratory Medicine*, *10*(1), 14. doi:10.118640248-015-0008-1 PMID:25874110

American Association of Cardiovascular & Pulmonary Rehabilitation. (2011). Guidelines for Pulmonary Rehabilitation Programs. In Human Kinetics (4th ed.). Author.

American College of Sports Medicine. (2009). American College of Sports Medicine position stand. Progression models in resistance training for healthy adults. *Medicine and Science in Sports and Exercise*, *41*(3), 687–708. doi:10.1249/MSS.0b013e3181915670 PMID:19204579

American College of Sports Medicine (2014). *Diretrizes do ACSM para os testes de esforço e sua prescrição* (9th ed.). Guanabara Koognan Ltda.

Araújo, R. B., Camisasca, M. T., Britto, R. R., & Parreira, V. F. (2017). O uso da ventilação não-invasiva na reabilitação pulmonar em pacientes portadores da doença pulmonar obstrutiva crônica: Uma revisão de literatura. *Fisioterapia em Movimento, 18*(1), 49–57.

Bach, J. R., & Martinez, D. (2011). Duchenne muscular dystrophy: Continuous noninvasive ventilatory support prolongs survival. *Respiratory Care, 56*(6), 744–750. doi:10.4187/respcare.00831 PMID:21333078

Balady, G. J., Arena, R., Sietsema, K., Myers, J., Coke, L., Fletcher, G. F., Forman, D., Franklin, B., Guazzi, M., Gulati, M., Keteyian, S. J., Lavie, C. J., Macko, R., Mancini, D., & Milani, R. V. (2010). Clinician's guide to cardiopulmonary exercise testing in adults. A scientific statement from the American Heart Association. *Circulation, 122*(2), 191–225. doi:10.1161/CIR.0b013e3181e52e69 PMID:20585013

Bohannon, R. W. (1995). Sit-to-stand test for measuring performance of lower extremity muscles. *Perceptual and Motor Skills, 80*(1), 163–166. doi:10.2466/pms.1995.80.1.163 PMID:7624188

Borg, G. A. (1982). Psychophysical bases of perceived exertion. *Medicine and Science in Sports and Exercise, 14*(5), 377–381. doi:10.1249/00005768-198205000-00012 PMID:7154893

Bott, J., Blumenthal, S., Buxton, M., Ellum, S., Falconer, C., Garrod, R., ... Potter, C. (2009). Guidelines for the physiotherapy management of the adult, medical, spontaneously breathing patient. *Thorax, 64*(Suppl 1), i1–i52. doi:10.1136/thx.2008.110726 PMID:19406863

Branco, P., Barata, S., Barbosa, J., Cantista, M., Lima, A., & Maia, J. (2012). *Temas de Reabilitação–Reabilitação Respiratória*. Servier.

Canteiro, M., & Heitor, M. (2003). Reabilitação respiratória. *Tratado de Pneumologia. lisboa: Sociedade Portuguesa de Pneumologia*, 1785-1896.

Conti, G., Costa, R., Craba, A., Festa, V., & Catarci, S. (2004). Non-invasive ventilation in COPD patients. *Minerva Anestesiologica, 70*(4), 145–150. PMID:15173688

Cordeiro, M. D. C. O., & Menoita, E. C. P. C. (2012). *Manual de boas práticas na reabilitação respiratória: Conceitos, princípios e técnicas*. Lusociência.

Corner, E., & Garrod, R. (2010). Does the addition of non-invasive ventilation during pulmonary rehabilitation in patients with chronic obstructive pulmonary disease augment patient outcome in exercise tolerance? A literature review. *Physiotherapy Research International, 15*(1), 5–15. PMID:20033880

Costa, M. F. D. L., Barros, M. P. D., & Lima, J. H. M. (2010). O Impacto do CPAP na Reabilitação Cardíaca de Pacientes com ICC: Relato de caso. *Arquivos Brasileiros de Cardiologia*, *95*(1), e7–e9. doi:10.1590/S0066-782X2010001100023 PMID:20694398

Costa-Dias, M.J.M.D., Ferreira, P.L., & Oliveira, A.S. (2014). Adaptação cultural e linguística e validação da Escala de Quedas de Morse. *Revista de Enfermagem Referência*, (2), 7-17.

DesJardins, T., Burton, G., & Timothy, P. (2015). Clinical manifestations and assessment of respiratory disease. Mosby Elsevier.

Direção-Geral da Saúde. (2009). Orientações técnicas sobre reabilitação respiratória na doença pulmonar obstrutiva crónica (DPOC). *Circular Informativa, 40.*

Ordem dos Enfermeiros. (2016). *Instrumentos de recolha de dados para a documentação dos cuidados especializados em Enfermagem de Reabilitação.* Ordem dos Enfermeiros.

Ordem dos Enfermeiros. (2018). *Guia Orientador de Boas Práticas – Reabilitação Respiratória.* Lisboa: Ordem dos Enfermeiros.

Dourado, V. Z. (2011). Equações de referência para o teste de caminhada de seis minutos em indivíduos saudáveis. *Arquivos Brasileiros de Cardiologia*, *96*(6), e128–e138. doi:10.1590/S0066-782X2011005000024 PMID:22262150

Dourado, V. Z., & Godoy, I. (2004). Recondicionamento muscular na DPOC: Principais intervenções e novas tendências. *Revista Brasileira de Medicina do Esporte*, *10*(4), 331–334. doi:10.1590/S1517-86922004000400010

Duiverman, M. L., Wempe, J. B., Bladder, G., Vonk, J. M., Zijlstra, J. G., Kerstjens, H. A., & Wijkstra, P. J. (2011). Two-year home-based nocturnal noninvasive ventilation added to rehabilitation in chronic obstructive pulmonary disease patients: A randomized controlled trial. *Respiratory Research*, *12*(1), 112. doi:10.1186/1465-9921-12-112 PMID:21861914

Dyer, F., Flude, L., Bazari, F., Jolley, C., Englebretsen, C., Lai, D., Polkey, M. I., & Hopkinson, N. S. (2011). Non-invasive ventilation (NIV) as an aid to rehabilitation in acute respiratory disease. *BMC Pulmonary Medicine*, *11*(1), 58. doi:10.1186/1471-2466-11-58 PMID:22177338

Fanelli, A., Cabral, A. L., Neder, J. A., Martins, M. A., & Carvalho, C. R. (2007). Exercise training on disease control and quality of life in asthmatic children. *Medicine and Science in Sports and Exercise, 39*(9), 1474–1480. doi:10.1249/mss.0b013e3180d099ad PMID:17805077

Felgueiras, J., Lohmann, C., Delerue, F., & Barata, J. (2006). Ventilação não invasiva numa unidade de cuidados intermédios. *Revue de Médecine Interne, 13*(21), 73–78.

Ferreira, S., Nogueira, C., Conde, S., & Taveira, N. (2009). Ventilação não invasiva. *Revista Portuguesa de Pneumologia, 15*(4), 655–667. doi:10.1016/S0873-2159(15)30162-8 PMID:19547897

Florence, J. M., & Hagberg, J. M. (1984). Effect of training on the exercise responses of neuromuscular disease patients. *Medicine and Science in Sports and Exercise, 16*(5), 460–465. doi:10.1249/00005768-198410000-00007 PMID:6513764

Garber, C. E., Blissmer, B., Deschenes, M. R., Franklin, B. A., Lamonte, M. J., Lee, I.-M., Nieman, D. C., & Swain, D. P. (2011). American College of Sports Medicine Position Stand. The quantity and quality of exercise for developing and maintaining cardiorespiratory, musculoskeletal, and neuromotor fitness in apparently healthy adults: Guidance for prescribing exercise. *Medicine and Science in Sports and Exercise, 43*(7), 1334–1359. doi:10.1249/MSS.0b013e318213fefb PMID:21694556

Garcia, S., Rocha, M., Pinto, P., Lopes, A. M., & Bárbara, C. (2008). Treino de músculos inspiratórios em doentes com DPOC. *Revista Portuguesa de Pneumologia, 14*(2), 177–194. doi:10.1016/S0873-2159(15)30229-4 PMID:18363017

Garrod, R., Bestall, J. C., Paul, E. A., Wedzicha, J. A., & Jones, P. W. (2000). Development and validation of a standardized measure of activity of daily living in patients with severe COPD: The London Chest Activity of Daily Living scale (LCADL). *Respiratory Medicine, 94*(6), 589–596. doi:10.1053/rmed.2000.0786 PMID:10921765

Gellish, R. L., Goslin, B. R., Olson, R. E., McDonald, A., Russi, G. D., & Moudgil, V. K. (2007). Longitudinal modeling of the relationship between age and maximal heart rate. *Medicine and Science in Sports and Exercise, 39*(5), 822–829. doi:10.1097/mss.0b013e31803349c6 PMID:17468581

Global Iniciative for Chronic Obstructive Lung Disease. (2019). *Global Strategy for the diagnosis, management and prevention of COPD-Pocket Guide to COPD Diagnosis, Management, and Prevention, 2019 Report*. Author.

Gosselink, R. (2003). Controlled breathing and dyspnea in patients with chronic obstructive pulmonary disease (COPD). *Journal of Rehabilitation Research and Development, 40*(5), 25-34.

Gosselink, R., De Vos, J., Van den Heuvel, S. P., Segers, J., Decramer, M., & Kwakkel, G. (2011). Impact of inspiratory muscle training in patients with COPD: What is the evidence? *The European Respiratory Journal*, *37*(2), 416–425. doi:10.1183/09031936.00031810 PMID:21282809

Granger, C. V., Hamilton, B. B., Keith, R. A., Zielezny, M., & Sherwin, F. S. (1986). Advances in functional assessment for medical rehabilitation. *Topics in Geriatric Rehabilitation*, *1*(3), 59–74. doi:10.1097/00013614-198604000-00007

Gulati, M., Shaw, L. J., Thisted, R. A., Black, H. R., Merz, C. N., & Arnsdorf, M. F. (2010). Heart rate response to exercise stress testing in asymptomatic women. The St. James Women Take Heart Project. *Circulation*, *122*(2), 130–137. doi:10.1161/CIRCULATIONAHA.110.939249 PMID:20585008

Hare, D.L., Ryan, T.M., Selig, S.E., Pellizzer, A.M., Wrigley, T.V., & Krum, H. (1999) Resistance exercise training increases muscle strength, endurance, and blood flow in patients with chronic heart failure. *Am J Cardiol. 83*(12), 1674–7.

Haskell, W. L., Lee, I. M., Pate, R. R., Powell, K., Blair, S. N., Franklin, B. A., Macera, C. A., Heath, G. W., Thompson, P. D., & Bauman, A. (2007). Physical activity and public health: Updated recommendation for adults from the American College of Sports Medicine and the American Heart Association. *Medicine and Science in Sports and Exercise*, *39*(8), 1423–1434. doi:10.1249/mss.0b013e3180616b27 PMID:17762377

Heuer, A., & Scanlan, C. L. (2013). *Wilkins' Clinical Assessment in Respiratory Care-E-Book*. Elsevier Health Sciences.

Hill, K., & Holland, A. E. (2014). Strategies to enhance the benefits of exercise training in the respiratory patient. *Clinics in Chest Medicine*, *35*(2), 323–336. doi:10.1016/j.ccm.2014.02.003 PMID:24874128

Holland, A. E., Wadell, K., & Spruit, M. A. (2013). How to adapt the pulmonary rehabilitation programme to patients with chronic respiratory disease other than COPD. Pulmonary Rehabilitation, 577-586. doi:10.1183/09059180.00005613

Hollandl, A. E., & Buttonl, B. M. (2006). Is there a role for airway clearance techniques in chronic obstructive pulmonary disease? *Chronic Respiratory Disease*, *3*(2), 83–91. doi:10.1191/1479972306cd097rs PMID:16729766

Hoo, G. W. S. (2003). Nonpharmacologic adjuncts to training during pulmonary rehabilitation: the role of supplemental oxygen and noninvasive ventilation. *Journal of rehabilitation research and development, 40*(5), 81-98.

Hough, A. (2001). *Physiotherapy in respiratory care: an evidence-based approach to respiratory and cardiac management.* Nelson Thornes.

Ides, K., Vissers, D., De Backer, L., Leemans, G., & De Backer, W. (2011). Airway clearance in COPD: Need for a breath of fresh air? A systematic review. *COPD, 8*(3), 196–205. doi:10.3109/15412555.2011.560582 PMID:21513439

Jones, P. W., Quirk, F. H., & Baveystock, C. M. (1991). The St George's Respiratory Questionnaire. *Respiratory Medicine, 85*(B), 25–27.

Keenan, S. P., Sinuff, T., Burns, K. E., Muscedere, J., Kutsogiannis, J., Mehta, S., ... Scales, D. C. (2011). Clinical practice guidelines for the use of noninvasive positive-pressure ventilation and noninvasive continuous positive airway pressure in the acute care setting. *Canadian Medical Association Journal, 183*(3), E195–E214. doi:10.1503/cmaj.100071 PMID:21324867

Kovelis, D., Segretti, N. O., Probst, V. S., Lareau, S. C., Brunetto, A. F., & Pitta, F. (2008). Validação do Modified Pulmonary Functional Status and Dyspnea Questionnaire e da escala do Medical Research Council para o uso em pessoas com doença pulmonar obstrutiva crónica no Brasil [Validation of the Modified Pulmonary Functional Status and Dyspnea Questionnaire and the Medical Research Council scale for use in Brazil patients with chronic obstructive pulmonary disease]. *Jornal Brasileiro de Pneumologia, 34*(12), 1008–1018. doi:10.1590/S1806-37132008001200005 PMID:19180335

Langer, D., Probst, V. S., Pitta, F., Burtin, C., Hendriks, E., Schans, C. P. V. D., ... Troosters, T. (2009). Guia para prática clínica: Fisioterapia em pacientes com Doença Pulmonar Obstrutiva Crônica (DPOC). *Brazilian Journal of Physical Therapy, 13*(3), 184–204. doi:10.1590/S1413-35552009005000034

Lee, C., Simmonds, M., Novy, D., & Jones, S. (2002). Functional self-efficacy, perceived gait ability and perceived exertion in walking performance of individuals with low back pain. *Physiotherapy Theory and Practice, 18*(4), 193–203. doi:10.1080/09593980290058553

Magano, C., Reis, M., Guedes, P. & Brito, R. M. (2007). Ventilação Não Invasiva. *Sinais Vitais, 72*, 13-19.

Mahoney, F. I., & Barthel, D. (1965). Functional evaluation: The Barthel Index. *Maryland State Medical Journal, 14*, 56–61. PMID:14258950

McCarthy, B., Casey, D., Devane, D., Murphy, K., Murphy, E., & Lacasse, Y. (2015). Pulmonary rehabilitation for chronic obstructive pulmonary disease. *Cochrane Database of Systematic Reviews*, (2), 1–22. doi:10.1002/14651858.CD003793.pub3 PMID:25705944

McHugh, M. P., & Cosgrave, C. H. (2010). To stretch or not to stretch: The role of stretching in injury prevention and performance. *Scandinavian Journal of Medicine & Science in Sports*, *20*(2), 169–181. PMID:20030776

Mendes, F. A., Almeida, F. M., Cukier, A., Stelmach, R., Jacob-Filho, W., Martins, M. A., & Carvalho, C. R. F. (2011). Effects of aerobic training on airway inflammation in asthmatic patients. *Medicine and Science in Sports and Exercise*, *43*(2), 197–203. doi:10.1249/MSS.0b013e3181ed0ea3 PMID:20581719

Moran, F., Bradley, J. M., & Piper, A. J. (2017). Non-invasive ventilation for cystic fibrosis. *Cochrane Database of Systematic Reviews*, (2), 1–21. PMID:28218802

Nápolis, L. M., Dal Corso, S., Neder, J. A., Malaguti, C., Gimenes, A. C. O., & Nery, L. E. (2011). Neuromuscular electrical stimulation improves exercise tolerance in chronic obstructive pulmonary disease patients with better preserved fat-free mass. *Clinics (São Paulo)*, *66*(3), 401–406. doi:10.1590/S1807-59322011000300006 PMID:21552662

Nelson, M. E., Rejeski, W. J., Blair, S. N., Duncan, P. W., Judge, J. O., King, A. C., Macera, C. A., & Castaneda-Sceppa, C. (2007). Physical activity and public health in older adults: Recommendation from the American College of Sports Medicine and the American Heart Association. *Medicine and Science in Sports and Exercise*, *39*(8), 1435–1445. doi:10.1249/mss.0b013e3180616aa2 PMID:17762378

Nici, L., Donner, C., Wouters, E., Zuwallack, R., Ambrosino, N., Bourbeau, J., & Garvey, C. (2006). American thoracic society/European respiratory society statement on pulmonary rehabilitation. *American Journal of Respiratory and Critical Care Medicine*, *173*(12), 1390–1413. doi:10.1164/rccm.200508-1211ST PMID:16760357

Pamplona, P., & Morais, L. (2007). Treino de exercício na doença pulmonar crónica. [English Edition]. *Revista Portuguesa de Pneumologia*, *13*(1), 101–128. doi:10.1016/S0873-2159(15)30340-8 PMID:17315093

Paranhos, W. Y., & Santos, V. L. C. G. (1999). Avaliação de risco para úlceras de pressão por meio da escala de Braden, na língua portuguesa. *Revista da Escola de Enfermagem da U S P.*, *33*(1), 191–206.

Peterson, M. D., Rhea, M. R., & Alvar, B. A. (2005). Applications of the dose-response for muscular strength development: A review of meta-analytic efficacy and reliability for designing training prescription. *Journal of Strength and Conditioning Research, 19*(4), 950–958. doi:10.1519/00124278-200511000-00038 PMID:16287373

Podsiadlo, D., & Richardson, S. (1991). The timed "Up & Go": A test of basic functional mobility for frail elderly persons. *Journal of the American Geriatrics Society, 39*(2), 142–148. doi:10.1111/j.1532-5415.1991.tb01616.x PMID:1991946

Rabinovich, R. A., & Vilaró, J. (2010). Structural and functional changes of peripheral muscles in COPD patients. *Current Opinion in Pulmonary Medicine, 16*(2), 123. doi:10.1097/MCP.0b013e328336438d PMID:20071991

Ram, F. S., Robinson, S. M., Black, P. N., & Picot, J. (2005). Physical training for asthma. *Cochrane Database of Systematic Reviews*, (4), CD001116. PMID:16235280

Ries. (2008). Pulmonary Rehabilitation in Emphysema. *American Thoracic Society Journal. 5*(4), 524–529.

Ries, A. L., Make, B. J., & Reilly, J. J. (2011). Pulmonary Rehabilitation. *Respiratory Journal, 38*, 971-975.

Ries, A. L., Bauldoff, G. S., Carlin, B. W., Casaburi, R., Emery, C. F., Mahler, D. A., Make, B., Rochester, C. L., ZuWallack, R., & Herrerias, C. (2007). Pulmonary rehabilitation: Joint ACCP/AACVPR evidence-based clinical practice guidelines. *Chest, 131*(5), 4S–42S. doi:10.1378/chest.06-2418 PMID:17494825

Rocha, S. M. P. (2017). *Impacto de um programa de reabilitação respiratória na qualidade de vida e nas atividades de vida diária de pessoas com doença pulmonar obstrutiva crónica* (Doctoral dissertation). Porto: Escola Superior de Enfermagem do Porto.

Sillen, M. J., Janssen, P. P., Akkermans, M. A., Wouters, E. F., & Spruit, M. A. (2008). The metabolic response during resistance training and neuromuscular electrical stimulation (NMES) in patients with COPD, a pilot study. *Respiratory Medicine, 102*(5), 786–789. doi:10.1016/j.rmed.2008.01.013 PMID:18294832

Silva, E. G. D., & Dourado, V. Z. (2008). Treinamento de força para pacientes com doença pulmonar obstrutiva crônica. *Revista Brasileira de Medicina do Esporte, 14*(3), 231–238. doi:10.1590/S1517-86922008000300014

Silva, L. C. (2012). *Validação do questionário clínico para a doença pulmonar obstrutiva crónica (CCQ) para a língua portuguesa.* Academic Press.

Simmonds, A. K. (2003). Home Ventilation. *The European Respiratory Journal, 22*(47, Supplement 47), 38–46. doi:10.1183/09031936.03.00029803

Society of Critical Care Medicine. (2008). Fundamental Critical Care Suporte (2nd ed.). São Paulo: AWWE.

Sousa, L., & Duque, H. (2012). Reabilitação respiratória na pessoa com Ventilação Não Invasiva. In *Manual de boas práticas na reabilitação respiratória – Conceitos* (pp. 211–225). Princípios e Técnicas. Lusociência.

Sousa, L., Duque, H., & Ferreira, A. (2012). Reabilitação respiratória na pessoa submetida a ventilação invasiva. In *Manual de boas práticas na reabilitação respiratória – Conceitos* (pp. 194–211). Princípios e Técnicas. Lusociência.

Spruit, M. A., Singh, S. J., Garvey, C., ZuWallack, R., Nici, L., Rochester, C., & Pitta, F. (2013). An official American Thoracic Society/European Respiratory Society statement: Key concepts and advances in pulmonary rehabilitation. *American Journal of Respiratory and Critical Care Medicine, 188*(8), e13–e64. doi:10.1164/rccm.201309-1634ST PMID:24127811

Tanaka, H., Monahan, K. D., & Seals, D. R. (2001). Age predicted maximal heart rate revisited. *Journal of the American College of Cardiology, 37*(1), 153–156. doi:10.1016/S0735-1097(00)01054-8 PMID:11153730

Troosters, T., Casaburi, R., Gosselink, R., & Decramer, M. (2005). Pulmonary rehabilitation in chronic obstructive pulmonary disease. *American Journal of Respiratory and Critical Care Medicine, 172*(1), 19–38. doi:10.1164/rccm.200408-1109SO PMID:15778487

Turner, S., Eastwood, P., Cook, A., & Jenkins, S. (2011). Improvements in symptoms and quality of life following exercise training in older adults with moderate/severe persistent asthma. *Respiration, 81*(4), 302–310. doi:10.1159/000315142 PMID:20501982

Tzeng, A. C., & Bach, J. R. (2000). Prevention of pulmonary morbidity for patients with neuromuscular disease. *Chest, 118*(5), 1390–1396. doi:10.1378/chest.118.5.1390 PMID:11083691

Van der Molen, T., Willemse, B. W. M., Schokker, S., ten Hacken, N. H. T., Postma, D. S., & Juniper, E. F. (2003). Development, validity and responsiveness of the Clinical COPD Questionnaire. *Health and Quality of Life Outcomes, 1*(1), 13. doi:10.1186/1477-7525-1-13 PMID:12773199

Velloso, M., & Jardim, J. R. (2006). Study of energy expenditure during activities of daily living using and not using body position recommended by energy conservation techniques in patients with COPD. *Chest*, *130*(1), 126–132. doi:10.1378/chest.130.1.126 PMID:16840392

Vieira, P. J., Chiappa, A. M. G., Cipriano, G. Jr, Umpierre, D., Arena, R., & Chiappa, G. R. (2014). Neuromuscular electrical stimulation improves clinical and physiological function in COPD patients. *Respiratory Medicine*, *108*(4), 609–620. doi:10.1016/j.rmed.2013.12.013 PMID:24418570

Vilaró, J., Resqueti, V. R., & Fregonezi, G. A. F. (2008). Avaliação clínica da capacidade do exercício em pacientes com doença pulmonar obstrutiva crônica. *Brazilian Journal of Physical Therapy*, *12*(4). Advance online publication. doi:10.1590/S1413-35552008000400002

Windisch, W., Walterspacher, S., Siemon, K., Geiseler, J., & Sitter, H. (2010). Guidelines for non-invasive and invasive mechanical ventilation for treatment of chronic respiratory failure. *Pneumologie (Stuttgart, Germany)*, *64*(10), 640–652. doi:10.1055-0030-1255558 PMID:20799159

Zhu, N., Suarez-Lopez, J. R., Sidney, S., Sternfeld, B., Schreiner, P. J., Carnethon, M. R., Lewis, C., Crow, R. S., Bouchard, C., Haskell, W. L., & Jacobs, D. R. Jr. (2010). Longitudinal examination of age-predicted symptom-limited exercise maximum HR. *Medicine and Science in Sports and Exercise*, *42*(8), 1519–1527. doi:10.1249/MSS.0b013e3181cf8242 PMID:20639723

Chapter 3
Non-Invasive Ventilation:
Adaptation of the Elderly Patients

Maria do Céu Mendes Pinto Marques
https://orcid.org/0000-0003-2658-3550
Universidade de Évora, Portugal

Ana Isabel Calha Mourato
Unidade Local de Saude do Norte Alentejano, Portugal

Gonçalo Batista
Unidade de Cuidados Continuados de Arronches, Portugal

Inês Trindade
Unidade de Cuidados Continuados de Arronches, Portugal

Joana Damasceno
Hospital de Abrantes, Portugal

Sara Abreu Nobre
Hospital do Espírito Santo de Évora, Portugal

Teresa Félix
Unidade Local de Saúde do Norte Alentejano, Portugal

ABSTRACT

The objective of this chapter is to analyze articles on the adaptation of the elderly to NIV. The methodology is integrative literature review, using the PICO methodology. After analyzing the content covered, the authors found that there are common factors regarding the adaptation of elderly users to NIV. COPD users are the main users of NIV. This technique promotes an improvement in the quality of life. The introduction of NIV in the user's daily life requires behavioral and lifestyle changes involving health professionals, the user, and caregivers. The choice of the type of ventilator and interfaces is important, in issues such as late assessment of the user's condition and the influence of external factors in adapting to NIV, such as the use of drugs. The adaptation of the elderly user to NIV is influenced by socio-demographic, pathological, anatomical, and associated factors.

DOI: 10.4018/978-1-7998-3531-8.ch003

Copyright © 2020, IGI Global. Copying or distributing in print or electronic forms without written permission of IGI Global is prohibited.

THEORETICAL FRAMEWORK

In Nursing Sciences, Research has been playing an important role since the second half of the 19th century, being that "it allows a systematic study of phenomena present in the field of nursing care, which leads to the discovery and development of knowledge specific to the discipline." (Fortin, 2009)

According to the General Directorate of Health [DGS] (2009) Respiratory Rehabilitation [RR] is an intervention based on the evidence implemented in users with chronic respiratory disease. "Integrated in the individualized treatment of the user, RR is designed to reduce symptoms, optimize functionality, increase social participation and reduce health costs, by stabilizing or regressing the systemic manifestations of the disease." (DGS, 2009).

According to data from the National Program for Respiratory Diseases [PNDR] 2012 - 2016, "the increase in life expectancy has an important impact on the morbidity and mortality of chronic respiratory diseases, and is expected to increase in the coming years." (DGS, 2012) In this program, from 2005 to 2016, it was found that the total number of hospitalizations for respiratory diseases increased by 35% and the episodes of users submitted to mechanical ventilation grew by 167%. This directive also states that "in Portugal, respiratory diseases are one of the main causes of morbidity and mortality, in particular chronic respiratory diseases, whose prevalence is around 40%, with a tendency to increase." (DGS, 2012)

The National Statistics Institute [INE], in the estimate of the population resident in Portugal in 2017, states that "the population aged 65 or over increased to 2 213 274 people (+36 634), representing, respectively, 13.8% and 21.5% of the total population; the oldest population (age 85 or older) was estimated at 297 538 (+11 922)."

This reality then constitutes a challenge for the National Health Service [SNS], which should be able to cope with these demographic and epidemiological changes, by reducing premature mortality (below 70 years of age) and increasing the years of healthy or disability-free lives. "Reducing the number of exacerbations, visits to the emergency department, hospitalizations and even their duration, as well as the intervention of respiratory rehabilitation, have a strong impact on costs."

(ONDR, 2017: 74) The document mentioned above also states that the offer of respiratory rehabilitation in Portugal is extremely scarce. It is in this sense, fundamental to increase the accessibility of the users and for that we suggest the creation of teams and specific physical structures for the provision of respiratory rehabilitation care.

López, Soto & Cruzdo (2009) cited by Pinto & Sousa (?) Noninvasive ventilation consists of a set of techniques that aim to increase alveolar ventilation without the need to use endotracheal intubation. NIV is a type of pressure ventilatory support that is increasingly used in urgent situations of respiratory failure. Historically, we have found two types of NIV, namely negative pressure ventilation (currently in disuse) and positive pressure ventilation.

The situations of chronic respiratory failure were pioneering in the use of NIV, however the application of this technique is also quite effective in acute cases. In view of this, it is extremely important that health professionals, particularly nurses, are familiar with the technique. It should be noted that "the user with NIV requires specific and complex care, of which nursing care is essential for the successful execution of this technique". (Pinto, 2013)

It should be noted, like all techniques, NIV has indications and contraindications, and it is not indicated for all types of pathology.

It is indicated, according to DGS (2015) in situations of chronic respiratory failure, sleep apnea, obesity / hypoventilation syndrome, neuromuscular diseases, chronic obstructive pulmonary diseases, including exacerbations of the same, respiratory failure after extubation, asthma and in the decompensations of cystic fibrosis.

"It can also be used in weaning from Invasive Ventilation, in patients who arc not candidates or who refuse Invasive Ventilation and in the treatment of some hypoxemic Acute Respiratory Failure pathologies, such as acute pulmonary edema, post-surgery respiratory failure, pneumonia and injury acute pulmonary disease." (Pinto, 2013: 3)

With regard to NIV contraindications, Blanco et al. (2011) refer as contraindications for the initiation of NIV, situations of cardio-respiratory arrest [CRP], in situations of hemodynamic instability, upper gastrointestinal bleeding and epistaxis. Its use should also be avoided in patients who have altered state of consciousness, inability to protect the airway with risk of aspiration or obstruction of the upper airway, excess of bronchial secretions, chest trauma, trauma, burns and/or surgical interventions on the face and nose, morbid obesity and myocardial infarction.

According to Pinto (2013) the main advantage of NIV is that it is more comfortable for users, it allows them to speak and make an oral feeding when ventilated with a nasal mask and in addition, the users preserve the cough reflex, humidify the airways and heating the inhaled air.

Regarding the complications related to NIV, these are generally of minor severity, such as injuries caused by contact with the interface, but may require the need to suspend the technique. Several authors describe comfort as a factor that interferes with the success of NIV affected mainly by synchrony with the ventilator, the interface, leaks, high pressures, positioning, mucosal dryness and communication. That is why the selection of the interface takes on a central role. Today, we have different models of interfaces, ensuring better adaptation and user comfort and reducing skin injuries.

According to the Regulation of the Order of Nurses published in Diário da República published in 2011, "Specialist is the nurse with an in-depth knowledge in a specific domain of nursing, taking into account human responses to life processes and health problems", which goes against the importance of continuous training for health professionals.

The skills acquired by nursing professionals, in addition to improving issues of a technical nature, increase trust in the relationship with the user and, consequently, their acceptance before NIV.

There is an awareness of the weight of professional experience around the relationship with the user / family and consequently the importance of informing and explaining to them the entire care process. The Order of Nurses, in the document referring to the definition of Quality Standards in Nursing Care, emphasizes the importance of professional experience when saying that "(...) in the scope of professional practice, nurses are distinguished by their training and experience it allows you to understand and respect others in a multicultural perspective (...) "(OE, 2001: 12). In this way, professional training and the user's relationship with the nurse has implications for the acceptance of treatments, namely NIV.

METHODOLOGY

The use of the PICOD format, in the formulation of the clinical question, leads to a literature search more oriented to the problem under study, being therefore the first step to follow. In the elaboration of this work, the following question was defined as a PICOD question: What are the factors that interfere in the elderly user's adaptation to NIV?

As an objective of this review it is intended to answer the question PICO, by identifying the factors that interfere in the adaptation to NIV (Outcomes) among the several studies found (Comparison), referring to the elderly user (Participant), with the presence of any intervention.

The election of studies, a posteriori, implies the definition of inclusion/exclusion criteria, namely the presence of elderly users with NIV, publication date between 2016 and 2018 and inclusion of all articles found, regardless of the type of study, provided that the full text is available.

In this line of reasoning we define as keywords "non-invasive ventilation", "geriatric" and "elderly". After this process, we verified its viability on the MESH and DESC platforms, respectively in the languages covered, and it was possible to verify that all of them fit into these platforms.

We carried out an integrative literature review through searches in the B-ON database. Using descriptors in English, the inclusion criteria in the selection of articles were those referred to in the previous table.

In the case of B-ON we use the combination of keywords with the Boolean operators AND and OR resulting in the combination: [("non-invasive ventilation" AND "elderly" OR "aged" OR "older" OR "elder" OR "geriatric")]. We also used the concepts of [("pediatrician; pediatric or child or children")] associated with the Boolean operator NOT, reducing the search to 149 articles.

In order to rigorously screen the results obtained from the initial research, full publications of academic journals, peer review, from 2016 to 2018, were accessed as accessors, accessing the Medline Complete and Complementary Index databases.

In view of the aforementioned items, we obtained 17 articles, of which, after reading the title and/or abstract, 8 articles were included in this integrative review, collected in the chosen database.

Figure 1. Article selection process

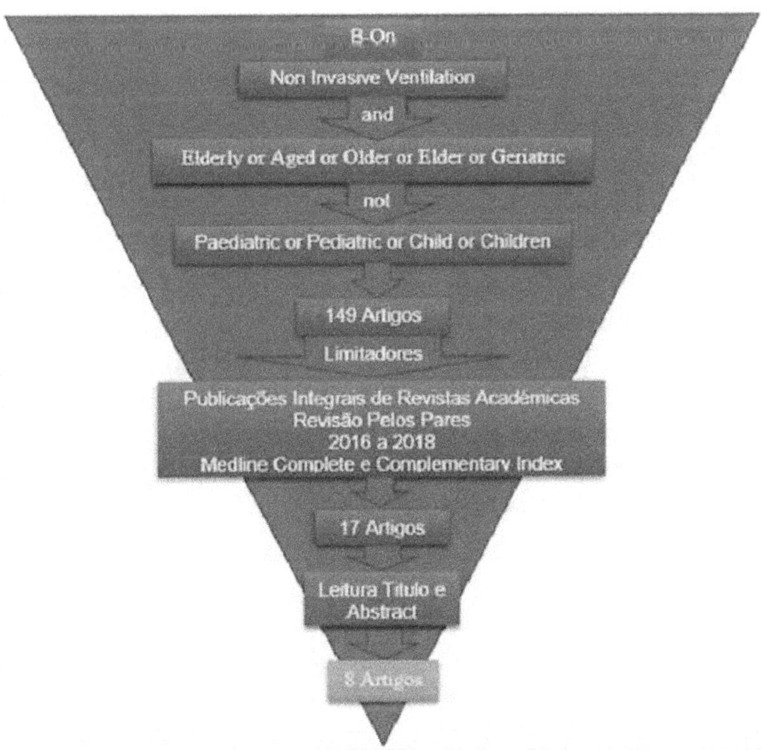

After selecting the articles, we proceed to their analysis from the point of view of the level of evidence and methodological quality.

According to the Integrative Systematic Bibliographic Review Manual, evidence-based research (2014): "Scientific evidence is formed by the set of information used to confirm or deny a scientific theory or hypothesis, taking place only through scientific research."

For inclusion in the study, each of the articles was subjected to a critical evaluation, using the definitions pointed out by the Joanna Briggs Institute [JBI], in order to find the level of evidence and the degree of recommendation of the referred articles.

We will then make an analogy between the number given to the articles and their title and later we present a table where we describe the level of evidence and the degree of recommendation of each one of them.

1. "A decade of domiciliary non-invasive ventilation in the west of Ireland" ;
2. "Impact of Non-Invasive Ventilation on Sympathetic Nerve Activity in Chronic Obstructive Pulmonary Disease";
3. "Long-term outcomes after acute hypercapnic COPD exacerbation: First-ever episode of non-invasive ventilation";
4. "Initiation of non-invasive ventilation in amyotrophic lateral sclerosis and clinical practice guidelines: Single-Centre, retrospective, descriptive study in a national reference Centre";
5. "A psychological intervention to promote acceptance and adherence to non-invasive ventilation in people with chronic obstructive pulmonary disease: study protocol of a randomized controlled trial";
6. "Factors predicting survival in amyotrophic lateral sclerosis patients on non-invasive ventilation";
7. "Home Non Invasive Ventilation (NIV) treatment for COPD patients with a history of NIV-treated exacerbation; a randomized, controlled, multi-center study";
8. "Effects of Provided Trainings Regarding Non-Invasive Mechanical Ventilation on the Knowledge Level of Nurses".

Table 1. Level of evidence and degree of recommendation

	Type of Study	Level of Evidence	Percentage	Degree of Recommendation
1	Longitudinal Section Study	3e	8/9 88,9%	Strong
2	Pseudo - RCT	1d	8/10 80%	Strong
3	RCT	1c	12/13 92,3%	Strong
4	Cross- Sectional Study	4b	6/8 75%	Strong
5	RCT	1c	11/13 84,6%	Strong
6	RCT	1c	11/13 84,6%	Strong
7	RCT	1c	12/13 92,3%	Strong
8	RCT	1c	9/13 69,2%	Strong

ARTICLE ANALYSIS

See Table 2.

DISCUSSION OF RESULTS

After reading the articles selected to carry out this integrative review, we performed a content analysis where, we can verify that there are common factors regarding the adaptation of elderly users to NIV and that lead us to the answer to the question PICO. This point was facilitated by the increase in the elderly population, namely in Portugal, as found by INE (2018) and which goes against what DGS (2012) analyzes, when referring that the increase in average life expectancy induces an increase in diseases chronic.

We found that the survival rate of COPD users using NIV is relatively short in contrast to users with other pathologies, as reported by the authors of article 1, P. Gouda et al. (2016). It also states that, regardless of the pathology, all users report an improvement in the quality of life after the introduction of NIV at home, preventing the recurrence of episodes of hypercapnia. (Article 7, N. Calzada et al. 2016) We can

Table 2.

	Study Objective and Design	Nº and Type of Participants	Intervention	Results	Conclusions
1	Longitudinal Cut Study that describes the evolution of home prescription and the benefits of NIV for the survival of users with respiratory pathologies from 2000 to 2012	161 users with home NIV, most of whom are obese, with Chronic Obstructive Pulmonary Disease [COPD], with two or more acute exacerbations associated with another type of pathology	Users of Galway University Hospital between 2000 and 2012, with NIV at home, approached to check the mortality rate and their experience with home NIV. The analyzed data include age, sex, indication for NIV, start date and mortality.	There were higher mortality rates in users with COPD and neuromuscular diseases in the first 3 years of the disease compared to other pathologies. The study included 161 users, 58 (36.3%) female, whose average age was 70 years. COPD was the most common indication for the prescription of NIV (n = 76, 48%), followed by the hypoventilation syndrome in obesity (n = 50.31%). Neuromuscular disorders were responsible for 21 prescriptions (12%).	The use of NIV at home increased from 2000 to 2012, as did the increase in NIV prescription for users with COPD. **The survival rate of these users under NIV is short in contrast to other pathologies. In the evaluation of the users, all refer to an improvement in the quality of life after the introduction of NIV at home, regardless of the pathology.**
2	**Pseudo-RCT Associate high sympathetic nervous activity with increased cardiovascular risk and muscle dysfunction due to increased vasoconstrictor stimulus.**	**5 COPD users with intermittent NIV and 11 COPD users in a control group without NIV**	**Performing handgrip exercises, before and after the beginning of NIV, in order to assess the influence of sympathetic nerve stimulation on adaptation to NIV**	Sympathetic Nerve Muscle Activity [AMNS] adjusted to heart rate did not differ between groups. NIV did not significantly affect AMNS levels at rest. During handgrip exercises directly after NIV, AMNS was lower than before, which was significant for dynamic handgrip movements. **ASNM increased in the control group during the dynamic static grip.** During dynamic gripping, the CO2 pressure [pCO2] was lower after NIV than before, while the blood pressure values did not change significantly.	**The authors concluded that NIV reduces sympathetic activation during the subsequent dynamic handgrip exercise and, therefore, can cause positive effects on the cardiovascular system, as well as on muscle function in patients with COPD.**
3	RCT Characterize long-term results and identify markers in COPD patients with NIV after the first episode of acute respiratory failure due to hypercapnia.	122 users, with an average age of 62 years, 52% of whom are female	Data collected between 2000 and 2012 to assess the reason for admission to hospital and subsequent application of NIV. These data were compared with 3 previous studies on the subject.	Advanced age, low body mass index [BMI] and persistent hypercapnia were risk factors for prescribing home NIV. Survival rates were 79% and 63% at 1 and 2 years after discharge, respectively.	COPD was regularly found as a co-morbidity and not as the main reason for admission, which leads to the exclusion of most cases. The reason for readmission to the services is mainly respiratory arrest and respiratory hypercapnia. The use of home NIV, age, cachexia and hypoxemia at admission are related to a higher probability of readmission. The use of NIV increased significantly over time, among hospitalized users, due to acute exacerbations of COPD, while the need for intubation and hospital mortality decreased.

continued on following page

Table 2. Continued

	Study Objective and Design	N° and Type of Participants	Intervention	Results	Conclusions
4	Descriptive quantitative study (Cross-sectional study). Describe NIP initiation practices according to French guidelines, in patients with Amyotrophic Lateral Sclerosis [ALS]	624 users with ALS started NIV between 2005 and 2013	For 568 (91%) of the 624 ventilated ALS users NIV was initiated according to guidelines, that is, in the presence of at least one symptom and an associated physiological criterion. The criteria used to initiate NIV include associated symptomatology, pCO2, maximum inspiratory pressures and time with measurement of peripheral oxygen saturation [SpO2] during the night.	At the time of onset, 90% of users reported a symptom and 57% of users reported three or more symptoms, corresponding to insomnia in 74% of cases, while the most common symptom reported was dyspnea. In the group of patients in whom NIV was started later, daytime hypercapnia was less identified as an indication for ventilation (43% before 2007 versus 31% from 2007 onwards), while symptoms related to sleep and poor quality of life (orthopnea, insomnia and morning headache) were most frequently identified.	This analysis suggests that NIV is started relatively late in the course of the disease, only when 70% of users report orthopnea, 74% report nocturnal symptoms related to breathing, and 58% have hypercapnia. However, several elements suggest that this late onset of NIV is due to poor surveillance from the clinical side and other factors may contribute to the increasing technical difficulty of performing pulmonary function tests due to the deterioration of the disease. and because, from the user's point of view, it may be difficult to accept the onset of NIV when based exclusively on functional abnormalities in the absence of symptoms.
5	Randomized controlled trial - clinical trial to analyze the effects of psychological support on NIV acceptance and adherence	150 COPD users for whom NIV was prescribed	The experimental group (40 participants) will receive a brief psychological support course that will include counseling, relaxation exercises and mindfulness. In some cases, it will also include neuropsychological rehabilitation exercises. An assessment of the change in quality of life will be made at 3, 6 and 12 months after the identification of psychological and clinical factors that predict rejection. Finally, semi-structured interviews will be conducted to obtain information about the perceptions of users submitted to NIV. Data analysis will be performed using the SPSS software.	Preliminary evidence suggests that it is necessary to pay attention to psychological factors in both treatment and rehabilitation. Psychological changes can be a consequence of physical symptoms, but they can also influence the course of the disease, like other chronic conditions. Clinical experience suggests that users with cognitive deficits or psychological problems, such as anxiety and depression, are less likely to accept and comply with NIV regimens. The few studies available have focused on early NIV failure. Previous studies suggest that users with COPD who have demonstrated a lower benefit with the use of NIV have the worst daily average of NIV use, due to the imbalance between restrictions imposed by NIV and the improvement that users perceive in their condition. The fan settings are not easy to adjust and influence the quality of sleep, which has side effects on daytime life.	The use of NIV requires that the user has to make some behavioral and lifestyle changes, such as changes in the daily routine, and this can reduce adherence to treatment. Adherence to treatment may also be adversely affected by the use of different drugs and devices, or because users have inadequate education about the disease and associated pathologies. The ventilator settings are not easy to adjust and influence the quality of sleep, which has an effect on daytime life.

continued on following page

Table 2. Continued

	Study Objective and Design	N° and Type of Participants	Intervention	Results	Conclusions
6	RCT - Intends to evaluate the factors that interfere in the survival time of patients with Amyotrophic Lateral Sclerosis [ALS] who undergo NIV	213 users who started NIV for more than 4 hours between 2000 and 2014	After diagnosis, users are evaluated every three months by all specialists during a home visit. The assessment of respiratory function includes a questionnaire about symptoms, the performance of arterial blood gas analysis, the control of cough effectiveness and the assessment of nocturnal oximetry. The interfaces used included a wide variety of nasal and oronasal masks. The ventilation parameters have been adjusted to achieve the greatest comfort. Changes to the ventilator or interface settings were made during the progression of the disease and, when necessary to optimize the comfort and effectiveness of NIV.	A total of 213 users were included in the study: 132 (62%) were male with an average age of 65 years. At the time of the initiation of NIV, 190 (98%) users were taking Riluzole and 14 (7.4%) had a nasogastric tube [SNG]. 9% of users used NIV at home, with the most widely used interface being the oronasal in about 59% of users. The results probably reflect poor prognosis and advanced disease, but this does not mean that NIV was not effective in these patients.	Better assessment, including assessment of the upper airway and careful titration of NIV are necessary to optimize treatment effectiveness. In users with significant bulbar dysfunction, there are major restrictions regarding the performance of NIV. Regarding survival, the results are consistent, showing a low survival after the beginning of NIV. Age at diagnosis and accumulation of mucus in the airways were factors for poor prognosis in patients treated with NIV. This is explained by the presence of mucus and saliva accumulated in the upper airway or in the destabilization / obstruction of the upper airway, which could cause glottis dysfunction in cases of severe bulbar involvement. A careful assessment of the upper part of the airways and an accurate titration of information about NIV should be considered as one of the factors of adaptation and effectiveness of NIV in these patients.
7	Randomized, multicenter, open-label study. To study whether the use of NIV can reduce mortality or repeat hypercapnic respiratory failure, reduce successive hospitalizations, exacerbations of the disease and improve the quality of life in users who have been admitted for long-term NIV treatment.	150 COPD users who survived admission and treatment with NIV. Included patients are randomized to the usual treatment or to continue NIV as long-term therapy, both with a follow-up period of one year.	Before discharge, the participant and caregivers are trained in handling and cleaning the ventilator, tubes, masks, etc. The participant is instructed to use the ventilator for a minimum of six hours daily, preferably during the hours of sleep. In home visits and consultations, NIV treatment is optimized according to the participant's requests or complaints. One month after discharge, participants who had only one episode of hypercapnic respiratory failure and who did not feel a subjective improvement are offered to discontinue treatment, provided that, after discharge, they have had no exacerbations, need for antibiotics, increased corticosteroids or inhaled medication, hospital stay or an emergency due to COPD, sputum or increased dyspnea for at least one day. Participants are randomized to long-term NIV treatment or usual care in a 1: 1 ratio.	The primary outcome is the difference in time to death or repeated acute respiratory failure between the two study groups. The secondary results are the differences in the following variables: • mortality in one year; • hospital admission for COPD; • hospitalization due to repetition of acute hypercapnic respiratory failure; • visits to the emergency department due to COPD; • exacerbations treated with oral corticosteroids or oral antibiotics; • changes in the body mass index • forced expiratory volume in one second.	This study assesses whether long-term NIV treatment can reduce mortality and prevent exacerbations of respiratory failure in patients with unstable COPD. Three previous studies evaluated long-term NIV for patients with COPD and the results were conflicting, as both showed that NIV could reduce the repetition of respiratory hypercapnia, while the other had no effect. It is documented that previous exacerbations of COPD predict new exacerbations and that these predict death. Based on this, it is concluded that long-term NIV can reduce mortality and repetition of cases of respiratory hypercapnia.

continued on following page

Table 2. Continued

	Study Objective and Design	Nº and Type of Participants	Intervention	Results	Conclusions
8	RCT - intends to determine the influence of the training of health professionals, nurses, on the effectiveness of treatment with NIV	70 nurses from a university hospital, with an average age of 33 years, in which 87.1% were female, 68.6% were bachelors and 47.1% worked in intensive care. 94.7% mentioned that they have no knowledge about the application of NIV.	4 weeks of training on the application of NIV, where knowledge about NIV indications, contraindications, complications, interfaces and success criteria were evaluated	The nurses' knowledge levels in relation to the evaluated points rose after the applied training. However, the levels of knowledge regarding the advantages of NIV did not show significant changes. It was determined that the nurses' knowledge levels regarding the problems of wearing a mask and airflow during NIV increased significantly after training.	Nurses' knowledge increased significantly after training on non-invasive applications. Through this they develop affective, cognitive and psychomotor skills allowing the increase of NIV success. Obtaining the user-ventilator interaction is the most important step to obtain positive NIV results. In addition to choosing an appropriate mask, the application of NIV according to the user's needs, the characteristics of the mask to be used, the mode and settings of the selected mask, the type of fan and the experience of the team members are also important for the management of the ventilation process. Training programs that aim to increase the knowledge and experience of members of the health team are believed to have positive effects in reducing complications associated with NIV.

also mention that the aspects found in the analysis of the chosen articles, coincide with the recommendations of the PNDR 2012-2016 created by DGS in 2012.

In turn, the authors of article 2, H. Haarmann et al (2016) adds that in users with this pathology, when practicing handgrip exercises, they verify a decrease in sympathetic nervous activation, which produces positive effects on the cardiovascular system and the consequent improvement of muscle function.

COPD is often associated with hospital readmission of patients with NIV, due to this pathology, there are other factors that lead to re-hospitalization, including respiratory hypercapnia and apnea, induced by age, cachexia and hypoxemia, which goes against the that the author Pinto (2013) mentions, as well as what the National Observatory for Respiratory Diseases [ONDR] indicates in 2017, which aims to "Reduce by 10% the number of people hospitalized for respiratory causes that can be prevented or treated in the centers during the 2014/2020 period. "

Several of the articles addressed refer to the use of NIV at home, thus showing its importance in improving quality of life, regardless of pathology. Over the years, there has been an increase in NIV prescription at home, with this adaptation being made gradually, without complications, which goes against what DGS (2009) recommends and which is described in the first phase of this document.

The introduction of NIV in the patient's daily life requires behavioral and lifestyle changes in order to allow time for this therapy, thus facilitating adaptation to treatment. This process can be affected by the therapy of each user, by their level of literacy and by the devices used in the use of NIV. It was demonstrated that the choice of interfaces according to the user's needs has an influence on their adaptation to NIV. The ventilation modes, the type of ventilator and the experience of the team members who manage the user's ventilation process, are simultaneously important factors in the process of adapting to NIV.

The sleep changes described in article 5, prepared by Eleonora Volpato et al. 2017 are a consequence of the choice of ventilator configurations and, in turn, responsible for the changes found in the user's life during the day.

In this follow-up and, after the evaluation of article 8, it was found that the training of Nursing professionals in this theme is correlated with the development of affective, cognitive and psychomotor skills, allowing the increase in the success of NIV and leading to the reduction of complications associated with this therapy. This analysis is corroborated by what is described by the Order of Nurses in 2001 in the document on Quality Standards in Nursing Care.

One of the factors that contribute to a low rate of adaptation to NIV is the late assessment of upper airway conditions as users with accumulation of secretions or intense sialorrhea condition asynchronism with the ventilator, causing additional discomfort and eventual rejection of the therapy. The authors of Article 4 report for this very reason, when they state that this late assessment leads to "increasing technical difficulty in carrying out pulmonary function tests with the deterioration of the disease" and also goes against what Sonay Göktaş et al. (2017), article 6, which shows the importance of age at diagnosis for adaptation to NIV. We can associate with this late assessment, the indications and contraindications of NIV described by Blanco (2011), which lead to the reticence of the application of this technique.

In this line of reasoning, the late onset of NIV is due to poor clinical surveillance, adding to the difficulty in accepting therapy when there are no associated symptoms.

FINAL NOTE

With this integrative literature review we can conclude that the adaptation of the elderly user to NIV is dependent on several factors, namely socio-demographic, pathological, anatomical and associated with devices.

The main factors that interfere in the adaptation of the elderly user to NIV, referred to in the articles studied are: the need for behavioral and lifestyle changes of the user, the influence of the low level of Body Mass Index, the therapy performed by the user and pathologies associated, low clinical surveillance and late assessment of the user's upper airway conditions as well as the need for monitoring by a multidisciplinary team with skills related to NIV. The appropriate choice in terms of interfaces, fans and ventilation modes.

As a difficulty in carrying out this integrative review, the fact that the adaptation of NIV is not exclusively associated with the elderly user can be highlighted in the articles. Most of the articles refer to adult users above a certain age group, later referring to the elderly user.

It is a suggestion to carry out studies aimed exclusively at the elderly population, considering the increase in average life expectancy and the comorbidities associated with the aging of the population. Another suggestion will be the investment in the training of health professionals in relation to non-invasive ventilation, given the growing number of users who need this therapy either in chronic situations at home or in hospital conditions.

REFRENCES

Ankjaergaard, K., Tonnesen, P., Laursen, L., Hansen, E., Andreassen, H., & Wilcke, J. (2016). *Home Non Invasive Ventilation (NIV) treatment for COPD patients with a history of NIV- treated exacerbation; a randomized, controlled, multi-center study.* BioMed Central. doi:10.118612890-016-0184-6

Blanco, J. B., Ribeiro, R., & Alves, I. (2011). Protocolo de Início da VMNI. In A. M. Esquinas (Eds.), Princípios da Ventilação Mecânica Não Invasiva – Do Hospital ao Domicílio. Vila do Conde: Gasin Médica.

Calzada, N., Soro, E., Gomez, L., Bulta, E., Izquierdo, A., Panades, M., Sargatal, J., & Muñoz, E. (2016). *Factors predicting survival in amyotrophic lateral sclerosis patients on non-invasive ventilation*. Taylor & Francis Group.

DGS. (2009). *Orientações Técnicas sobre Reabilitação Respiratória na Doença Pulmonar Obstrutiva Crónica (DPOC)*. Circular Normativa nº: 40A/DSPCD de 27/10/09. Acedido a 19 de Novembro de 2018. Disponível em: https://www.dgs.pt/directrizes-da- dgs/normas-e-circulares-normativas.aspx

DGS. (2012) *Programa Nacional para as Doenças Respiratórias*. Acedido a 17 de Novembro de 2018. Disponível em: https://www.dgs.pt/pns-e-programas/programas-de- saude-prioritarios/doencas-respiratorias.aspx

DGS. (2015) Norma 022/2011, actualizada a 11/09/2015: *Cuidados Respiratórios Domiciliários: Prescrição de Ventiloterapia e outros Equipamentos*. Acedido a 09 de Dezembro de 2018. Disponível em: https://www.dgs.pt/directrizes-da-dgs/Fnormas-e- circulares-normativas/norma-n-0222011-de-28092011-jpg.aspx

Diário da República. (2011). Regulamento das Competências Comuns do Enfermeiro Especialista. *Regulamento, 122*.

Fazekas, A., Aboulghaith, M., Kriz, R., Urban, M., Breyer, M., Kohansal, R., Burghuber, O., Harti, S., & Funk, G. (2017). *Long-term outcomes after acute hypercapnic COPD exacerbation – first-ever episode of non-invasive ventilation*. The Central European Jounal of Medicine. Taylor & Francis Group.

Fortin. (2009). Fundamentos e etapas do processo de investigação. Lisboa: Lusodidacta.

Georges, M., Goldmard, J., Llontop, C., Shoukri, A., Salachas, F., Similowski, T., … Bermejo, J. (2017). *Initiation of non-invasive ventilation in amyotrophic lateral sclerosis and clinical practice guedelines: Single-centre, retrospective, descriptive study in a national referece centre*. Academic Press.

Göktas, S., Kiraner, E., Dogan, P., & Tunali, B. (2017). *Effects of Provided Trainings Regarding Non-Invasive Mechanical Ventilation on the Knowledge Level of Nurses*. Eurasian Pulmonol. doi:10.5152/ejp.2016.05706

Gouda, P., Chua, J., Langan, D., Hannon, T., Scott, A., & O'Regan, A. (2016). *A decade of domiciliary non-invasive ventilation in the west of Ireland*. Royal Academy of Medicine in Ireland.

Grupo Anima Educação. (2014). *Manual de Revisão Bibliográfica Sistemática Integrativa: A Pesquisa Baseada em Evidências*. Grupo Anima Educação.

Haarmann, H., Folle, J., Nguyen, X., Herrmann, P., Heusser, K., Hasefub, G., … Raupach, T. (2016). *Impact of Non-Invasive Ventilation on Sympathetic Nerve Activity in Chronic Obtrutive Pulmunary Disease.* Springer Science + Business Media.

Instituto Nacional de Estatística. (2018). *Estimativas de População Residente - A redução da população residente atenuou-se - 2017.* Acedido a 7 de Dezembro de 2018. Disponível em: https://www.ine.pt/xportal/xmain?xpid=INE&xpgid=ine_destaques&DESTAQUESdest_boui=315156710&DESTAQUESmodo=2&xlang=pt

Ordem Dos Enfermeiros. (2001). *Padrões de Qualidade dos Cuidados de Enfermagem - enquadramento conceptual enunciados descritivos.* Acedido a 9 de Dezembro de 2018. Disponível em: https://www.ordemenfermeiros.pt/media/8903/divulgar-padroes-de-qualidade-dos-cuidados.pdf

Pinto. (2013). Ventilação Não Invasiva – Uma prática fundamentada em evidência científica. *Revista Nursing Edição, 25*(288).

Respiratorias Observatório Nacional Das Doenças. (2017). *Relatório de 2017.* Acedido a 19 de Novembro de 2018. Disponível em: http://respirarmelhor.pt/wp-content/uploads/2017/11/Relat%C3%B3rio-Completo-ONDR-2017.pdf

The Joanna Briggs Institute. (n.d.a). *Critical Appraisal Tools.* The University Adelaide. 2014. Acedido a 8 de Novembro de 2018. Disponível em: https://joannabriggs.org/research/critical-appraisal-tools.html

The Joanna Briggs Institute. (n.d.b). *Levels of Evidence.* The University Adelaide. 2014. Acedido a 8 de Novembro de 2018. Disponível em: http://joannabriggs.org/jbi- approach.html#tabbed-nav=Levels-of-Evidence

The Joanna Briggs Institute. (n.d.c). *Grades of Recommendations.* The University Adelaide. 2014. Acedido a 8 de Novembro de 2018. Disponível em: http://joannabriggs.org/jbi-approach.html#tabbed-nav=Grades-of-Recommendation

Volpato, E., Banfi, P., & Pagnini, F. (n.d.). *A psychological intervention to promote acceptance and adherence to non-invasive ventilation in people with chronic obstrutive pulmonary disease: study protocol of a randomised controlled trial.* BioMed Central.

Chapter 4
Early Weaning of the Person Undergoing Invasive Mechanical Ventilation:
Impact of Rehabilitation Nursing Interventions

Raquel Cruz Amorim
Hospital Center of Setúbal, Portugal

Ana Daniela Costa
Hospital Center of Setúbal, Portugal

Rogério Ferrinho Ferreira
https://orcid.org/0000-0001-5180-2036
Polytechnic Institute of Beja, Portugal

João Vitor Vieira
https://orcid.org/0000-0002-3905-4802
Polytechnic Institute of Beja, Portugal

ABSTRACT

The use of invasive mechanical ventilatory support has been increasingly used in the treatment of respiratory insufficiency, since it replaces the respiratory work while reversing the pathological processes that led to its necessity, allowing the recovery of respiratory function. The critical patient's ventilatory weaning requires a rigorous assessment by qualified professionals to reduce complications and the eventual need for (re) intubation, referring to the design and implementation of rehabilitation nursing programs. The nurse specialist in rehabilitation nursing intervenes in an early, autonomous, and differentiated way, avoiding complications and incapacities, promoting effective ventilatory weaning. This integrative review of the literature made evident the gains obtained in the critical patient undergoing invasive mechanical ventilation and included in an early rehabilitation program, revealing significant impact for both the patient and the hospital institution.

DOI: 10.4018/978-1-7998-3531-8.ch004

Copyright © 2020, IGI Global. Copying or distributing in print or electronic forms without written permission of IGI Global is prohibited.

INTRODUCTION

Scientific and technological advances in medicine have resulted in the ability to prolong life. One of the consequences of this progress is the significant increase in patients requiring prolonged invasive mechanical ventilation (IMV), which is defined by the need to maintain mechanical ventilatory support for 21 days or more for more than six hours daily (MacIntyre, Epstein, Carson, Scheinhorn, Christopher & Muldoon, 2005).

Ventilatory weaning corresponds to a gradual reduction of ventilatory support until it is no longer necessary, and this process is considered a priority, taking into account that, although it is a fundamental technique for maintaining life, it can cause physiological and psychological complications that should be minimized (Cederwall, Plos, Rose, Dübeck & Ringdal, 2014). In this context, it is important to perform an early ventilatory weaning, either to promote the occurrence of spontaneous ventilation after extubating or to avoid the occurrence of complications associated with this therapy.

In general, for all persons undergoing invasive mechanical ventilation, 40% to 50% of the total time of this ventilatory support is spent in the ventilatory weaning process (Cederwall et al., 2014). This period contributes significantly to the total cost of intensive care hospitalization, with some authors pointing to around 50% of the total costs of an ICU (Cederwall et al., 2014). This factor raises questions regarding occupancy rates, use of resources and, consequently, costs for hospital institutions. The attempt to reduce and minimize the impact caused by these aspects should be taken into account as a matter of priority, both for health professionals and for those institutions.

The negative consequences associated with immobility are commonly associated with patients who require IMV and are widely recognized. The establishment of early rehabilitation protocols are reported as evident in reducing length of stay in the intensive care unit (ICU), increasing muscle strength and functional capacity, as well as reducing the duration of effective ventilatory weaning (Dunn, Quinn, Corbrigde, Eldeirawi, Kapella & Collins, 2017).

The need for ventilatory weaning protocols is transversal to several authors, advocating the implementation of strategies aimed at decreasing IMV time, its pathophysiological consequences and its hospital cost (MacIntyre et al., 2005).

Associated with the implementation of early ventilatory weaning protocols, rehabilitation programs aimed at patients, hospitalized in the ICU; aim to improve residual capacity, preventing complications associated with decreased muscle strength due to ventilatory dependence and prolonged immobility. The application of these rehabilitation protocols also aims to reduce the need for rehospitalization and contributes to a lower functional deficit after hospital discharge (Ambrosino, Venturelli, Vagheggini & Clini, 2012).

It is in this sense that the presence of specialized multidisciplinary teams is pointed out as these professionals have the competencies to perform, implement and evaluate autonomous and differentiated care plans to intervene in the real and potential problems of patients. Their knowledge enables them to act in an early manner, implementing preventive measures, in order to avoid complications and disabilities. It also allows therapeutic interventions aimed at regaining independence in the various functions of the body, namely respiratory function (Order of Nurses, 2011).

Nursing Rehabilitation at Early Ventilatory Weaning

As mentioned previously, one of the main reasons for hospitalization in the ICU is the need for IMV. Prolonged mechanical ventilation presupposes the existence of an artificial airway, in particular through an endotracheal tube or a tracheostomy cannula, in the patient considered in a critical condition, requiring a ventilator (which generates a positive pressure, allowing air to be blown into the lungs of the patient periodically, through the inspiratory circuit, and air outlet through the expiratory circuit). IMV aims to improve gas exchange and restore alveolar ventilation, thereby preventing complications when spontaneous ventilation is not adequate or ineffective (Severino, 2016).

Mechanical ventilation is a therapeutic process that allows spontaneous breathing to be assisted, or sometimes replaced, when it is affected, to a greater or lesser degree (Cordeiro & Menoita, 2014). Despite the benefits of this technique in the stabilization of the critical patient, there are some side effects that can be corrected or minimized by the intervention of the Specialist Nurse in Rehabilitation Nursing (SNRN).

It can thus be affirmed that SNRN intervention in Respiratory Functional Reeducation (RFR) can be developed in the various stages of the IMV process. Interventions in RFR should begin before oral-tracheal intubation in an attempt to avoid this technique or in the preparation of the patient for the invasive technique (Cordeiro & Menoita, 2014). The ventilation phase can occur either in the controlled modes (controlled volume, pressure controlled volume control and pressure controlled) or assisted modes (support pressure, support volume, pressure support / continuous pressure in the airways). As the next-to-last phase of intervention, weaning occurs (Severino, 2016). The SNRN also acts in the post-invasive mechanical ventilation phase and in the preparation of ICU discharge / discharge.

The RFR in the patient submitted to IMV is appropriate in the preparation and adjustment of the ventilator, during intubation, during invasive ventilation, ventilatory weaning and extubation (Cordeiro & Menoita, 2014).

The person undergoing IMV and during hospitalization in the ICU can frequently present atelectasis, ineffective airway clearance, and decreased respiratory muscle strength. These factors will condition ventilatory weaning and may increase the likelihood of (re) intubation (Cordeiro & Menoita, 2014). Therefore, it is imperative to establish an RFR program for the patient considered critical, in order to prevent and minimize such complications.

RESPIRATORY FUNCTIONAL RE-EDUCATION BEFORE MECHANICAL VENTILATION

There are objectives to take into account before submitting the patient to IMV, from the RFR:

- Reduce fear and anxiety with emotional support for the person and family;
- Decrease respiratory work through rest and relaxation positions, with relaxation at the level of the cervical and scapula-humeral muscles;
- Optimize gas exchange by performing breathing control exercises;
- Mobilizing and eliminating secretions through instruction and training of the active cycle of respiratory techniques and forced expiration, used alone with or without the open glottis, directed and assisted cough (Cordeiro & Menoita, 2014).

The objectives of the RFR at this stage are:

- Prevention and correction of ventilatory defects;
- Improve the performance of respiratory muscles;
- Maintain airway permeability (including mobilization and elimination of bronchial secretions);
- Prevention and correction of musculoskeletal disorders;
- Reeducate in the effort;
- Promote ventilatory weaning (Severino, 2016).

When the patient is submitted to IMV, the ventilatory weaning program is started immediately, and there are essential criteria for initiating this program:

- Ventilation in assisted mode for 48 hours;
- Full or partial recovery of the cause that led to IMV;
- Body temperature below 39 ° C;
- No signs of infection;
- Acceptable renal function;
- Neurological status compatible with spontaneous ventilation;
- Metabolic balance;
- Hemoglobin> 8 g / dL;
- No signs of heart failure;
- Ability to cough;
- Reduced amount of bronchial secretions;
- Absence of arrhythmias or conduction disturbances (Severino, 2016).

RESPIRATORY FUNCTIONAL RE-EDUCATION DURING MECHANICAL VENTILATION

The complications of IMV are described and recognized, such as alterations in the mechanisms of tracheobronchial hygiene (increase and alteration of secretion characteristics, muco-ciliary dysfunction and ineffective coughing), decreased thoracic expansion capacity, altered ventilation / perfusion ratio, (presence of the orotracheal tube and barotrauma), increased risk of respiratory infection and alteration in respiratory muscles (Cordeiro & Menoita, 2014).

The objectives of RFR defined in this phase are to promote synchronization and adaptation to the ventilator (improving ventilation / perfusion ratio and maintaining airway permeability), mobilizing and eliminating secretions, and preventing and correcting vicious and anti-allergic positions (Cordeiro & Menoita, 2014).

In order to achieve these objectives, the SNRN should take into account the interventions presented in Table 1.

Table 1. Techniques that optimize IMV

Techniques that promote synchrony and adaptation to the ventilator	• Relaxation technique and rest positions; • Teaching and control of breathing in synchrony and according to the ventilatory modality, accompanying the costal dynamics. • Respiratory re-education exercises of the abdomino-diaphragmatic type and costal (selective and global).
Techniques that improve the ventilation / perfusion ratio	• Recruitment techniques of volumes through voluntary hyperinflation, with manual resuscitator or with volumetric ventilator; • Provide teachings of flexibilization exercises and increase of thoracic expandability through the control and dissociation of breathing times with emphasis on inspiration, abdominal-diaphragmatic re-education, directed ventilation and selective and global costal opening with and without a stick (if patient collaboration is involved).
Techniques that maintain airway permeability	• Hydration and humidification of secretions; • Administer inhaled therapy; • Encourage deep breathing, pulmonary expansion / re-expansion (if appropriate for ventilatory modality).
Techniques that promote the mobilization and elimination of secretions	• Postural drainage; • Accessory maneuvers: compression, percussion and vibration; • Aspiration of secretions; • Aspiration (open and closed system); • Manual overflight or mechanical fan.
Techniques that prevent and correct vicious and anti-allergic positions	• Selective and global costal opening with staff (if patient collaboration exists); • Postural correction sitting on a chair in front of a grid mirror (if patient collaboration exists); • Position therapy.
Techniques that improve mobility, strengthening and re-adaptation to the effort	• Positioning and postural correction techniques; • Passive mobilization exercises; • Exercises of active mobilization (in the absence of contraindications, progressing to the active-resistive mobilization for reactivation and muscular reinforcement and self-mobilization in the bed); • Transfer training and early release; • Static and dynamic balance training in sitting and orthostatic position; • Gait; • Other activities of daily living.

(Cordeiro & Menoita, 2014)

RESPIRATORY FUNCTIONAL RE-EDUCATION DURING VENTILATORY WEANING

Ventilatory weaning should be a gradual technique, and it is essential to observe step by step the adaptation of the person to spontaneous breathing and the monitoring of signs of fatigue (Severino, 2016).

In order to perform effective ventilatory weaning, the determining cause of mechanical ventilation should be known and respiratory stimulus considered normal should be present. The patient should present a state of consciousness that allows collaboration, and the sedative therapy should be suspended. Effective cough reflex ability should also be present in order to mobilize secretions, and hemodynamic stability should be verified and maintained (Cordeiro & Menoita, 2014).

There are five criteria for the disconnection decision of the IMV:

- Presence of effective respiratory stimulus;
- The need for an aid pressure of less than 12 cmH2O;
- Volume less than 10L / min (or 12L / min if the patient's body area is elevated);
- the PaO2 greater than 60mmHg (90% Saturation) for a FiO2 of less than 45%;
- Respiratory rate less than 30 cycles / min (Severino, 2016).

The most frequently used ventilatory modalities during the ventilatory weaning period include Assisted Pressure and Synchronized Intermittent Mandatory Ventilation. Simultaneously, periods of spontaneous ventilation with T-piece should be instituted, which should be associated with RFR techniques, especially respiratory muscle strengthening therapy, diaphragmatic re-education, in order to increase tidal volume and promote alveolar expansion, and training of airway cleansing techniques, mainly through the use of assisted and assisted cough technique (Cordeiro & Menoita, 2014).

Noninvasive ventilation appears as adjuvant therapy in the weaning process of IMV as well as in the subsequent extubating process. It appears as an effective method in reducing IMV time in patients with difficult ventilatory weaning, reducing the risk of complications inherent to this procedure (Suzuki, T., Kurazumi, T., Toyonaga, S., Masuda, Y., Morita, Y., Masuda, J., 2014)

RESPIRATORY FUNCTIONAL REEDUCATION AFTER MECHANICAL VENTILATION AND THE USE OF NONINVASIVE VENTILATION

The noninvasive strategy has been initiated as a strategy associated to the VMI decision protocol, as is the process of restoring the effective physical inspiration in IMV time in patients who are submitted to extubation breathing (Epstein, SK. & Durbin, CG, 2010.)

The objectives of the SNRN at this stage of ventilatory weaning are to reduce anxiety and fear, decrease respiratory work, maintain airway permeability, prevent and correct vicious and anti-anxiety positions, and focus on stress re-education techniques (Cordeiro & Menoita, 2014).

In order to achieve these objectives, the following interventions must be carried out:

- Emotional support for the patient / family;
- Resting and relaxation positioning technique, massage in the cervical muscles and mobilization of the scapula-humeral joint, associated with breath control;
- Incentive to deep inspirations and abdominal-diaphragmatic re-education, postural drainage, forced expiration technique, active cycle of respiratory techniques, strengthening of effective cough teaching, directed and assisted coughing, humidification of secretions if necessary, aspiration of secretions;
- Positioning technique with alternating decubitus, positional therapy, postural correction in the sitting position and orthostatic position;
- General exercises with therapeutic ball, pedal, gait training and climbing and descending stairs (Cordeiro & Menoita, 2014).

The intervention of the SNRN in an ICU aims to improve the quality of life by improving the functional capacity, tolerance to the effort, reduction of complications of IMV and success in ventilatory weaning, contributing consecutively to the reduction of the period of hospitalization and to the decrease of reinstatement rates.

Impact of Rehabilitation Nursing Interventions

The integrative literature review has become an appropriate method to synthesize the information of studies that address it, allowing the analysis of the scientific evidence around the central question of this investigation. This study involved the definition of the objective, formulation of the research question, methodology, results and discussion and main conclusions.

Objective

To identify the impact of Rehabilitation Nursing interventions in the early weaning of the person submitted to Mechanical Invasive Ventilation.

Research Question

For the selection of articles and formulation of the research question, the PI [C] OD methodology was used, being the target population (P), the type of Intervention (I), the comparisons (C), the outcome - outcome (O) and the type of study - design (D). The following question was elaborated to answer the objective outlined and that served as the guiding thread for this integrative review of the literature: What is the impact of Intervention Nursing interventions in the early weaning (Outcomes) of the person undergoing Mechanical Ventilation Invasive (Population)?

Methodology

After the formulation of the question of departure, a research was done on the topic under study. The EBSCOHOST database was used and in this the MEDLINE COMPLETE and CINHAL COMPLETE databases were selected, with the following descriptors:

- "Rehabilitation", "Rehabilitation nursing", "Early mobilization", "Intensive Care Unit", "Artificial respiration", "Mechanical ventilator", "Respiratory care", "Respiratory", "Ventilator weaning" and "Weaning".

The descriptors were searched at EBSCO in the following order:

- [(rehabilitation) OR (rehabilitation nursing)] AND
- [(early mobilization)] AND
- [(intensive care unit)] AND
- [(artificial respiration or mechanical ventilator)] AND
- [(respiratory care) or (respiratory)] AND
- [(ventilator weaning) or (weaning)].

The descriptors were searched in full text and researched retrospectively until 2014.

The inclusion and exclusion criteria to be used during the research were defined. As inclusion criteria, articles with quantitative and / or qualitative, full-text methodologies that focused on the subject of study, from academic journals (analyzed by specialists), with available references and with date published between January 2014 and September 2018 were prioritized.

In the exclusion criteria, all articles with ambiguous methodology, repeated in both databases, without correlation with the object of study and with dates below 2014 were considered.

The selection of articles involved the evaluation of the title and analysis of the summary to verify that the articles met the criteria of inclusion and exclusion. When the title and the abstract were not illuminating, the article was read in its entirety to minimize the loss of important studies for the accomplishment of this integrative review of the literature.

95 articles were identified from the databases, MEDLINE COMPLETE and CINHAL COMPLETE. Of these, eight were removed because they were duplicates.

This evaluation was carried out in two phases: in the first phase, 34 articles were maintained after the titles were read and in a second phase after the abstracts were read, the potential interest for 22 articles was justified. From these, seven articles were selected as a result of the analysis of the methodological quality, after reading the article.

Given the selected articles, the critical analysis of methodological quality focused on the assessment of the levels of evidence of each article. We used the contributions of Melnyk and Fineout-Overholt (2005), in order to identify the types of production of knowledge implicit in it. These authors considered the following levels of evidence:

- Level I- Systematic reviews (meta-analyzes, guidelines for clinical practice based on systematic reviews);
- Level II - Experimental studies;
- Level III - Quasi-experimental studies;
- Level IV - Non-experimental studies;
- Level V- Program evaluation reports / literature reviews;
- Level VI - Opinions of authorities / consensus panels.

In the evaluation of methodological quality, two researchers were involved, using the tools recommended by Joana Briggs Institute (2014), which determined the incorporation of articles that obeyed more than 50% of the quality criteria. Where necessary, a third researcher was used to analyze the articles.

In this process, two synthesis tables were constructed: the first to describe the studies and the second one to synthesize the results. These synthesis tables were constructed jointly by the researchers, culminating in the incorporation of seven articles in this integrative review of the literature.

RESULTS

With the purpose of answering the question of departure, several articles were read, aiming the analysis of its content. The results obtained are summarized in Table 2.

Discussion

Following the analysis carried out, five categories emerged, supported by the indicators systematized in Table 3.

Table 2. Results of bibliographic research

Authors/ Method/ Level of Evidence	Objectives	Results
Dong, Yu, Sun, Fang & Li (2014) **Method:** Experimental study, with participants randomly assigned to two groups (experimental group and control group). **Level of evidence:** II **Participants:** 60 patients under IMV with endotracheal intubation or tracheostomy with more than 48 hours and less than 72 hours upon admission to the ICU of the Affi Medical School Hospital of Qingdao University from May 2010 to May 2012 and were randomly assigned in the experimental group and control group, with 30 people in each group.	To investigate the feasibility, efficacy and safety of the early implementation of rehabilitation techniques in patients with mechanical ventilation.	This study suggested that early rehabilitation therapy is feasible, safe and effective to improve patient outcomes under IMV. He pointed out the relation between the decrease of the time in relation to the first lift, with the early ventilatory weaning and the reduction of the time of permanence in the ICU. The remaining variables studied (body mass index, APACHE II - Acute Physiologic Assessment and Chronic Health Evaluation II score - higher FiO2, lower PaO2 / FiO2 and hospital mortality) did not present significant differences between the two groups analyzed. There are no adverse effects resulting from early rehabilitation interventions.
Albuquerque, Machado, Carvalho & Soares (2015) **Method:** Systematic Review of Literature **Level of evidence:** I	To evaluate the impact and safety of the implementation of programs of early mobilization in patients hospitalized in ICUs.	There is evidence that mobilization programs, when applied early, are safe, improve functional performance after ICU discharge, reduce the incidence of delirium, decrease IMV time, and length of hospital stay. The level of evidence regarding the impact of early mobilization on long-term outcomes, such as hospital mortality, is low and limited.
Hashem, Nelliot & Needham (2016) **Method:** Prospective observational study. **Level of evidence:** IV **Participants:** 122 patients hospitalized in a medical-surgical ICU with a need for IMV equal to or greater than four days, with no cognitive or neuromuscular antecedents and with muscle weakness acquired in the ICU.	To prove that early mobilization and rehabilitation in patients hospitalized in an ICU prevent respiratory and muscular complications, with an impact on physical condition and quality of life. It also intends to prove that muscle weakness acquired in the ICU is associated with the need for longer IMV, longer hospital stay (with associated hospitalization costs), and increased morbidity and mortality.	Three months after application of the ICU protocol there was a significant decrease in the use of sedative medication, with a considerable increase in the period in which the patients were conscious (66% vs. 29%) and without delirium (53% vs. 21%). There was a significant decrease in the number of days that patients with criteria for rehabilitation did not (7% vs 41%). Compared to the same period of the year prior to the study, there was a 30% decrease in ICU with an increase of 20% of service admissions. After this study, there was an increase in the number of rehabilitation professionals in the service, and an early rehabilitation program was created in patients hospitalized in the ICU. A new sedation protocol was also instituted. Thus, it was concluded that early mobilization and rehabilitation are safe and reliable interventions, and there is evidence that improves the results obtained by decreasing IMV time and increasing physical condition. It is understood that through the creation of a multidisciplinary team there may be a change in the culture of ICUs, leading to the implementation of a rehabilitation plan and early mobilizations.
Lai et al. (2016) **Method:** Retrospective observational study, with participants randomly assigned to two groups (pre-protocol group and post-protocol protocol group). **Level of evidence:** IV **Participants:** 63 patients in the pre-application protocol group and 90 in the post-application protocol group. Inclusion criteria included patients submitted to IMV using endotracheal tube for 48 hours and who presented criteria for extubation between January 1, 2014 and December 31, 2014 (the study period was divided into three phases).	To evaluate the effects of a quality improvement program to introduce early mobilization in patients with invasive mechanical ventilation (IMV) in intensive care units (ICUs).	After the implementation of the early mobilization program, the clinical results observed were different for the two groups: the IMV time was 4.7 days after protocol vs. 7.5 days pre-protocol; time of ICU stay was 6.9 days after protocol application. 9.9 days prior protocol. The length of stay in the ICU and associated hospital costs decreased from the first phase of implementation of the protocol to the third and last phase of the intervention period. The data obtained showed that the duration of IMV affects both the APACHE II score and some analytical results under study; the association between early rehabilitation and IMV duration was inversely proportional (there was no significant relationship between IMV duration with age, sex, body mass index, analytical data, vital signs, or ventilatory parameters of the patients under study). A logical regression was observed for a number of factors that predicted IMV duration of less than seven days (a lower score on the Glasgow Coma Scale and increased PaCO2 were significantly associated with IMV greater than seven days). The risk of IMV greater than seven days was lower in patients who participated in the early rehabilitation program.

continued on following page

Table 2. Continued

Authors/ Method/ Level of Evidence	Objectives	Results
Cameron, et al. (2015) **Method:** Systematic literature review. **Level of evidence:** I	Demonstrate the effectiveness of an early rehabilitation program as well as its impact on the critical illness recovery process.	Active mobilization in patients admitted to an ICU is indicated as effective and recommended in international guidelines. Early mobilization can be initiated safely on the first day of admission to the ICU, and during IMV, administration of vasopressors, dialysis therapy and with femoral catheters placed. The rate of adverse events is between 0% and 3% (and reported adverse events are not usually severe, and rarely result in the need for treatment or additional costs). Passive exercise can be used in patients who do not collaborate in rehabilitation programs, and is also safe when used in patients under IMV. This type of mobilization demonstrates an increase in the functional capacity, muscular strength and reduction of the score in the pain scales. Patients who received an early rehabilitation program were able to perform the first lift faster (five days vs. 11 days), had significantly shorter ICU admissions (5.5 days vs. 6.9 days), and even fewer length of hospital stay (11.2 days vs.14, 5 days). There is also a reduction in the duration of delirium (two vs. four days), a greater number of days without connection to IMV (23.5 vs. 21.1 days) and improvement in functional capacity at hospital discharge (59% vs. 35%).
Dunn, et al. (2017) **Method:** Integrative literature review **Level of evidence:** I	Evaluate the existence of publications that determine whether rehabilitation interventions in patients under prolonged IMV improve functional capacity, how they influence the rates of ventilatory weaning, and what hospital outcomes are obtained.	There is heterogeneity regarding the rates of ventilatory weaning; studies indicate better successful weaning outcomes in early mobilized patients. The hospitalization period and survival rate after hospital discharge is about 70% of the patients who were included in an early rehabilitation program. After the implementation of physical and mobility training, an increase in inspiratory and expiratory maximum volume is reported, an indicator of the criterion for ventilatory weaning. Patients who participated in this type of rehabilitation program had a shorter hospitalization time, a lower mortality rate, and a higher survival rate after hospital discharge.
Ntoumenopoulos (2015) **Method:** Literature review **Level of evidence:** V	Discuss the role of rehabilitation interventions in the patient under IMV.	Improvements in muscle strength, functional capacity, successful outcomes in ventilatory weaning, reduction in length of stay and stay in an ICU, and hospital admission have been reported as a result of a variety of intensive care rehabilitation interventions. Studies show that when an early rehabilitation protocol was applied, and referring to a prospective study of 103 patients with respiratory failure under IMV, there was a significant increase in the level of early mobilizations that resulted, for most patients, in the ability to wander an average distance of 65 meters after discharge from the ICU. There is also a reference to a total of 1449 rehabilitation programs, where less than 1% of adverse events occurred. Another clinical trial, which investigated the impact of the application of an early mobilization protocol, states that of 330 patients in respiratory failure, and compared with data obtained from patients who did not have access to the same protocol, early mobilization interventions were used safely and progressively applied in the first 48 hours of endotracheal intubation (IMV), even with patients under sedation and unconscious. In an initial phase, there were no significant differences in ventilatory weaning in the two groups; however in the patients with access to the intervention protocol, they performed the first lift about five days earlier, compared to 11.3 days in the first rise of the control group. Compared with the control group, the intervention group had a significant reduction in ICU stay (5.5 vs. 6.9 days) and subsequent hospital stay (11.2 vs. 14.5 days). Another randomized clinical trial involved 104 patients under IMV who had access to an early, daily, and interrupted sedation program. When compared, this group of patients did not gain muscle strength, but a significant number of patients in this group achieved functional independence at discharge from the control group. Patients in the intervention group had a mean of more than 2.4 days of early ventilatory weaning, compared with patients in the control group. The duration of delirium was reduced by about 50%.

Table 3. Synthesis of the impact of rehabilitation nursing interventions on early weaning of the person submitted to IMV

Categories	Indicators
Physical capacity and control of the patient's symptoms	• Decrease in time for the 1st lift: Dong et al. (2014); Cameron et al. (2015); Ntoumenopoulos (2015). • Improvement of functional capacity: Cameron et al. (2015); Albuquerque et al. (2015), Ntoumenopoulos (2015). • Improvement of the patient's physical condition: Hashem et al. (2016). • Increased muscle strength: Cameron et al. (2015); Ntoumenopoulos (2015). • Decreased pain: Cameron et al. (2015). • Increased patient awareness period: Hashem et al. (2016). • Decreased use of sedative medication: Hashem et al. (2016). • Reduction in incidence and duration of delirium: Albuquerque et al. (2015), Hashem et al. (2016); Cameron et al. (2015); Ntoumenopoulos (2015). • Improvement of inspiratory and expiratory volume: Dunn et al. (2017).
Period of hospitalization and rehabilitation in the ICU	• Improvement of the number of days with criteria for rehabilitation: Hashem et al. (2016). • Improvement of the number of days without connection to IMV: Cameron et al. (2015). • Decrease in IMV time: Albuquerque et al. (2015), Hashem et al. (2016); Lai et al. (2016). • Decreased length of stay in the ICU: Dong et al. (2014); Hashem et al. (2016); Lai et al. (2016); Cameron et al. (2015); Ntoumenopoulos (2015). • Decreased length of hospital stay: Albuquerque et al. (2015); Cameron et al. (2015); Dunn et al. (2017); Ntoumenopoulos (2015).
Creation of programs, protocols and recommendations	• Creation of an early rehabilitation program for patients admitted to the ICU: Hashem et al. (2016). • Creation of sedation protocol: Hashem et al. (2016). • Recommendation on the active mobilization of patients admitted to the ICU by international guidelines: Cameron et al. (2015).
Mortality rate	• Reduction of mortality rate: Dunn et al. (2017). • Improvement in survival rate after hospital discharge: Dunn et al. (2017).
Health expenses	• Reduction in hospital costs: Lai et al. (2016).

Physical Capacity and Control of the Patient's Symptoms

Mobilization is physical activity that exerts effects on physiological functions such as ventilation, central and peripheral perfusion, circulation, muscle metabolism and alertness. It also contravened phenomena related to venous stasis and deep vein thrombosis (Cameron et al., 2015). Still according to these authors, early mobilization is the term referred to the application of physical activity between the first two to five days of illness or critical accident.

In order to prevent physical and psychological disorders, early interventions are necessary. In this sense, early rehabilitation programs in critically ill patients present as a valid therapeutic resource in the restoration of functional capacity (Albuquerque et al., 2015).

A rehabilitation program is tailored to the interventions required of the patient admitted to the ICU, based on factors such as physical strength and functional capacity. The level of collaboration of the same (evaluating indices of consciousness and presence of delirium) and the presence of equipment devices, namely endotracheal tube, IMV or tracheostomy, are also taken into account in the elaboration of the same (Ntoumenopoulos, 2015).

Although studies show that early mobilization of the patient promotes a decrease in the side effects of immobility, providing a better clinical outcome, some health professionals are reluctant to apply this type of protocols and programs in patients undergoing IMV, eventually restricting these patients to inactivity (Albuquerque et al., 2015).

An early rehabilitation program may be applied to all patients admitted to the ICU as long as they maintain hemodynamic stability, including patients who are unable to follow instructions or actively collaborate (Cameron et al., 2015). These authors also make reference to the fact that, even when evaluating the possibility of performing only passive exercises, functional capacity is increased, with improvements in functional status, which conditions an increase in muscle strength, decreasing pain. Ntoumenopoulos (2015) corroborates this idea, emphasizing the continuity of passive exercise as an intervention that minimizes loss of muscle fiber, improving functional capacity, including at the time of hospital discharge, and exerting beneficial systemic effects, such as reduction of inflammatory processes.

In the patients included in this type of rehabilitation programs, there is still evidence of an improvement in pulmonary mechanics, in which there is an increase in inspiratory and expiratory volumes and pressures, indicative of the phase of ventilatory weaning (Dunn et al., 2017).

The date of the first rise, duration of IMV and length of stay in the ICU is given as significantly lower in patients enrolled in an early rehabilitation program (Dong et al., 2014).

The first uptake and out-of-bed rehabilitation interventions can safely be initiated in patients undergoing IMV, with data demonstrating that the results obtained in these patients translate into shorter periods of need for IMV and a decrease in the incidence of delirium (Ntoumenopoulos, 2015). Cameron et al. (2015), also point to this point, stating that patients who are included in a rehabilitation program perform the earliest early release and have a significantly shorter ICU stay and hospital stay compared to patients who do not have access to the interventions contemplated in this type of program.

The most common interventions of the generalist nurse applied to the critical patient promote immobility and administration of analgesic and sedative therapy in order to facilitate the process of mechanical ventilation, reduction of pain, agitation and / or anxiety (Cameron et al., 2015).

The continued use of intravenous sedation is associated with prolonged IMV. Daily discontinuation of sedation in critically ill patients submitted to IMV may result in a decrease in extubation time, thereby influencing the length of hospital stay in the ICU. Deep sedation and immobility may potentiate the process of atrophy / neuromuscular weakness associated with ICU, and the use of lighter sedation may reduce this factor (Dong et al., 2014).

The rehabilitation program may also lead to a reduction in the duration of the delirium period, since increasing the frequency of time intervals without administration of sedative medication modifies the risk factors associated with the occurrence of this factor (Cameron et al., 2015). In this sense, Hashem et al. (2016) present data showing an increase in the proportion of the number of days in which patients improve their state of consciousness (no delirium), with a ratio directly proportional to the implementation of early rehabilitation programs, including the reduction of sedative therapy.

The daily discontinuation of sedation associated with an early mobilization and occupational therapy protocol is an effective strategy in the functional improvement of critically ill patients undergoing IMV, particularly highlighted by Albuquerque et al. (2015). These authors demonstrate that the duration of the delirium and the time required for ventilatory weaning are clearly diminished when this program is implemented, and also affirm that this type of non-pharmacological protocol, associated to an early and intensive rehabilitation program, produces gains in reducing the delirium rate of patients hospitalized in the ICU, with gains in functional independence at the time of hospital discharge, improvements in cognitive function, increase in palmar grip strength and decrease in hospitalization time.

The combination of discontinuation of the administration of sedative medication with rehabilitation intervention in critically ill patients is an intervention strategy advocated by Ntoumenopoulos (2015). It is fundamental in the process of returning to functional independence at the time of hospital discharge, as well as in reducing the delirium period and decreasing the time of ventilatory weaning.

Clinical, cognitive and physical status of patients should be monitored frequently for gains in a safe and effective early rehabilitation program. The daily interruption of sedative medication, except in cases where there is contraindication, will allow the evaluation of cognitive status and functional capacity of the patient to participate in the program, as well as allowing the multidisciplinary team to evaluate the risk / benefit of the implementation of the same (Ntoumenopoulos, 2015).

Period of Hospitalization and Rehabilitation in the ICU

The use of IMV induces improvement in lung capacity and reduces cardiac output, but mechanical ventilation can inevitably cause side effects in patients hospitalized in the ICU context, with an incidence in the development of neuromuscular problems, namely in the pathological process called atrophy / acquired neuromuscular weakness in ICUs (Dong et al., 2014). This pathology can lead to the permanence of symptoms, affecting the quality of life of these patients, so that nursing rehabilitation interventions should start as early as possible, as it may affect the health condition of the patients involved.

The consequences associated with immobility are widely recognized as being frequently associated with the critical patient, requiring IMV (Dunn et al., 2017).

The return to functional independence at hospital discharge is significantly higher in patients enrolled in an early rehabilitation program, with age, absence of sepsis and early mobilization, variables associated with success in acquiring functionality (Albuquerque et al., 2015). There is a need for early interventions to prevent physical and psychological disorders. Therefore, there is a need to establish early rehabilitation protocols in critically ill patients, including patients undergoing IMV, which include reduction of sedation, broadening the mobilization approach, and functional physical training as early as possible in these patients (Albuquerque et al., 2015).

After application of an early mobilization protocol during the first three days of ICU stay in a patient submitted to oral-tracheal intubation for IMV, the capacity of muscular activity of the extremities is evident and it is possible to interact with the conscious patient in several aspects (Lai et al., 2017).

Through early rehabilitation interventions it is possible to achieve the improvement of functional capacity and potentiation of muscle strength, which leads to superior effective weaning success rates, thus reducing the permanence in the ICU and subsequent hospitalization in the destination hospital after high of the ICU (Ntoumenopoulos, 2015).

The existence of multiple investigations that refer to the period of reduction of hospitalization in the ICU and hospital stay after investing in the functional capacity gain of these patients is highlighted by Dunn et al. (2017). The reduction of the IMV period and the decrease in the duration of the ventilatory weaning process is a result of the early intervention in the critical patient (less than 21 consecutive days). Lai et al. (2017) corroborate the use of these intervention strategies, since the effects of a rehabilitation program with early interventions applied to patients submitted to IMV are positive in relation to the decrease in the duration of the need for IMV and consequently of the stay in the ICU.

An early rehabilitation program is safe and effective in critically ill patients, including patients undergoing IMV, conscious or unconscious, with measurable results in reducing ICU stay, reducing delirium, decreasing IMV time and ventilatory weaning and greater functional capacity at the time of hospital discharge (Cameron et al., 2015). This idea is corroborated by Albuquerque et al. (2015), when affirming that early rehabilitation programs are safe and that the evidence points to a better functional performance of patients admitted to the ICU, reducing the incidence of delirium, as well as reducing the time needed for IMV and hospital stay. In this sense, the early mobility of patients under IMV is understood as safe and effective, with no adverse effects of such intervention, but a reduction in the number of complications associated with immobility (Hashem et al., 2016).

Creation of Programs, Protocols and Recommendations

Acute respiratory failure is one of the most common causes for admission to an ICU, and IMV is an extremely important intervention in maintaining vital capacity in critically ill patients with this pathology. However, during this acute condition, and as previously reported, the neuromuscular system of most patients undergoing IMV is negatively affected by the prolonged process of immobility, which may result in muscle atrophy, neuromuscular dysfunction and even system paralysis skeletal muscle. Associated with these facts, there is still to be taken into account psychological processes such as depression and anxiety, after the occurrence of a critical situation or prolonged IMV (Lai et al., 2017).

In order to answer the question of the physical and psychological sequelae associated with a process of immobility and prolonged IMV, there is a need to implement an early rehabilitation protocol (Lai et al., 2017).

Thus, the concept of active mobilization in critically ill patients hospitalized in ICU emerges, proving to be effective and recommended in international guidelines. A variety of early mobilization protocols have been advocated, including passive, active or active-resistive mobilizations (Cameron et al., 2015), and this has been a recent focus on the importance of applying standardized protocols and the development of new measuring instruments in order to evaluate the functional results obtained in the critical patient submitted to IMV and under the application of these same protocols (Dunn et al., 2017).

As mentioned earlier, the interventions most often associated with early mobilization are the three types of mobilizations, early release, tidal volume increase, respiratory muscle strengthening, respiratory training and airway clearance (Hashem et al., 2016). The elaboration of these protocols is a defended necessity, since it leads to a decrease in ventilation time, a higher rate of ventilatory weaning (75% vs. 53.3%) and a decrease in hospitalization time (Hashem et al., 2016). These authors present data that combine a rehabilitation program that includes early mobilization, establishment of sedation protocols (in which periods of cessation of any type of sedative agent are established, leading to spontaneous arousal), combined with attempts at spontaneous ventilation and monitoring / management of delirium. After the application of this program, the data showed that the patients had a longer period of time without IMV, a higher incidence of out-of-bed mobilization (at least once a day), and a decreased probability of experiencing delirium at any time during hospitalization in the ICU. It also notes that the implementation of this type of program implies the need to coordinate the multidisciplinary team to achieve effectiveness and overcome the barriers of deep sedation and delirium, allowing patients to benefit from early rehabilitation interventions.

It is necessary to emphasize the importance of having a specialized multidisciplinary rehabilitation team so that this early rehabilitation care can be widely promoted (Dong et al., 2014), providing a more effective application of these (Cameron et al., 2015).

The results in critical patients are usually measured through mortality rates and organic and physiological dysfunction (Ntoumenopoulos, 2015). Care models that include a multidisciplinary team focusing on ventilator weaning health professionals achieve significant quality of care outcomes, which are reflected in the gains achieved with patients, as well as cost reduction data for hospital institutions. A team of differentiated professionals has the skills to evaluate the clinical situation and, in this sense, in the culture of general care to the critical patient submitted to IMV, the shortage of specialized professionals can impose limits to the application of early mobilization protocols, not being the viability of this is evident because of the allocation of priorities other than early mobilization.

Taking into consideration the previous analysis, the existence of a greater number of specialized professionals is considered a necessity for the realization of an early ventilatory weaning. The integration of the interventions of a multidisciplinary team is essential to its success (Hashem et al., 2016). This idea is conveyed by Lai et al. (2017), considering that the implementation of these programs through a specialized multidisciplinary team is feasible, safe and effective in critically ill patients, since this team is responsible for the frequent evaluation of patients submitted to IMV, including weaning phases and spontaneous ventilation. In this evaluation is implied the frequent evaluation of hemodynamic parameters, as well as in the level of consciousness compatible with spontaneous respiration, hemodynamic stability, respiratory stability, as well as in the control of gasimetric values.

An early rehabilitation program is attainable, safe and effective and produces results in patients undergoing IMV (Dong et al., 2014). There is a significant increase in the functional capacity of these patients, and the APACHE II score - Acute Physiologic Assessment and Chronic Health Evaluation II, reflects the fact that patients submitted to IMV and included in an early rehabilitation program survive the state of critical health, initiating a period of physical stability during the remaining hospitalization (Dunn et al., 2017).

Mortality Rate

As mentioned previously, and by multiple authors, it is stated that the success rate of ventilatory weaning is directly proportional to the decrease in the length of time related to hospital admission.

Patients enrolled in an early rehabilitation program have shorter hospitalization time and, in terms of long-term data, there is evidence that only a small percentage of the patients have suffered invalidity or death (Albuquerque et al., 2015).

A significant survival rate (70%) is indicated after hospital discharge in patients enrolled in the early rehabilitation program (Dunn et al., 2017).

Health Expenses

The effects of an early rehabilitation program on patients undergoing IMV are recognized and broadly referenced, both in the length of time that mechanical ventilation is required and in the ICU stay, and the length of hospital stay required in hospital services that welcome patients after the ICU discharge.

This fact allows Lai et al. (2016) affirm that these early rehabilitation programs are associated with a reduction in the risk of maintaining IMV for a period of more than or equal to seven days, which refers to a shorter hospitalization, presenting data compatible with a success rate of upper respiratory weaning (98.9%) and, consequently, a reduction in associated hospital costs.

CONCLUSION

The conclusions of this study point to the evaluation of the impact of the interventions obtained through the application of a rehabilitation program in early ventilatory weaning, since in the ICU setting, immobility is still common practice, especially in mechanically ventilated patients, incurring in short, medium and long term sequelae.

In view of the objective of this study and based on the data analyzed, a great variety of studies are available that refer to the existence in patients considered critical and submitted to IMV, high risk of developing physical and psychological complications, which may influence the duration of the recovery period.

The application of protocols for early rehabilitation in critically ill patients is considered safe and effective, with beneficial implications, and evidencing the reduction of time under IMV, a decrease in the incidence of delirium, an increase in muscular strength and capacity and functional autonomy at the time of hospital discharge, thus reducing the length of stay in the ICU and consequently associated costs.

Noninvasive ventilation emerges as a therapeutic approach described as feasible in reducing the complications associated with re-intubation of patients who presented acute respiratory failure after applying the extubation protocol.

However, there is a need to make changes within the overall care of critically ill patients. What is verified by this study is that this practice is not widely valued in the context of ICU, which can be justified by the shortage of specialized health professionals, the undervaluation of the consequences of prolonged immobility and the prioritization attributed to other aspects in the approach the critical patient. One of the changes considered necessary includes the development of multidisciplinary teams aimed at achieving goals in terms of early rehabilitation, optimizing the functional gains in these patients and stipulating protocols that include the reduction of administration of sedative medication, promoting early rehabilitation interventions and, consequently, the process of ventilatory weaning.

The vast majority of the data analyzed and included in this study refers to the need to recognize that early rehabilitation programs are understood and included as a crucial process in the recovery of critical patients. To this end, and as previously mentioned, the formation of multidisciplinary health teams, the formulation and structuring of protocols in which the target time of application, intensity, frequency and duration of the application are identified, as well as the continuous demonstration of benefits of early, short, medium and long-term rehabilitation may be feasible strategies to promote such change in care provided.

The research carried out to highlight the importance of the Specialist Nursing Rehabilitation Nursing, in the process of early weaning of the critical patient submitted to invasive mechanical ventilation, emerges as essential and fundamental, undoubtedly contributing to the development of knowledge related to nursing care, in this field of knowledge in Nursing.

Given the relevance of the SNRN intervention in the development of specialized care for these people, it is essential that health institutions value their skills in preventing complications and rehabilitation of people, in a dynamic multidisciplinary team.

The professional development of Rehabilitation Nurses should involve a continuous learning process in programs and strategies of professional intervention that ensure gains in the care of critical patients submitted to invasive mechanical ventilation and with criteria to perform an early ventilatory weaning. It is a process that must reconcile the needs and interests of the People, from the organizational perspective, with the motivations of these professionals specialized in rehabilitation nursing.

This path will be decisive for the development of the nursing discipline and profession, in order to improve the care of critical patients undergoing invasive mechanical ventilation.

REFERENCES

Albuquerque, I., Machado, A., Carvalho, M., & Soares, J. (2015). Impact of early mobilization in Intensive care patient. *Salud(i)Ciencia, 21*, 403-406. Retrieved from: https://www.siicsalud.com/dato/sic/214/146066.pdf

Ambrosino, N., Venturelli, E., Vagheggini, G., & Clini, E. (2012). Rehabilitation, weaning and physical therapy strategies in chronic critically ill patients. *The European Respiratory Journal, 39*(2), 487–492. doi:10.1183/09031936.00094411 PMID:22135278

Cameron, S., Ball, I., Cepinskas, G., Choong, K., Doherty, T. J., Ellis, G. C., Martin, C. M., Mele, T. S., Sharpe, M., Shoemaker, J. K., & Fraser, D. D. (2015). Early mobilization in the critical care unit: A review of adult and pediatric literature. *Journal of Critical Care, 30*(4), 664–672. doi:10.1016/j.jcrc.2015.03.032 PMID:25987293

Cederwall, C., Plos, K., Rose, L., Dübeck, A., & Ringdal, M. (2014). Critical care nurses management of prolonged weaning: An interview study. *Nursing in Critical Care, 19*(5), 236–242. doi:10.1111/nicc.12092 PMID:24809683

Cordeiro, M. & Menoita, E. (2014). *Manual de boas praticas na reabilitação respiratória. Conceitos, princípios e técnicas*. Loures: Lusociência.

Dong, Z., Yu, B., Sun, Y., Fang, W., & Li, L. (2014). Effects of early rehabilitation therapy on patients with mechanical ventilation. *World Journal of Emergency Medicine, 5*(1), 48–52. doi:10.5847/wjem.j.issn.1920-8642.2014.01.008 PMID:25215147

dos Enfermeiros, O. (2011). *Regulamento dos Padrões de Qualidade dos Cuidados Especializados em Enfermagem de Reabilitação*. Retrieved from: https://www.ordemenfermeiros.pt/colegios/documents/pqceereabilitacao.pdf

Dunn, H., Quinn, L., Corbridge, J. S., Eldeirawi, K., Kapella, M., & Collins, G. E. (2017). Mobilization of prolonged mechanical ventilation patients: An integrative review. *Heart & Lung, 46*(4), 221–233. doi:10.1016/j.hrtlng.2017.04.033 PMID:28624337

Epstein, S. K., & Durbin, C. G. (2010). Should a patient be extubated and placed on noninvasive ventilation after failing a spontaneous breathing trial? *Respiratory Care, 55*(2), 198–206. PMID:20105345

Hashem, M. D., Nelliot, A., & Needham, D. (2016). Early Mobilization and Rehabilitation in the ICU: Moving Back to the Future. *Respiratory Care*, *61*(7), 971–979. doi:10.4187/respcare.04741 PMID:27094396

Joana Briggs Institute. (2014). *Joana Briggs Institute Reviewers' Manual* (2014 edition). Joana Briggs Institute.

Lai, C., Chou, W., Chan, K., Cheng, K., Yuan, K., Chao, C., & Chen, C. (2016). Early Mobilization Reduces Duration of Mechanical Ventilation and Intensive Care Unit Stay in Patients with Acute Respiratory Failure. *Archives of Physical Medicine and Rehabilitation*, *98*(5), 931–939. doi:10.1016/j.apmr.2016.11.007 PMID:27979608

MacIntyre, N. R., Epstein, S. K., Carson, S., Scheinhorn, D., Christopher, K., & Muldoon, S. (2005). Management of patients requiring prolonged mechanical ventilation: Report of a NAMDRC consensus conference. *Chest*, *128*(6), 3937–3954. doi:10.1378/chest.128.6.3937 PMID:16354866

Ntoumenopoulos, G. (2015). Rehabilitation during mechanical ventilation: Review of the recent literature. *Intensive & Critical Care Nursing*, *31*(3), 125–132. doi:10.1016/j.iccn.2015.02.001 PMID:26026495

Severino, S. (2017). Enfermagem de Reabilitação à Pessoa submetida a Ventilação Mecânica. In. C. Marques Vieira & L. Sousa (Eds.), Cuidados de Enfermagem de Reabilitação à Pessoa ao Longo da Vida (pp. 365-380). Loures: Lusodidacta.

Suzuki, T., Kurazumi, T., Toyonaga, S., Masuda, Y., Morita, Y., Masuda, J., Kosugi, S., Katori, N., & Morisaki, H. (2014). Evaluation of nonivasive positive pressure ventilation after extubation from moderate positive end-expiratory pressure level in patients undergoing cardovasicular surgery: A prospective observational study. *Journal of Intensive Care*, *2*(1), 5. Advance online publication. doi:10.1186/2052-0492-2-5 PMID:25520822

Section 2

Elderly People in VNI Programs and Comorbities

Chapter 5
Noninvasive Ventilation in the Elderly Patient With COPD

Maria do Céu Mendes Pinto Marques
https://orcid.org/0000-0003-2658-3550
Universidade de Évora, Portugal

Ana Patricia Miguel
Centro Hospitalar Universitário do Algarve, Portugal

Carla Pinho
Centro Hospitalar Universitário do Algarve, Portugal

Solange Vieira Mega
Centro Hospitalar Universitário do Algarve, Portugal

Sónia Isabel Carmo
Suporte Imediato de Vida de Loulé do Instituto Nacional de Emergência Médica, Portugal

Marlene Silvestre
Centro Hospitalar Universitário do Algarve, Portugal

ABSTRACT

The objective of this chapter is to identify the latest evidence on the elderly critical patient with chronic obstructive pulmonary disease. Nine articles were analysed. The effectiveness of NIV has been demonstrated in cases of elderly critically ill patients with acute COPD. Evidence has been shown to decrease hospital stay and mortality, although long-term survival has been shown to be short. The prediction of NIV failure is multifactorial, including very old age, comorbidities, low analytical values of albumin, simplified severity index II, pH < 7.3 of arterial blood, PaCO2 (Carbon Dioxide Pressure) < 45 mmHg, CAT (COPD Assessment Test) elevated, Glasgow Coma Scale < 11, and APACHE II (Acute Physiology and Chronic Health Evaluation) 29. NIV has demonstrated efficacy in elderly patients in situations of acute COPD.

DOI: 10.4018/978-1-7998-3531-8.ch005

Copyright © 2020, IGI Global. Copying or distributing in print or electronic forms without written permission of IGI Global is prohibited.

THEORETICAL FRAMEWORK

Currently, there is an increase in the number of people over the age of 65 worldwide, especially in developed countries where there is already an aging population, that is, an inversion in the demographic pyramid. To mark World Population Day (11 July 2015), the National Statistics Institute (INE) elected the analysis of some demographic indicators related to the aging of the population in Portugal and in the context of the European Union. In terms of the global proportion of people over 60 years of age, there was an increase from 9.2% in 1990 to 11.7% in 2013 and it is expected to continue to increase, reaching 21.1% in 2050. In absolute figures, the United Nations projections indicate that the number of people aged 60 or over will rise to more than two billion by 2050 and the number of people aged 80 or over may more than triple, reaching 392 million in 2050 (INE, 215).

In Portugal, as a result of the drop in birth rates and the increase in longevity in recent years, there was a decrease in the young population (0 to 14 years old) and in the working age population (15 to 64 years old), in simultaneously with the increase in the elderly population (65 years of age or older) (INE 2015). The aging index, which reflects the relationship between the number of elderly people and the number of young people, reached 141 elderly people for every 100 young people in 2014. In the same year, the resident population in Portugal was made up of 14.4% of young people, 65.3% of people of working age and 20.3% of the elderly (INE, 2015).

According to the World Health Organization (WHO, 2002), the elderly can be defined chronologically as the person aged 60 years or older in developing countries and 65 years old or older in developed countries. The WHO Annual Report on Aging and Health also states that:

As the evidence shows, the loss of abilities commonly associated with aging is actually only loosely related to people's chronological age. There is no such thing as a "typical" elderly person. The diversity of the capacities and health needs of older adults is not random but comes from events that occur throughout the course of life and are often modifiable, highlighting the importance of the life cycle approach to understand the process of aging. (Chan, 2015, p. 3).

All of this leads to the observation of a population that is weaker and more vulnerable to the development of diseases, essentially chronic pathologies. The European Respiratory Society (ERS, 2013) estimates that about one billion of the world population suffers from chronic respiratory diseases and that four million will die for that reason, with an impact on health, society and the world economy.

If we speak at the national level, the same situation is verified, with the number of people with respiratory pathology on the rise, largely due to the older age groups

(65 years of age or older), with 18% as having chronic obstructive pulmonary disease (COPD) (DGS, 2015). In this age group, respiratory diseases are the third leading cause of death, after cardiovascular disease and tumours, the fifth leading cause of hospitalization and the first cause of mortality (ONDR, 2017). In the Report of the National Program for Respiratory Diseases (2017), in 2015, the mortality rate of the group of diseases in which COPD was inserted was 20.92%, with the latter in second place in the list of hospitalizations, with 14.04%. Respiratory failure is responsible for 33% of hospitalizations due to respiratory disease and 12% of the mortality rate associated with this pathology (British Thoracic Society / Intensive Care Society Guidelines for the Ventilatory Management of Acute Hypercapnic Respiratory Failure in Adults, 2016).

COPD corresponds to the set of two situations such as chronic bronchitis and pulmonary emphysema, which cause obstruction or a sensation of tightness at the bronchial level (DGS, 2016). Acute respiratory failure (ARF) is associated with exacerbation of COPD, in which gas exchange is not carried out effectively and, consequently, the respiratory system is unable to maintain adequate pressures of oxygen and carbon dioxide in the body. This situation is urgent whenever the patient does not receive adequate and timely treatment. The rapid deterioration of respiratory function allows the appearance of severe clinical manifestations and gasimetric changes in the acid-base balance, alkalosis or respiratory acidosis are common (Ferreira, 2017).

Non-Invasive Ventilation (NIV) is a form of administration of positive pressure in the airways, through an interface or facial mask, without resorting to an endotracheal tube or tracheostomy (Pinto & Sousa, 2016). NIV has been an alternative to conventional mechanical ventilation in patients with ARF associated with exacerbation of COPD (Saraiva, Moreira, Santos, & Martins, 2014). In addition to respiratory failure associated with COPD, it is also used successfully in situations of sleep apnoea, neuromuscular diseases, diseases associated with alteration of the rib cage, in weaning from Invasive Ventilation, in patients who are not candidates or who refuse Invasive Ventilation and in treatment of acute pulmonary edema, pneumonia and acute lung injury.

According to Ferreira, Nogueira, Conde & Taveira (2009), the objectives of NIV are to decrease respiratory work, rest the respiratory muscles, improve gas exchange and, in COPD patients, decrease self-peep (positive expiratory end pressure). The application of positive pressure in the airways causes changes both at the respiratory level and at the hemodynamic level. Continuous positive pressure has positive effects on cardiac performance, through the reduction of preload, through the reduction of venous return, and the reduction of afterload, through the reduction of left ventricular transmural pressure (Ferreira & Santos, 2008).

The use of NIV is contraindicated in cardio-respiratory arrest, in hemodynamic instability, in situations of upper gastrointestinal bleeding, uncontrollable epistaxis, in patients who are unable to protect the airway with risk of aspiration, upper airway obstruction, excess secretions bronchial tubes with inability to eliminate them, undrained pneumothorax or pneumomediastinum, trauma, burns and/or surgical interventions on the face and nose, decreased state of consciousness (Glasgow score less than 10), little collaboration and agitation, morbid obesity and myocardial infarction (Pinto, 2013).

The following factors have been described as predictors of NIV failure in hypercapnic respiratory failure: Glasgow Coma Scale Score less than 11; tachypnoea above 35 cycles per minute; the absence of patient-ventilator synchrony; excessive escape; agitation; abundant secretions; intolerance to the interface; no improvement after two hours of treatment; no improvement in pH, persistent tachypnoea and maintained hypercapnia. While in hypoxemic acute respiratory failure the predictors of failure are: diagnosis of Acute Respiratory Difficulty Syndrome or Pneumonia; age over 40; hypotension; metabolic acidosis (pH <7.25); low PaO2 / FiO2 ratio; SAPS II (Simplifield Acute Physiology Score)> 34; inability to improve oxygenation in the first hour of NIV: PaO2 / FiO2 (Partial Arterial Oxygen Pressure / Inspired Oxygen Fraction Ratio)> 175 mmHg (Hess, 2013).

Its application is associated with the fact that it substantially reduces complications associated with mechanical ventilation, such as the mortality rate, infections and associated costs (Balachandran, D'Souza, Radhakrishnan & Venkatesaperumale, 2013). Scientific evidence states that, due to its effectiveness and applicability, it must be part of the understanding of all health professionals who care for patients with these pathologies (Hess, 2013), namely in the area of nursing, with them assuming themselves as dedicated and experienced in NIV, this factor being a predictor of success (Pinto, 2013).

OBJECTIVE/QUESTION

After an initial research was carried out to analyse the existing literature on the theme, it was found that NIV is increasingly used, in the hospital context, in the treatment of symptoms associated with exacerbation of COPD. These factors, associated with the existing data that prove the aging of our population and the ever-higher rate of elderly people with this pathology, led us to reflect on how effective NIV would be in these situations. Therefore, this integrative review aims to analyse the effectiveness of non-invasive ventilation in elderly critically ill patients with COPD, based on the question "What is the effectiveness of non-invasive ventilation in elderly critically ill patients with COPD?". The research question was constructed according to the PICOD format:

P - Critical elderly patient aged 65 or over,
I - NIV effectiveness,
C - Critical hospital situation,
O - NIV effectiveness in treating acute COPD in critical elderly patients,
D - Mixed studies and articles by research published in full.

METHODOLOGY

To answer the question under study, it was necessary to conduct a search of the existing literature on the subject, using search engines - B-on and EBSCOhost - where all databases associated with both were used.

Literature published in the last five years that evidenced the benefit of NIV in elderly patients with worsening COPD was searched. The research was based on full texts of free access, in the English language. As it presents a structured vocabulary, we use Health Sciences Descriptors (DeCS) to help define keywords and research information sources.

The research was carried out during November 2018 with the descriptors Non-invasive Ventilation, COPD/Chronic Obstructive Pulmonary Disease, aged/elderly/senior/older adults/elderly/senior/geriatric. In the B-on search engine, 33092 studies emerged from which, through the application of Booleans, inclusion and exclusion criteria, limiting factors, reading the abstract and conclusions, six studies were selected (Flowchart 1). In the search engine EBSCOhost 288 studies appeared. Through the application of Booleans, inclusion and exclusion criteria, limiters, reading the abstract and conclusions, five studies were selected (Flowchart 2).

The total number of studies obtained on the two platforms was 11 studies, which were subsequently evaluated for their level of evidence and recommendation strength, according to the tables by Joanna Briggs (2014) (Table 1). After this evaluation, two studies were discarded, due to their weak scientific evidence, leaving nine studies. The studies considered in the review all had a recommendation strength with a percentage equal to or greater than 50%, according to the checklists by Joanna Briggs.

Figure 1. Flowchart of the search methodology in the B-on search engine.
Source. Self-Elaboration.

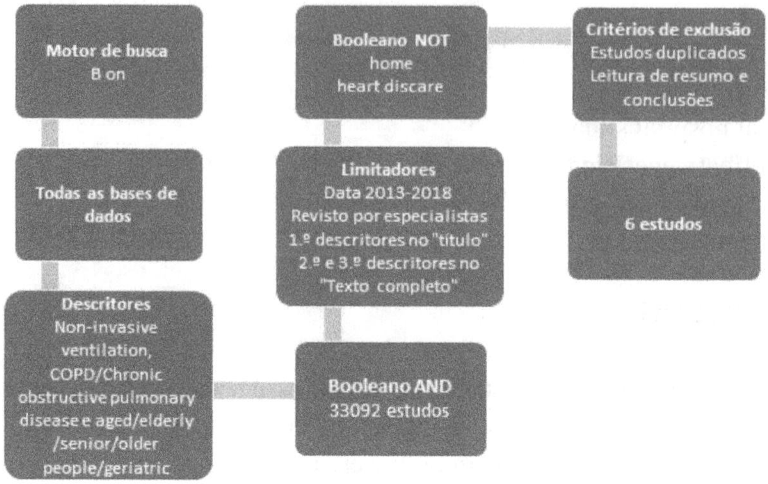

Figure 2. Flowchart of the search methodology on the EBSCOhost search engine.
Source. Self-Elaboration.

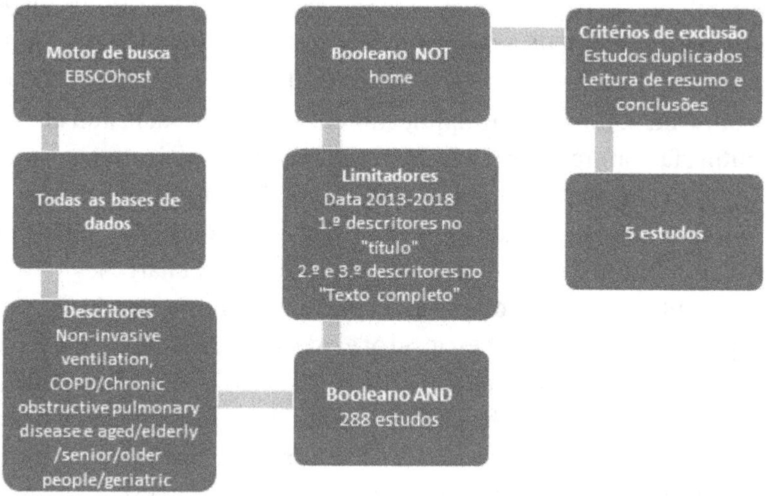

Table 1. Level of evidence, methodological quality of studies and strength of studies according to JBI (2014)

Identification of Study	Level of Evidence According to JBI	Recommendation Strength According to JBI
Perrin et al. (2015)[1]	3.e	50% - STRONG - DEGREE A
Moxon et al. (2015)[2]	3.e	75% - STRONG - DEGREE A
Domínguez et al. (2015)[3]	3.e	62,5% - STRONG - DEGREE A
Çiftci et al (2017)[4]	3.c	81% - STRONG - DEGREE A
Akyil et al. (2016)[5]	3.c	81% - STRONG - DEGREE A
Ou et al. (2016)[6]	1.c	77% - STRONG - DEGREE A
Lun et al. (2013)[7]	1.c	77% - STRONG - DEGREE A
Soleimanpour et al. 2014)[8]	2.c	55% - STRONG - DEGREE A
Nicolini et al. (2014)[9]	4.c	100% - STRONG - DEGREE A

Source. Self-Elaboration.

1. 1. Non-invasive ventilation in acute respiratory failure in the pulmonology department.
2. Non-invasive ventilation in the emergency department for patients in type II respiratory failure due to COPD exacerbations.
3. 3. Characterization of non-invasive ventilation in patients with acute chronic obstructive pulmonary disease.
4. Non-invasive ventilation for acute hypercapnic respiratory failure in older patients.
5. Patient outcome after COPD exacerbations requiring non-invasive ventilation during hospitalization.
6. Efficacy of non-invasive ventilation as a rescue therapy for relieving dyspnoea in patients with stable severe COPD.
7. A pilot randomized study comparing two methods of non-invasive ventilation withdrawal after acute respiratory failure in chronic obstructive pulmonary disease.
8. Rapid shallow Breathing Index Survey, a predictor of non-Invasive Ventilation Necessity in Patients with Chronic Obstructive Pulmonary Disease Exacerbation: An Analytical Descriptive Prospective Study.
9. The use of non-invasive ventilation in very old patients with hypercapnic acute respiratory failure because of COPD exacerbation.

RESULTS

After the critical analysis of the studies, we found that all of them present relevant information for the answer to the starting question, presenting not only data about the sample that interested us, but success rates of NIV in the worsening of COPD in elderly critically ill patients. Table 2 shows the data from the analysed studies.

DISCUTION

In order to objectify the research question initially stated, a reflection is made on the conclusions obtained from the analysis of the studies selected for the integrative review. It is intended, then, to analyse the main results and their applicability.

After analysing the sample of the studies, it was found that the average age of the population studied was greater than or equal to 65 years, with associated basic lung diseases, with an emphasis on COPD. These data are in accordance with what was reported by Andretta and Genske (2018, pp. 59-67), when they concluded that "the profile of patients submitted to NIV, are elderly, of both sexes, white, with pulmonary diseases, followed by heart disease ".

While conducting this integrative review, we were able to confirm the scientific evidence already described by Hess (2013) that demonstrates the benefit of using NIV in patients with exacerbation of COPD and EAP. But and Masip (2014) also consider COPD to be one of the situations most proven by scientific evidence for the implementation of NIV. According to Çiftci et al (2017) we found validation for this reality, since it was identified that the highest success rate of NIV is associated with patients with COPD or cardiogenic EAP. The successful application of NIV was also demonstrated in dyspnoea, a characteristic of respiratory failure in COPD. Regarding the failure of NIV, in one of the articles the percentage was high in patients older than 65 years, but with the association of infections.

Regarding the failure of NIV, in one of the articles the percentage was high in patients older than 65 years, but with the association of infections.

In all studies, the importance of using NIV in acute COPD is emphasized, compared with oxygen therapy and/or orotracheal intubation in hospitalized patients, concluding that the early use of this technique is extremely relevant, avoiding its failure, since its failure leads to an increase in the mortality rate of patients. For the success of this technique, an appropriate selection of patients to initiate NIV is important.

Table 2. Analysis of the selected articles

Identification of the Study	Objective of the Study	Study Design	Sample	Interventions	Results	Conclusions
1. (2015) Perrin et al. Perrin et	-Assess the evolution of acute respiratory failure (ARI) treated with NIV; -Putting out the predictive criteria for NIV failure	Primary, quantitative, retrospective, observational, without control group	- 49 patients who needed NIV in a period of 1 year were studied at the Pulmonology Service of Hospital de Cannes, which were divided into 2 groups: 10 patients with PaCO2 <45 mmHg and 31 patients with PaCO2 ³45 mmHg -Average age: 66 years	Study states that the nursing team had specific training in NIV and 1h of monthly training given by the service doctors	-NIV used in 46.5% of cases of acute respiratory failure, with a success rate of 73.5% and a failure rate of 26.5% -The group with PaCO2 <45 mmHg had a higher failure rate, longer treatment time and longer hospital stay -Training allowed nurses to participate in the preparation of material and in monitoring the patient	There is efficacy in the use of NIV in acute respiratory failure, such as exacerbation of COPD, but there are factors associated with failure: the simplified severity index II, the pH <7.3 of arterial blood and PaCO2 <45 mmHg; the training in the area by nurses allows them to have a more active intervention, in the early detection of failures, functioning as a predictor of success
2. (2015) Moxon et al.	-Perceive the benefit of NIV in improving blood gas analysis -Note if the action of the Emergency Department follows the guidelines for obtaining measurements within 15 minutes after the arrival and start of NIV within 1 hour after -Observing health professionals who started NIV	Primary, quantitative, observational retrospective	- 49 patients who needed NIV in a period of 1 year were studied at the Pulmonology Service of Hospital de Cannes, which were divided into 2 groups: 10 patients with PaCO2 <45 mmHg and 31 patients with PaCO2 45 mmHg; -Average age: 66 years	- Not applicable	-The 2nd evaluation took place between 30-60 min after the beginning of NIV, with significant improvements in the values of respiratory rate (RR), SPO2, pH, PaCO2 and PaO2; -From 48 patients, 89% harvested blood gas in 30 min, among which 50% harvested in 15 min -The nursing team was the one who started NIV early, and 15 nurses made the decision individually	The performance of blood gas analysis, the early onset of NIV and the experience of the nursing team are predictors of the success of the technique

continued on following page

Table 2. Continued

Identification of the Study	Objective of the Study	Study Design	Sample	Interventions	Results	Conclusions
3. (2015) Domínguez et al	Identify / describe the importance of using NIV in acute COPD, compared to conventional oxygen therapy and / or orotracheal intubation.	Primary, quantitative, observational, descriptive, and cross-sectional	98 users with acute COPD, with NIV in emergency Intensive Care, in the Intensive Care Unit (ICU) and Intermediate Care Unit (UCIM) (with the same sociodemographic, clinical, ventilatory and hematogasometric variables), of the Provincial Hospital de Clínica e Cirurgia "Saturnino Lora Torres" from Santiago de Cuba, for 1 year -Age of age:> 65 years	NIV was applied through face masks, with CPAP (Continuous positive airway pressure) fans and support pressure. They evaluated RF, Heart Rate (HR), Blood Pressure, Glasgow Scale and blood gas analysis, at the time of entry and at 2 hours -Patients who did not tolerate NIV were considered to have an unfavourable outcome and invasive MI mechanical ventilation was started	-67.3% used CPAP -The unfavourable evolution was higher than world statistics (63.3%), in which 82.3% of users were aged> 65 years and 86.7% had infection as the main triggering factor of failure -In 56.2% of cases, NIV was applied every 4 hours, but there was no direct relationship between its frequency and failure. - Favourable evolution: 72.2% after receiving NIV in less than 48 hours; 77.8% with hospital stay <7 days; significant 2h improvement in pH, decreasing of HR and RF and increase in the Glasgow Scale -Unfavourable evolution: no changes before and 48h after NIV; pH had no significant improvement; increased HR, RR and decreased Glasgow Scale -The failure in the NIV technique is directly related to the increase in mortality	-NIV is used in the treatment of exacerbated COPD and decreases hospital mortality, but in cases of failure, mortality increases, so the criteria for NIV must be strict -There is no direct relationship between failure and ventilatory modes - Greater success of NIV associated with early onset before severe acidosis, to prevent invasive intubation and longer hospital stay, and avoided interruptions in the first hours -Higher failure rate with very low pH -The Glasgow Scale is a predictor of success if> 11. -Internment <5 days leads to favourable evolution
4. (2017) Çiftci et al	Analyse the effectiveness of NIV in Hypercapnic Acute Respiratory Failure	Primary, Prospective, Interventional	162 ICU patients at the University Hospital in Ankara, for 4 years and 8 months, aged> 65 years - 90 with COPD, 31 with cardiogenic acute lung edema (EAP), 19 with community-acquired pneumonia, 15 with exacerbation of bronchiectasis and 7 with kyphoscoliosis. -From the 162 patients 71 were aged 65-74 years, 70 between 75-84 years and 21 aged> 85 years; - Inclusion criteria: increased dyspnoea and tachypnoea, respiratory acidosis and hypercapnia	-NIV sessions were started with an oronasal mask and ventilator in support pressure mode continuously, except during feeding and therapy -Arterial blood gas results were analysed immediately before the beginning of NIV and 1h, 2h, 12h, 24h after NIV	-NIV treatment had a success rate of 73.5%, which had no significant difference between age groups -NIV had a higher success rate in patients with COPD (60.5%) and EAP (19.3%) -After evaluating the success and failure of NIV treatment, the GCS, APACHE II and PaO2 / FiO2 were very different in the groups -The analysis reveals that GCS <11, high CAT and APACHE II> 29 are predictors of NIV failure	-VNI success is independent in different age groups> 65 years old -NIV has higher success rate in patients with COPD or EAP cardiogenic cause - Predictors of failure in NIV in COPD were identified: CAT, GCS and APACHE II

continued on following page

Table 2. Continued

Identification of the Study	Objective of the Study	Study Design	Sample	Interventions	Results	Conclusions
5.(2016) Akyil et al.	To determine predictors of in-hospital mortality and survival in hospitalized patients with COPD with acute hypercapnic respiratory failure undergoing NIV	Primary, Retrospective, Observational Cohort	Study carried out in the Emergency Department of the Research and Training Hospital in Istanbul, for 2 years, with 574 patients submitted to NIV in the emergency department and later transferred to inpatient services - Of the total of 574 patients included in the study, 357 were men with an average age of 68 +/- 11 years	- For the study of the predictive factors of mortality, they performed laboratory and gasimetric analyses at admission of the SU, at 24h, 48h and before discharge -Acute response to NIV treatment was assessed after 2 hours of treatment	-The average survival time was 27 months -Mortality at 3 and 6 months and 1 year were 14.5%, 19.5% and 30% respectively, with an average in-hospital mortality time of 8.5 +/- 6 days -Reduced survival time is related to older age, higher Charlson index, lower hematocrit and albumin analytical values and lower 24-hour pH value	- Survival time of the patient with COPD exacerbation undergoing NIV in the hospital is short (27 months) -Indicators of worst outcome in intrahospital mortality: higher analytical values of leukocytes, lower hematocrit and serum albumin at the time of admission and lower pH values, and higher PaCO2 at 24 hours of treatment; Indicators of worst long-term outcome: old age and low analytical albumin values
6. (2016) Ou et al	To determine the effectiveness and the respiratory mechanism of NIV with oxygen as a rescue therapy for the relief of dyspnoea after exercise in patients with severe COPD	Primary, quantitative, prospective, randomized crossover	-18 patients, with an average age of 69 years, from Guangzhou Medical University Hospital, chosen for 1 year, with severe COPD, with the following inclusion criteria: expected volume of forced expiration <50%, in a stable situation in the last month, on long-term medication for at least 3 months, dyspnoea as the main daily symptom	In the 1st phase, we collect patient data and explain test or test. In the 2nd phase, an evaluation was carried out, up to the maximum tolerance point, through bicycle exercise, with 5L / min of oxygen in progress. 9 patients were given only oxygen, the other 9 were given NIV with associated oxygen. On the 2nd visit made in the same test but crossed by the patients. During testing, patients were monitored at various levels until they recovered	-Compared with oxygen, it was found that NIV with oxygen results in a greater increase in tidal volume and ventilation, a greater decrease in the intensity of dyspnoea and a lesser need for time to recover from it, although not statistically significant - Patients with faster response to NIV had poorer lung function, probably associated with increased expiratory flow	-NIV as a rescue therapy may help to alleviate dyspnoea after exercise in patients with severe COPD - Patients with severe COPD and poorer respiratory function respond better to NIV
7. (2013) Lun et al	Compare two methods of weaning from non-invasive ventilation in a patient with acute COPD	Primary, Quantitative, Randomized controlled study	-Sample of 60 patients, with 35 in the weaning non-invasive ventilation group in stages and 25 patients in the non-phased NIV removal group -1st group: average age of 75.3 years -2nd group: average age of 73.9 years	In the immediate withdrawal group from NIV, it was suspended as soon as the patient was defined for that group. In the group, the NIV was removed in stages, the time was reduced to 16h on day zero. Subsequently reduced to 12h on day 1, to 8h on day 2 and to zero hours on the third day	There was no statistically significant difference in the success rate of weaning from non-invasive ventilation. NIV was suspended in 74.3% and 56% in the groups of gradual and immediate withdrawal, respectively	The immediate removal of NIV in COPD patients, recovered from acute respiratory failure with hypercapnia, did not show better results than the removal of NIV in stages. Therefore, the best strategy cannot be defined based on this study (small sample)

continued on following page

Table 2. Continued

Identification of the Study	Objective of the Study	Study Design	Sample	Interventions	Results	Conclusions
8. (2014) Soleimanpour et al.	To verify the viability of RSBI, as a factor to predict the need for NIV in patients with acute COPD	Primary, quantitative and qualitative, prospective, quasi-experimental, controlled	The sample presents 98 users over 40 with acute COPD - Average age: 68.4 years	In the patients selected for the study, three scales were applied, RSBI, ABG (arterial blood gas) and APACHE II. The data were collected (quantitative and qualitative) and were treated statistically	-From total patients, 43.9% needed NIV -From the three scales applied, RSBI (Rapid Shallow Breathing Index) and APACHE II demonstrated that 94.8% and 72%, respectively, of patients would need NIV. ABG has not shown a significant role in predicting the need for NIV	The application of the RSBI and APACHE II index in patients with acute COPD, has the ability to predict the need for NIV, as a decisive factor in its implementation
9.(2014) Nicolini et al	Realize the viability of using NIV to treat patients over the age of 75 years in acute respiratory failure	Quantitative Primary Case series	207 users, 121 over the age of 75 and 86 under the age of 75	Data collection for two years, dividing into 2 groups: patients aged> 75 years and patients aged <75 years. Documented data on patient changes after 2 hours of NIV; the cases in which NIV was unsuccessful; the duration of NIV and length of stay. A follow-up was carried out after discharge, which lasted 6 months	All patients were treated with NIV and were only intubated when their respiratory function worsened. The intubation rate was similar in both groups. Data collected at 6 months after discharge revealed that the group of patients aged> 75 years had a higher mortality rate. The data collected demonstrated that the NIV success rate is inversely related to the severity of the disease and associated comorbidities.	The use of NIV in patients aged> 75 years was effective in several cases. It was found in this study that the use of NIV in patients aged> 75 years did not significantly change the mortality and intubation rates, when compared with the group of patients aged <75 years. Thus, the success of NIV is related to the comorbidities of patients, the level of consciousness and the resolution of the problem that caused respiratory failure.

Source. Self-Elaboration

According to Khan (2011), NIV should be used in carefully selected patients, to avoid the appearance of complications and possible increase in mortality. Blanco, Ribeiro and Imelda (2011), states that the person proposing to start NIV must be vigilant, with spontaneous breathing, with dyspnoea secondary to hypoxic, hypercapnic or mixed respiratory failure, with signs of fatigue, presenting an RF> 25 cycles/minute, with the airway protected and collaborating.

Ferreira et al. (2009) says that there are several factors that influence the success of NIV, among them: the absence of pneumonia, a lower initial severity, small secretions, less age, capacity for cooperation / good patient-ventilator synchrony, better neurological status, good adaptation to the interface / without significant leaks, blood gas analysis with pH values between 7.0 and 7.35 and partial pressure of carbon dioxide between 45 mmHg and 92 mmHg, clinical improvement and gas exchange in the first 2 hours of NIV .

In the study by Perrin, Rolland, Berthier, Duval & Jullien (2013) it was found that the effectiveness of NIV depends directly on the arterial pH, in which a pH <7.3 is associated with a greater probability of treatment failure. This factor had already been mentioned by Hess (2013), when he addresses that metabolic acidosis with pH <7.25 was a predictor for the failure of NIV in respiratory failure. In the same study, it was concluded that a PaCO2 <45 mmHg (respiratory acidosis) is associated with a higher failure rate of NIV, longer treatment time and longer hospital stay.

The article previously referenced by Çiftci et al (2017) points out the COPD Assessment Test (CAT), the Glasgow Coma Scale and the APACHE II Scale, as factors to consider in the patient's prognosis, being that are predictive factors for NIV failure if the CAT is high, the Glasgow Scale is less than 11 and the APACHE II Scale is greater than 29.

The study by Ou, Lin, Wu, Luo & Chen (2016) describes that the use of NIV with associated oxygen is more effective in the recovery of dyspnoea than the administration of oxygen alone, by reducing the response time, increasing the tidal volume and improve lung ventilation. However, the effectiveness of NIV is not the same in all patients with COPD. The response was more significant in patients who had weaker lung function, which may be associated with increased expiratory flow.

Another factor mentioned as influencing the improvement of patients with acute COPD is related to the rapid assessment of the patient, namely blood gas analysis, as early as possible and after one hour of starting NIV. It was found that the analysis of early arterial blood gas analysis was performed, with advantages for the early onset of NIV and thus the best success of it. The assessment of patients with worsening COPD does not only involve blood gas analysis, but also the assessment of RF, HR, PA and Glasgow Coma Scale. Regarding this conclusion, Ozyilmaz, Ugurlu, & Nava (2014), report that the failure of NIV occurs in the first hour and the following 48 hours, although in cases of COPD an improvement in the pH value, reduction in RF and in PaO2 / FiO2 in the first time are significant factors for the success of NIV.

One of the articles analysed shows that patients with AKI associated with COPD who underwent NIV in the hospital had an average survival time of 27 months, which demonstrates how short the survival is (Akyil et al., 2016). The same authors explored which indicators were associated with this long-term mortality, having been associated with advanced age and with analytical albumin values below normal reference values. Finally, the indicators that are associated with the worst results related to in-hospital mortality were identified, these being the higher analytical values of leukocytes, lower hematocrit and serum albumin at the time of admission, lower pH values, and higher levels of PaCO2 at 24 hours of treatment.

Regarding the use of NIV in patients after the use of Mechanical Ventilation, it is concluded that this did not significantly change the mortality and intubation rates, previously mentioned by the authors Balachandran et al (2013). Thus, the success of NIV is related to patients' comorbidities, the level of consciousness and the resolution of the problem that caused respiratory failure.

Regarding the application of RSBI and APACHE II scales during the practice of using NIV, the results obtained were clear as predictors of success / failure in the use of NIV, being an added value for the care provided to elderly patients. In another study, immediate removal of NIV or in stages does not differ, given that the sample was small, making the results inconclusive.

Another point of interest in one of the studies was in relation to the nurses' intervention in the early onset of NIV, as a determining factor for its success. The importance of this intervention had already been reported by Pinto (2016), when he states that despite NIV being initiated by medical prescription, its monitoring and consequent success depends deeply on nursing care.

In the study by Perrin et al (2013) it was explained that the nursing professionals had training on NIV given by the service physicians. Thanks to the experience they acquired, nurses detected and acted earlier when there were changes in the patient, reducing the rate of intubation and, therefore, the failure of NIV. This conclusion is in line with the definition of the specialist nurse, when he mentions that one of his competencies is precisely to prevent complications and to identify early onset of instability (DR, 2018). Their experience will allow them to master the practice of care, generating so-called "experts", which will lead to gains in the quality of care provided and consequently in the recovery of patients (Benner, 2001).

CONCLUSION

Based on the PICOD question "How effective is non-invasive ventilation in elderly critically ill patients with COPD?", Through the integrative literature review, the research allowed us to make final assessments through the evidence found.

In a first line, we found that there are no primary studies on this theme carried out in Portugal. All the research found referred us to studies carried out abroad, showing the interest and concern in this theme.

Currently, NIV is a therapeutic method used both in the hospital and in the community, with benefits already evident, namely in length of hospital stay and mortality, although it has been shown that the long-term survival time of the patient is 27 months, being considered short.

It is a technique that is increasingly seen as a first-line therapeutic option in the treatment of acute and chronic respiratory failure, with increasing utility in several pathologies or only in the relief of symptoms. It has been an increasingly studied theme, but it is still a challenge that health professionals face.

It is worth highlighting the fundamental role that the nurse plays in the implementation and surveillance during the technique, becoming a predictive factor of success, together with the early initiation of NIV and the laboratory and gasimetric analyses at appropriate and recommended times.

Although it has been shown that NIV treatment is effective at ages older than 65 years, failure factors were considered not only to very advanced age, but also to comorbidities, low analytical values of albumin, simplified severity index II, pH <7, 3 arterial blood and PaCO2 <45 mmHg, elevated CAT, Glasgow Scale <11 and APACHE II Scale> 29.

The elderly patient in an acute COPD situation is one of the situations with the highest incidence in the implementation of the NIV technique. The scientific evidence found in this integrative review was transversal and global, in which all studies demonstrate the effectiveness of NIV in a critical patient with COPD over the age of 65 years.

REFERENCES

Akyil, F. T., Gunen, H., Agca, M., Gungor, S., Yalcinsoy, M., Sucu, P., Akyil, M., & Sevim, T. (2016). Patient outcome after COPD exacerbations requiring non-invasive ventilation during hospitalization. *Archivos de Bronconeumologia*, *52*(9), 470–476. doi:10.1016/j.arbr.2016.03.012 PMID:27156204

American Psychological Association. (2010). *Publication Manual of the American Psychological Association* (6th ed.). Author.

Andretta, G., & Genske, J. H. (2018). Índice de sucesso da ventilação não invasiva em um hospital universitário e o perfil desses pacientes. *Revista Varia Scientia: Ciências da Saúde, 1*(4), 1–9.

Balachandran, S., D'Souza, M., Radhakrishnan, J., & Venkatesaperumal, R. (2013). Role of a nurse in non-invasive positive Pressure ventilation: A conceptual model for clinical practice. *International Journal of Nursing Education, 1*(5), 119–123.

Benner, P. (2001). *De iniciado a perito: excelência e poder na prática clínica de enfermagem*. Quarteto Editora.

Blanco, J. B., Ribeiro, R., & Alves, I. (2011). Protocolo de início da VMNI. In A. M. Esquinas (Ed.), *Princípios da Ventilação Mecânica Não Invasiva - Do Hospital ao Domicílio* (pp. 173–185). Gasin Médica.

Chan, M. (2015). Prefácio. In Organização Mundial de Saúde (Ed.), Relatório Mundial de Envelhecimento e Saúde, (p. vii). Genebra: Autor.

Çiftci, F., Çiledağ, A., Erol, S., & Kaya, A. (2017). Non-invasive ventilation for acute hypercapnic respiratory failure in older patients. *Wiener klinische Wochenschrift. Central European Journal of Medicine, 129*, 680–686. PMID:28283771

Davidson, A. C., Banham, S., Elliot, M., Kennedy, D., Gelder, C., Glossop, A., Church, A. C., Creagh-Brown, B., Dodd, J. W., Felton, T., Foëx, B., Mansfield, L., McDonnell, L., Parker, R., Patterson, C. M., Sovani, M., & Thomas, L.BTS Standards of Care Committee Member, British Thoracic Society/Intensive Care Society Acute Hypercapnic Respiratory Failure Guideline Development Group. (2015). BTS/ICS guideline for the ventilatory management of acute hypercapnic respiratory failure in adults. *Thorax Journal, 71*, 1–35. PMID:26976648

Direção Geral da Saúde. (2015). *A Saúde dos Portugueses: perspetiva 2015*. Autor.

Direção Geral da Saúde. (2016). *Aprenda a viver com a DPOC: Doença Pulmonar Obstrutiva Crónica*. Autor.

Direção Geral da Saúde. (2017). *Programa Nacional para as Doenças respiratórias*. Autor.

Domínguez, R. S., Rodríguez, Z. N., & Mendoza, Y. L. (2015). Caracterización de la ventilación no invasiva en pacientes con enfermedad pulmonar obstructiva crónica agudizada. *Medisan (Santiago de Cuba), 18*(9), 1085–1092.

European Respiratory Society. (2013). *Respiratory disease in the world*. Autor.

Ferreira, C. A. C. (2017). Um percurso de especialização em urgência e cuidados intensivos: relevância da ventilação mecânica no tratamento da insuficiência respiratória (Relatório de estágio não publicado). Escola Superior de Enfermagem de São José de Cluny, Funchal.

Ferreira, H., & Santos, F. (2008). *Aspectos Gerais da Ventilação Não-Invasiva*. Disponível em http://www.hce.eb.mil.br/rev/rev2008/aspectosgerais.pdf

Ferreira, S., Nogueira, C., Conde, S., & Taveira, N. (2009). Ventilação Não Invasiva. *Revista Portuguesa de Pneumologia*, *4*(15), 655–667. doi:10.1016/S0873-2159(15)30162-8 PMID:19547897

Hess, D. R. (2013). Noninvasive ventilation for acute respiratory failure. *Respiratory Care*, *58*(6), 950–969. doi:10.4187/respcare.02319 PMID:23709194

Instituto Nacional de Estatística. (2015). *Envelhecimento da população residente em Portugal e na União Europeia*. Autor.

Joanna Briggs Institute. (2014). *Joanna Briggs Institute Reviewers' Manual* (2014 edition). Autor.

Khan, M. U. (2011). Noninvasive positive pressure ventilation in hospital setting. *JPMA. The Journal of the Pakistan Medical Association*, *61*(6), 592–597. PMID:22204218

Lun, C. T., Chan, V. L., Leung, W. S., Cheung, A. P. S., Cheng, S. L., Tsui, M. S. N., & Chu, C. M. (2013). A pilot randomized study comparing two methods of non-invasive ventilation withdrawal after acute respiratory failure in chronic obstructive pulmonary disease. *Respirology (Carlton, Vic.)*, *18*(5), 814–819. doi:10.1111/resp.12080 PMID:23490403

Mas, A., & Masip, J. (2014). Noninvasive ventilation in acute respiratory failure. *International Journal of COPD*, *9*, 837–852. PMID:25143721

Moxon, A., & Lee, G. (2015). Non-invasive ventilation in the emergency department for patients in type II respiratory failure due to COPD exacerbations. *Elsevier: International Emergency Nursing*, *23*(3), 232–236. doi:10.1016/j.ienj.2015.01.002 PMID:25665756

Nicollini, A., Santo, M., Ferrera, L., Ferrari-Bravo, M., Barlascini, C., & Perazzo, A. (2014). The use of non-invasive ventilation in very old patients with hypercapnic acute respiratory failure because of COPD exacerbation. *International Journal of Clinical Practice*, *68*(12), 1523–1529. doi:10.1111/ijcp.12484 PMID:25283150

Norma 028/2011. (2013). *Norma do Diagnóstico e Tratamento da Doença Pulmonar Obstrutiva Crónica*. Lisboa: Direção Geral de Saúde.

Observatório Nacional das Doenças Respiratórias. (2017). *Relatório do Programa Nacional para as Doenças Respiratórias*. Autor.

Organização Mundial de Saúde. (2009). *World Health Organization Guidelines on Hand Hygiene in Health Care*. Autor.

Ou, Y., Lin, Z., Wu, W., Luo, Q., & Chen, R. C. (2016). Efficacy of non-invasive ventilation as a rescue therapy for relieving dyspnea in patients with stable severe COPD. *Elsevier: Respiratory Medicine*, *121*, 74–80. PMID:27888995

Ozyilmaz, E., Ugurlu, A. O., & Nava, S. (2014). Timing of noninvasive ventilation failure: Causes, risk factors and potential remedies. *BMC Pulmonary Medicine*, *14*(19), 1–10. doi:10.1186/1471-2466-14-19 PMID:24520952

Perrin, C., Rolland, F., Berthier, F., Duval, Y., & Jullien, V. (2015). Ventilation non invasive dans l'insuffisance respiratoire aiguë en service de pneumologie. *Elsevier Masson: Revue des Maladies Respiratoires*, *32*(9), 895–902. doi:10.1016/j.rmr.2015.03.002

Pinto, C. J. C., & Sousa, P. M. L. (2016). *Ventilação Não Invasiva: desenvolvimento de linhas orientadoras recorrendo à metodologia Delphi* (Artigo baseado em Dissertação de Mestrado). Leiria: Instituto Politécnico de Leiria.

Pinto, C. J. C., & Sousa, P. M. L. (2016). *Ventilação não invasiva: uma revisão integrativa da literatura* (Artigo baseado em Dissertação de Mestrado). Leiria: Instituto Politécnico de Leiria.

Pinto, S. (2013). Ventilação Não Invasiva: Uma prática fundamentada em evidência científica. *Nursing Magazine Digital*, *288*, 1–14.

Saraiva, P., Moreira, M. H., Santos, R., & Martins, R. (2014). Qualidade de Vida do Doente Submetido a Ventilação Não Invasiva. *Millenium*, *46*, 179–195.

Soleimanpour, H., Taghizadieh, A., Salimi, S., Golzari, S. E., Mahmoodpoor, A., Safari, S., Esfanjani, R. M., & Heshmat, Y. (2014). Rapid shallow Breathing Index Survey, a predictor of non-Invasive Ventilation Necessity in Patients with Chronic Obstructive Pulmonary Disease Exacerbation: An Analytical Descriptive Prospective Study. *Red Crescent Medical Journal*, *16*(2), 1–6. doi:10.5812/ircmj.13326 PMID:24719729

World Health Organization. (2002). *Active Ageing: a police framework*. Contribuição na 2.ª Assembleia das Nações Unidas sobre o Envelhecimento, Madrid.

Chapter 6
Non-Invasive Ventilation in People With Acute Lung Edema

Pedro Nunes Raposo
https://orcid.org/0000-0002-0836-0217
Hospital Professor Doutor Fernando Fonseca, Portugal

Isabel Pedrosa Simões
Hospital Egas Moniz, Portugal

Catarina Varão Simão
Hospital Egas Moniz, Portugal

ABSTRACT

The objective of this study is to identify the health gains obtained with the use of non-invasive ventilation in patients with acute lung edema. A narrative review of the literature was carried out with bibliographic research carried out in the CINAHL, MEDLINE, and COCHRANE databases, in May 2019, with defined inclusion criteria and descriptors. This review highlighted a set of conclusive studies on the place of operation as the first line, as well as the contribution to the reduction of mortality, the need for endotracheal intubation, and a reduction in hospital stay. These results can contribute to the improvement of healthcare, practices, and patient satisfaction.

INTRODUCTION

Noninvasive ventilation (NIV) consists of ventilator support that depends on the interface between the ventilator and the patient, dispensing with invasive methods such as the use of tracheal prostheses (Mendes, 2015). Its use has progressively

DOI: 10.4018/978-1-7998-3531-8.ch006

Copyright © 2020, IGI Global. Copying or distributing in print or electronic forms without written permission of IGI Global is prohibited.

increased in interest, and in the past two decades it has become essential for the treatment of acute respiratory insufficiency (ARI) (Digby et al., 2015).

NIV allows providing physiological benefits similar to ventilator support by invasive mechanical ventilation, namely in reducing respiratory work and gas exchange (Didby et al., 2015). In this sense, its use has been fundamental in different intra-hospital contexts such as in intensive care units, emergency services and in the infirmary. (Digby et al., 2015; Ugurlu et al., 2015), with strong evidence in the treatment of exacerbation of chronic obstructive pulmonary disease (COPD), and in cardiogenic acute pulmonary edema (APE) (Demoule et al., 2016; Masa et al., 2016; Mendes, 2015). Additionally, with less evidence, benefits are also reported in the treatment of respiratory failure in the context of immunosuppression or installed after abdominal and lung surgery, in neuromuscular respiratory failure, in prophylaxis of reintubation in patients at risk of recurrent respiratory failure, moderate to severe asthma attacks, community-acquired pneumonia and adult respiratory distress syndrome (Hoo, 2016; Mendes, 2015).

Compared to invasive mechanical ventilation, this ventilation mode allows the person greater autonomy and comfort, ensuring adequate oxygenation, reducing hypercapnia and respiratory acidosis. The main advantages come from a reduction or even abolition of the need for intubation, considerably reducing the complications resulting from this procedure such as airway trauma, infections associated with health care and the need for sedation, reflected in the decrease in ventilation and hospitalization days, in the reduction of mortality rates and, concomitantly, in the global decrease in health costs (Costa et al., 2018; Digby et al., 2015; Mendes, 2015; Santos et al., 2017).

NIV is not exempt from complications, assuming that they are less severe or have less impact, which usually includes eye irritation due to air leakage through the interface, facial discomfort, risk of loss of integumentary integrity, gastric distension, hemodynamic changes resulting from positive intrathoracic pressure, dryness of mucous membranes and consequent secretion retention. Due to its use, the highest mortality risk report is associated with excessive delay in intubation (Mendes, 2015).

In clinical practice, when using NIV, positive pressure is applied to the patient's airway, generated by the ventilator, coupling an interface to the patient's nose, mouth, entire face or head. The two most commonly used basic ventilatory modalities are: continuous positive airway pressure (CPAP) where pressure is applied continuously throughout the entire respiratory cycle and bilevel positive airway pressure (BPAP) with two pressure levels, one during inspiratory phase - IPAP - higher than that applied during the expiratory phase - EPAP (Mendes, 2015, Pereira, Sequeira, Marques, Oliveira & Realista, 2016).

One of the main causes of acute respiratory failure is cardiogenic APE (Demoule et al., 2016; Masa et al., 2016). In an APE situation there is a compromise in gas exchange caused by alveolar collapse resulting from pulmonary congestion. Medical treatment includes a reduction in preload and afterload through vasodilator and diuretic therapy when this fluid overload occurs. In order to provide better alveolar recruitment, positive pressure is applied through NIV, improving the ventilation / perfusion ratio (Maraffi, Brambilla & Cosentini, 2018). This positive pressure allows a decrease in venous return, aiding cardiac function in this type of patients with heart failure, as well as reducing inspiratory effort by reducing negative pleural pressure in the inspiratory phase (Maraffi et al., 2018; Pereira et al., 2016). Recently, the CPAP modality has been the most used for its simplicity and low cost (Mendes, 2015).

This is a recurrent situation in patients with heart failure, due to the physiological deterioration of the heart and the consequent decrease in pumped blood flow. It is considered an epidemic that continues to progress, reflecting high rates of hospitalization and mortality (Sousa et al., 2017). More prevalent in the elderly population, its poor prognosis has hospital mortality between 4 and 7% and a re-hospitalization in 60 to 90 days of 25 to 30%, determining high health costs (Farmakis, Parissis, Lekakis & Filippatos, 2015).

With the undertaking of this study, it is intended to:

Evidence of health gains from the use of non-invasive ventilation in patients with acute pulmonary edema;

METHODOLOGY

The narrative review of the literature consists of the traditional or exploratory review, in which the state of the art is described and discussed in a contextual perspective. Without explicit criteria and a random selection of articles, the author includes documents according to his perspective and there is an interpretation and personal critical analysis of the author (Camargo et al., 2017; Ferenhof & Fernandes, 2016). Its steps are the selection of a review theme; literature search; literature collection, reading and analysis, review writing and references (Sousa, Firmino, Marques-Vieira, Severino & Pestana, 2018).

The formulation of the question uses the acronym PICO: In patients with acute pulmonary edema (Population) what are the health gains (Results / Outcome) with the use of non-invasive ventilation (Intervention)?

In order to give a better answer to this question, the following keywords were defined, previously validated by the Health Sciences and Medical Subject Headings Descriptors (MeSH): noninvasive ventilation, pulmonary edema e pulmonary edema therapy. The survey was conducted on May 25, 2019 through the EBSCO Host platform by accessing the CINAHL Plus with Full Text, MEDLINE with Full Text and Cochrane Database of Systematic Reviews databases.

The selection was initially carried out by reading the title and the abstract, which should include the expression non-invasive ventilation while the expression acute pulmonary edema should simultaneously be present in any part of the articles. Only articles available in full and in the time between January 2015 and May 2019 would be of interest.

DISCUSSION OF RESULTS

By analyzing the selected articles, it is possible to verify the various advantages that NIV presents to people in the context of APE.

A concern presented by different authors focused on what would be the best time to start NIV. Thus, Demoule et al. (2016), carried out a comparative study in three different clinics in the years 1997, 2002 and 2010. From the results demonstrated, he stated that NIV was frequently initiated before admission to the intensive care units (ICU), such as in ambulances and in emergency departments. More used in 2010/11 than in 2002 and 1997 ($P < 0.05$), it was assumed as a first stable line of action in the APE, with no increase in mortality recorded, showing success rates of 56% and 70% in 2002 and 2010/11 respectively (Demoule et al., 2016). Digby et al. (2015) in his study carried out in 11 care centers in Canada, he made reference to the place where NIV was started, verifying that it was in the emergency department where Nipples started to 50% of patients, with one third (35, 5%) had an indication to discontinue, which contributed to a decrease in the rates of endotracheal intubation and mortality (Digby et al., 2015). The beginning of NIV in emergency departments was strongly advocated by Ugurlu et al. (2015) when, in their cohort study, I concluded that the cases of APE that started NIV in these locations were 77% successful and when they were managed exclusively in these departments they obtained an 88% success rate, arguing that the place where NIV starts is determinant in reducing hospital mortality. People who started NIV in the emergency department had the lowest mortality rate with 12% and the shortest hospital stay with five days (Ugurlu et al., 2015).

Regardless of whether NIV was started in the emergency department, in the ICU or in a general ward, several authors are unanimous in considering NIV as an advantage, as it allows the reduction of invasive mechanical ventilation and its complications. Demoule et al. (2016) defends in his study that NIV is associated with a decrease in mortality ($p < 0.0001$), and that even in cases of failure, these were not correlated with a higher mortality rate. The average time of need for ventilatory support has also progressively decreased with a need from approximately three days in 1997 and 2002 to approximately two days in 2010/11 (Demoule et al., 2016). Ugurlu et al. (2016), reinforces in its study the benefits of NIV with an in-hospital mortality rate of 18% when compared to the mortality rate of the person undergoing mechanical ventilation, of 32% (Ugurlu et al., 2016). Melo et al. (2015) in his observational and prospective study of 37 people submitted to NIV, he found that it was possible to prevent orotracheal intubation in 18 people, which corresponds to 48.6% of success. This result reinforced the idea of previous authors in reducing hospital stay and consequently lowering hospital costs. In cases of unsuccessful NIV, with APE as the main cause of ARI, mortality rates of 73.8% were registered compared to the 16.7% observed in the group submitted to NIV (Melo et al., 2015).

Ugurlu and collaborators, in their two studies, refer to the characteristics of patients who underwent NIV and invasive mechanical ventilation, observing that the first group comprises a higher percentage of patients with an indication not to intubate / an indication not to resuscitate. This therapy was assumed in these patients as their therapeutic ceiling or palliative measure. Regardless of status, low hospital mortality rates were obtained, which the authors related to the type of diagnoses, such as the case of APE (Ugurlu et al., 2015; Ugurlu et al., 2016).

Digby et al., in a descriptive analysis carried out in Canadian care centers, reports that the bilevel was the most used ventilator mode, although there is reference in some centers to the use of CPAP as a start of treatment. Demoule and collaborators corroborate this same idea, stating an increasing use of the bilevel at the progressive detriment of the CPAP mode (Demoule et al., 2016; Digby et al., 2015). The application of the bilevel mode is as effective as the application of CPAP according to Maraffi and collaborators, arguing that the literature assumes CPAP as the preferred mode due to the better ease of handling and the request for less technical equipment (Maraffi et al., 2018).

Regardless of the ventilation modality, the use of the full facial and facial interface overrides the use of the nasal interface due to the effectiveness of ventilation in this type of patient (Demoule et al., 2016; Digby et al., 2015). The choice of the interface is decisive in the success of NIV, and the different types of interface (nasal mask, oronasal, full face and helmet) must be adapted to the different characteristics of the person, safeguarding comfort and minimizing leakage. Maraffi and collaborators defend as a first choice the total oronasal and facial interface for the successful use of the NIV level. In CPAP mode, the first choice falls on the use of the helmet due to greater long-term tolerance (Maraffi et al., 2018).

In the analysis presented by Masa and collaborators, the duration of NIV action in alveolar recruitment and relaxation of respiratory muscles in APE is dependent on the pharmacological treatment used, such as steroids and diuretics, which require time for its action (Masa et al., 2016).

For Maraffi and collaborators, the use of NIV has benefits in the normalization of peripheral oxygen oximetry (SpO2), in decreasing the respiratory rate and in the signs of breathing difficulties (Maraffi et al., 2018). The benefits are not only limited to the registration of vital signs but also in terms of blood gas analysis with an initial improvement in the assessment of oxygenation (an assessment to be made under the terms PaO_2/FiO_2). The values of pH as well as PaCO2 may not show a clear improvement in the first hour of evaluation, but should not be worsened (Maraffi et al., 2018). Within this reading, Melo et al. (2015), demonstrated in his group of success significant improvements in the stabilization of vital signs, namely in the values of systolic and diastolic blood pressure, in the normalization of heart rate and respiratory rate immediately before the last use of NIV. These improvements were also significant in the values shown by the gas analysis, presenting an average record of 97.1% of SpO_2; pH of 7.43; PaO_2 of 115.7 mmHg and $PaCO_2$ 34.3 mmHg. In your study it is possible to verify that the water balance parameter was also evaluated, noting that the successful group had negative water retention values or close to zero (-448.9ml and 125.6ml at 24 hours and 72 hours respectively) (Melo et al., 2015), strengthening the affirmation of Massa and collaborators regarding the complementation of the pharmacological intervention in the period of time gained by the action of NIV (Masa et al., 2016). Ugurlu and collaborators report that patients subject to NIV present a stabilization in the values of respiratory and heart rate, blood pressure, pH and $paCO_2$ (Ugurlu et al., 2015; Ugurlu et al., 2016). In both studies, it was possible to verify the contribution and benefit that NIV obtained in stabilizing the values presented by these patients.

On the other hand, the application of NIV is based on a set of factors that, through evaluation, can contribute to its success or failure. Demoule and collaborators state that from 1997 to 2010/11 there has been a progressive increase in the success of this therapy, basing that same success on a more careful selection of patients, changes in practices and available devices, as well as changes and advances in the types of existing masks (Demoule et al., 2016). Melo et al. (2015) concluded that ARI and low levels of consciousness were the reasons that justify the need to move towards endotracheal intubation. For the success of NIV it is necessary to take into account the level of experience of the team as well as to establish strategies based on protocols (Melo et al., 2015). Çiftci, Çiledağ, Erol & Kaya (2017) considered that there were no significant differences between different age groups with regard to NIV success ($p = 0.803$). However, in the group aged 65 and over, the complications that arises from the invasive mechanical ventilation procedure increase. In the analysis of their study, they assume a set of factors responsible for the lack of success of NIV such as the Glasgow Coma Scale, the Acute Physiology, Age, Chronic Health Evaluation II (APACHEII), the Charlson Comorbidity Index (CCI), initial value pH, PaO2 / FiO2 and C-Reactive Protein (CRP) (Çiftci et al., 2017). The experimental study conducted by Masa et al. (2016) consisted of understanding the influence of the pH value in the NIV intervention by assigning a group without severe acidosis (pH $\geq$7.25) and another with severe acidosis (pH <7.25). In the results obtained, there was no difference between the different patients in the failure of NIV; there was only a need for more time to normalize the pH of the most acidotic group, which did not give a difference in the total hospitalization time in both groups (Masa et al., 2016).

CONCLUSION

In patients with APE, the institution of NIV has demonstrated effectiveness in its performance as a first line. The reduction in mortality and the need for endotracheal intubation are identified as its main benefits, resulting from the progressive increase in its use in pre-hospital situations and in emergency departments. The reduction in hospital stay and associated hospital costs are gains that can be obtained with the use of NIV.

The use of NIV presents itself as a treatment option that promotes the reduction of mortality rates in patients with orders not to intubate / resuscitate and in patients older than 65 years, avoiding invasive mechanical ventilation and consequent complications.

In patients in the context of APE, the success of NIV allows pharmacological measures to be taken, translating gains in vital parameters such as heart and respiratory rate, blood pressure, SpO2, gas values, symptomatic control and water balance.

In the ventilatory modes most used in the context of APE, the bilevel is currently the most successfully used. However, CPAP mode is also an option for easy handling, parameterization and simplicity of equipment.

The success of NIV depends on the existence of extrinsic and intrinsic factors to patients. The experience and training of professionals, the existence of protocols and criteria for patient selection, the renewal of equipment and the application of the total oronasal and facial interface are identified as extrinsic factors. As intrinsic factors are identified the scores of the APACHE II, CCI and Glasgow coma scale, as well as the gasimetric values, namely the severity of pH, PaCO2 and the analytical value of CPA.

As a limitation of this narrative review, we mention that ARI in need of NIV was mostly addressed in the set of different pathologies that characterize it, making it difficult to differentiate between patients with APE from other associated pathologies, such as COPD.

We recommend a greater differentiation between the different pathologies, namely the APE of COPD and Pneumonia acquired in the community, as well as a better characterization of the different ventilation modes indicated for the treatment of the patient with APE.

REFERENCES

Camargo, F. C., Iwamoto, H. H., Galvão, C. M., Monteiro, D. A. T., Goulart, M. B., & Garcia, L. A. A. (2017). Modelos para a implementação da prática baseada em evidências na enfermagem hospitalar: Revisão narrativa. *Texto & Contexto Enfermagem*, *26*(4), 1–12.

Çiftci, F., Çiledağ, A., Erol, S., & Kaya, A. (2017). Non-invasive ventilation for acute hypercapnic respiratory failure in older patients. *Wiener Klinische Wochenschrift*, *129*(19-20), 680–686. doi:10.100700508-017-1182-2 PMID:28283771

Costa, J. C., Machado, J. N., Costa, J., Fortuna, J., Gama, J., & Rodrigues, C. (2018). Ventilação Não Invasiva: Experiência de um Serviço de Medicina Interna. *Medicina Interna*, *25*(1), 18–22. doi:10.24950/rspmi/original/78/1/2018

Demoule, A., Chevret, S., Carlucci, A., Kouatchet, A., Jaber, S., Meziani, F., ... Rabbat, A. (2016). Changing use of noninvasive ventilation in critically ill patients: Trends over 15 years in francophone countries. *Intensive Care Medicine*, *42*(1), 82–92. doi:10.100700134-015-4087-4 PMID:26464393

Digby, G. C., Keenan, S. P., Parker, C. M., Sinuff, T., Burns, K. E., Mehta, S., ... Berthiaume, L. R. (2015). Noninvasive ventilation practice patterns for acute respiratory failure in Canadian tertiary care centres: A descriptive analysis. *Canadian Respiratory Journal*, *22*(6), 331–340. doi:10.1155/2015/971218 PMID:26469155

Farmakis, D., Parissis, J., Lekakis, J., & Filippatos, G. (2015). Insuficiencia cardiaca aguda: Epidemiología, factores de riesgo y prevención. *Revista Espanola de Cardiologia*, *68*(3), 245–248. doi:10.1016/j.recesp.2014.11.009 PMID:25659507

Ferenhof, H. A., & Fernandes, R. F. (2016). Desmistificando a revisão de literatura como base para redação científica: Método SSF. *Revista ACB*, *21*(3), 550–563.

Hoo, G. W. S. (2016). Determinants of Utilization of Noninvasive Mechanical Ventilation in Hospitals: Key Technical and Nontechnical Issues. In *Noninvasive Mechanical Ventilation* (pp. 839–850). Springer. doi:10.1007/978-3-319-21653-9_97

Maraffi, T., Brambilla, A. M., & Cosentini, R. (2018). Non-invasive ventilation in acute cardiogenic pulmonary edema: How to do it. *Internal and Emergency Medicine*, *13*(1), 107–111. doi:10.100711739-017-1751-4 PMID:28952011

Masa, J. F., Utrabo, I., de Terreros, J. G., Aburto, M., Esteban, C., Prats, E., ... Farrero, E. (2016). Noninvasive ventilation for severely acidotic patients in respiratory intermediate care units. *BMC Pulmonary Medicine*, *16*(1), 97. doi:10.118612890-016-0262-9 PMID:27387544

Mendes, J. (2015). Ventilação Mecânica Não Invasiva. In P. Ponce (Ed.), *J. Mendes. Manual de Medicina Intensiva* (pp. 113–122). Lidel.

Pereira, J., Sequeira, R., Marques, M. D. C., Oliveira, N., & Realista, S. (2016). Ventilação não-invasiva: opção terapêutica nos cuidados ao doente com dispneia em contexto pré-hospitalar. *Nursing Magazine Digital*. Available in: http://hdl.handle.net/10174/20492

Santos, L. A., de Oliveira Sanchez, M., Pinto, R. G. S., da Luz Filho, A. C., Luz, K. R. G., & Soares, J. L. (2017). Efeitos da ventilação não invasiva em pacientes com insuficiência respiratória aguda: Uma revisão integrativa. *Revista Ciência & Saberes-Facema*, *3*(3), 642–648.

Sousa, L. M. M., Severino, S., & Pestana, H. C. F. C. (2018). Revisões da literatura científica: tipos, métodos e aplicações em enfermagem. *Rev Port Enferm Reabil*, 46-55. Disponível na Internet: https://www.aper.pt/ficheiros/revista/rpern0.pdf

Sousa, M. M. D., Oliveira, J. D. S., Soares, M. J. G. O., Bezerra, S. M. M. D. S., Araújo, A. A. D., & Oliveira, S. H. D. S. (2017). Associação das condições sociais e clínicas à qualidade de vida de pacientes com insuficiência cardíaca. *Revista Gaúcha de Enfermagem*, *38*(2). Advance online publication. doi:10.1590/1983-1447.2017.02.65885 PMID:28700025

Souza deMelo, F. E., Nogueira, I. D. B., Felismino, A. S., dosSantos Vicente, R. N. I., & Soares daSilva, I. (2015). Use of noninvasive ventilation for acute respiratory failure in intensive care unit. *Manual Therapy, Posturology & Rehabilitation Journal= Revista Manual Therapy*, 13.

Ugurlu, A. O., Sidhom, S. S., Khodabandeh, A., Ieong, M., Mohr, C., Lin, D. Y., ... Hill, N. S. (2015). Where is noninvasive ventilation actually delivered for acute respiratory failure? *Lung*, *193*(5), 779–788. doi:10.100700408-015-9766-y PMID:26210474

Ugurlu, A. O., Sidhom, S. S., Khodabandeh, A., Ieong, M., Mohr, C., Lin, D. Y., ... Hill, N. S. (2016). Use and outcomes of noninvasive ventilation for acute respiratory failure in different age groups. *Respiratory Care*, *61*(1), 36–43. doi:10.4187/respcare.03966 PMID:26374908

Chapter 7
Formal and Informal Care:
Home Care in the Elderly With Obstructive Sleep Apnea

Sagrario Gomez-Cantarino
https://orcid.org/0000-0001-6894-2270
University of Castilla-La Mancha. Spain

Patricia Dominguez-Isabel
https://orcid.org/0000-0001-6894-2270
University of Castilla-La Mancha, Spain

Blanca Espina-Jerez
https://orcid.org/0000-0001-9961-072X
University of Castilla-La Mancha, Spain

Mª Carmen Bouzas-Mosquera
University of Castilla-La Mancha, Spain

M. Teresa Agullo Ortuño
University of Castilla-La Mancha, Spain

Maria de las Mercedes de Dios-Aguado
Service of Castilla-La Mancha (Sescam), Spain

Manuel Carlos Rodrigues Fernandes Chaves
https://orcid.org/0000-0002-8018-9581
Nursing School of Coimbra, Portugal

ABSTRACT

Due to the increase in life expectancy and therefore the prevalence of chronic pathologies, health services have required a change, as well as healthcare. One of

DOI: 10.4018/978-1-7998-3531-8.ch007

Copyright © 2020, IGI Global. Copying or distributing in print or electronic forms without written permission of IGI Global is prohibited.

these chronic pathologies is obstructive sleep apnea syndrome (OSAS), which is a disorder characterized by an occlusion of the upper airway, an issue that causes an interruption of breathing inducing transient asphyxia. The treatment of this disease is based on continuous positive airway pressure devices (CPAP), but the main caregiver faces problems of adherence to this treatment, causing a deterioration both physically, socially, and psychologically. Therefore, the objective of this present work is to 1) identify the characteristics of OSAS, 2) describe adherence to treatment, and 3) detail the biopsychosocial deterioration of the main caregiver of this pathology in the elderly.

INTRODUCTION

Caring for the elderly has been a challenge for the health community. Currently, the population's framework means that health care takes great responsibility in the ageing process in order to address the problems related to this segment of the population (Bielicki, Byskniewicz, Kumor, Korczynski, & Chazan, 2006; Ganga, Thangaraj, & Puppala, 2009; Onen & Onen, 2010; Parra et al. 2015).

Ageing is a progressive and universal process that takes place in every living being, generating a series of changes of a physical, psychological and social type, producing modifications which do not originate from an illness (Leiton, 2016). Even so, there seems to be a tendency of the appearance of diseases when people are in old age, an issue that produces incapacitating diseases or geriatric syndrome, which leads to an impairment in the quality of life and even leads to a decrease in life expectancy at this age (Salech, Jara, & Michea, 2012).

According to the WHO, active ageing is a process that unifies health, safety and participation, with the purpose of increasing the quality of life as they age. In other words, it gives the elderly with an active and healthy life the opportunity to achieve their physical, psychological and social well-being throughout their life trajectory and be able to participate in society by fulfilling their desires, needs and capacities (Ortiz, Aguilera & Hernández, 2016).

The most prevalent chronic processes found in the elderly are related to the cardiovascular system, an example of which is arterial hypertension or ischemic cardiopathy (Cantero, 2011; Jackson & Wenger, 2011). As for the respiratory system, one of the issues we find as a pathology in elderly people is the obstructive sleep apnea syndrome (OSAS), also known as obstructive sleep apnea-hypoapnea syndrome (OSAHS), which is a disorder characterized by an obstruction of the upper airway which is why breathing is interrupted causing a transient asphyxia (Bronc, 2005; Nogueira et al., 2013). We found this pathology as a notable interest due to the high prevalence in the elderly, as well as the clinical characteristics, being very different from young adults (Egía & Cascante, 2007; Gabbay & Lavie, 2012; Launois, Pepín, & Levi, 2007; Naresh & Punjabi, 2008).

This pathology must take into account the family environment and especially the person within this nucleus that is performing as the main caregiver.

Therefore, the magnitude of family care greatly exceeds the time spent on the person suffering from OSA by the informal carer, as opposed to a rather scarce and very reduced time spent by the formal system that is generally institutional (De la Cuesta, 2005; Falque-Madrid, 2014).

Dependent elderly people need to be cared for, a fact that is carried out by both the informal and formal carer. Although it is true that there is a clear question regarding public coverage, which is very basic while the private coverage is mostly unreachable mainly due to its high cost, families are forced to perform this care within their own home. Therefore, the people dedicated to the care of these elderly will be known as informal carers (ICs). (Crespo & López, 2007; Carreño & Chaparro, 2016).

Dependent persons can reside in their habitual domicile or even move to the carer's domicile, as the care demanded by these persons is carried out by relatives and even friends of relatives (García, Sala, & Coscolla, 2009). In most cases, this situation results in the necessary health activities carried out by non-professional carers with the possibility of receiving training from specialist nursing staff and even financial compensation for these activities (De la cuesta, 2005; Crespo & López, 2014).

OBJECTIVES

1. Identify the characteristics of OSAS
2. Describe adherence to treatment
3. Detail the biopsychosocial deterioration of the main caregiver of this pathology in the elderly.

METHODOLOGY

A narrative review of the evidence available in the last 10 years was carried out, although it was necessary to have information prior to the period indicated by the importance of the subject, being reviewed in databases: PubMed, Dialnet, Cuiden, IME, LILACS, Cochrane Library Plus, ENFISPO, Medline, Elsevier. The following descriptors have been used as search limiters: "apnea", "obstructive sleep apnea", "treatment", "aging", "elderly", "formal caregiver", "informal caregiver". These same terms were included in English for database searches. Free natural language was used, combined with Boolean operators ("y/and", "o/or", "no/not"). In all cases, the type of font selected was scientific journals. A review of the repository of books located at the University of Castilla-La Mancha was also carried out. To help in this selection, a series of inclusion criteria were established: 1) articles referring to the human species; 2) studies carried out in Europe, the United States and Latin America; 3) articles whose full text is in English or Spanish; 4) articles referring to the subject of study; 5) full text articles. As exclusion criteria: 1) articles written in languages not controlled by the researchers were discarded; 2) articles with incomplete texts; 3) information that did not deal with the topic of study. On the other hand, a filter was introduced for the date of publications referring to socio-health behavior and informal care: from 1990 to 2018, a new temporary filter was also carried out only for articles published between 2005 and 2018. Only full text articles were chosen.

BACKGROUND

In Spain, epidemiological studies establish that people over the age of 65 may present some sleep-related disorder (Schubert, Cruickshanks, Dalton, Klein, & Nondahl, 2002), due to the fact that the aging process is associated with a deterioration of sleep, with the presence of an increase in superficial sleep and a decrease in deep sleep. All of this is the result of physiological processes subject to neurohormonal changes associated with the alteration of endocrine secretion in the hypothalamus-pituitary-adrenal axis, as well as neurological activity (Basheer & Shiromani, 2001; Shiromani, Lu & Wagner, 2000), accompanied by a decrease in growth hormone, alteration in melatonin secretion, and an increase in cortisol at night. This means that there is a decrease in the time of total sleep and its effectiveness, with the person being able to wake up fifteen times during the night, an issue that leads to a deterioration both in the elderly person who suffers it and therefore in the main caregiver (De la Cuesta, 2005).

In addition to neurohormonal changes, the elderly suffer from anatomical modifications, favoring the appearance of chronic diseases and syndromes. With respect to the upper airway, specifically in the oropharynx, there is a collapse that leads to apnea. The factors that favor collapse include the previous narrowing of these pathways (anatomic factor), an excessive loss of muscle tone (muscular factor) and defect in the protective reflexes (neurological factor) (García & Martínez, 2015). Therefore, the stability of its calibre depends on the action of the oropharyngeal dilator muscles and abductors, which are normally activated rhythmically during each inspiration, issues that to a greater or lesser extent they produce pluripathology which must be addressed by a multidisciplinary health team (García and Martínez 2015; Wilkinson et al. 2017).

All these characteristics are causes of the aging process and, therefore, give an increase in the number of syndromes of obstructive sleep apnea physiologically with age due to a greater tendency of the upper airway to collapse, which corresponds to several factors of great heterogeneity in elderly individuals. Without forgetting that factors such as environmental factors, diet and physical activity (Duffy, et al., 2002; Kendall, Lewy & Sack, 2001), will give rise to sleep disturbances producing insomnia, an increase in the number of respiratory disorders during sleep; a very frequent issue in advanced ages (Bloom, et al., 2009; Collop, 1997).

OSAS is defined as "a condition characterized by excessive daytime sleepiness, cognitive-conceptual disturbances, respiratory (lack of alveolar ventilation causes oxygen desaturation), cardiac, metabolic or inflammatory disturbances secondary to repeated episodes of airway obstruction during sleep" (Eguía and Casante, 2007; p.54). These episodes cause repeated transient awakenings (called aurosals or microdespertares) (García and Martínez 2015) that lead to unrepairable sleep and decreases in oxygen saturation (Martínez et al., 2018).

This context extrapolated to the family home and added to people in a situation of dependency under the care of an informal caregiver will produce an impact on sleep of both the person who suffers it and the caregiver itself, as a consequence of the demand and needs suffered by people with OSAS at night. Therefore, the main carer will experience repercussions in their daily activities and even in their devoted time used to interact with other people, as well as in their moments of leisure, being the emotional support of vital importance for the informal carer (CI) (López, et al., 2009).

Informal carers (IC) are those people with an affective bond at a family or friendship level, dedicated to the care for dependent people, who may or may not receive economic remuneration (Crespo and López, 2007). It cannot be ignored how at the labor level, these IC are more affected, because they face conflicts since they lack sufficient time to coordinate work and care. This situation sometimes leads to a lack of concentration, sick leave, and even loss of employment, and therefore causes major economic problems within the family structure (Inoye, Silva, Iost and Yoshie, 2009). Henceforth, one could speak of the caregiver overload syndrome, also known as being burnt out, which presents a characteristic symptomatology: emotional exhaustion, stress and fatigue (Molina, Iáñez and Iáñez, 2005), an issue that increases when the person to be cared for suffers from chronic diseases such as OSAS.

About an Underdiagnosis: Typical Signs and Symptoms in the Elderly

Typical symptoms and signs of elderly people with OSAS that aid medical diagnosis are snoring, daytime sleepiness, overweight and obesity, a high basal metabolic rate, large neck circumference, and craniofacial and respiratory tract abnormalities (García & Martínez, 2015). But an objective study such as polysomnography will be necessary, which consists of a study of the patient's sleep to record, among other parameters, the level of oxygen in the blood, heart rate, respiratory rate, respiratory effort and snoring or any other sound produced by the patient during rest. On the other hand, a subjective study is necessary, such as the Epword Test, which consists of a scale that assesses situations associated with drowsiness (from 1 to 24 points) and a score obtained through of a series of questions (0-3 points) asked to the patient (Martínez et al., 2018). The interpretation of this test is established at 1-6 points, referring to normal sleep; while the score between 7-8 points indicates average drowsiness; and finally, a score between 9-24 points informs us of an anomalous and possibly pathological drowsiness (Molina, Iáñez, & Iáñez, 2005).

In order to diagnose this pathology, it is necessary to observe an apnea-hypoapneas index (AHI) through polysomnography. Accordingly, the sum of apneas and hypoapneas are divided by hours of sleep to make up the AHI (García & Martínez, 2015). An AHI greater than 5 associated with symptoms and clinical signs of the disease is considered pathological in this type of patients (Eguía & Cascante, 2007).

There are various studies that have demonstrated that there is no significance of the signs and symptoms mentioned previously with AHI higher than 5. Therefore, it is necessary to explore and confirm other signs and symptoms, such as detailed enuresis and secondary nocturia, cognitive impairment, ophthalmic conditions, cardiovascular diseases, diurnal hypersomnia and falls as possible main complaints of OSAS in elderly subjects (Launois, et al., 2007) and furthermore suffered and also manifested by IC.

Bwilise in 2011 highlights a theory that suggests a heuristic model with two forms of OSAS, on the one hand, that of a pathological nature that would appear in the middle ages of life and on the other hand, that which would appear from the age of 60, with some overlap with the previous one, and which would be caused physiologically by the aging process itself and the consequent increase in pharyngeal collapsibility. That is to say, the OSAS detected in the elderly population could represent the people who suffered in their middle ages of life in a pathological way or on the contrary, be appearing in the elderly age due to the physical, physiological and psychological alterations typical of the age, being a less clinical relevance, although it must be made clear that this double model is still under study (Martínez, et al., 2010).

The lack of knowledge of OSAS in the elderly is due to the fact that we are faced with an underdiagnosed pathology (Onen & Onen, 2010). The low relevance of detected cases has meant that at the health level, it does not have the repercussion it should have, an issue that produces a low level of training of the main carer for the direct care of the relative. Therefore, formal caregivers have an important role in the process of health education (EHEA) (Gómez, Duque & Sukkarieh, 2015).

The overload borne by the caregiver has a negative impact on their physical and mental health, without forgetting the social aspect, as the quality of life will be diminished and the economic sphere may also be affected (López, Domínguez & Ochoa, 2010). The observable overload is usually in accordance with the physical load, the time of occupation and delivery without forgetting the stress produced by the care needed by this type of patients suffering from OSAS. But there is also a subjective overload, which is related to the emotional response shown by the caregiver (Lara, González & Blanco, 2008), as they manage to leave themselves aside producing negative consequences at the mental level (Lara, et al., 2008; López, et al., 2010), even leading to a lack of sleep or appetite and great tiredness (González & Reyes, 2012).

The Elderly Patient and the Difficulties Presented in Adherence to Treatment

On the one hand, we have surgical treatments such as tonsillectomy and uvulopalatopharyngoplasty, although these treatments are not the first choice in the elderly (Antonio & Gómez, 2016). On the other hand, we have treatments focused on the application of hygienic-dietary measures, such as weight loss and postural correction, which diminishes apneas. Finally, the therapy of initial choice is carried out with continuous positive airway pressure devices (CPAP) (González & Reyes, 2012), in a non-invasive and effective manner that was developed in the eighties (Sullivan, et al., 1981). These devices have the advantage of being a home treatment.

This CPAP generates a continuous flow of nasal, oronasal and oral air that, through a tubing and mask, reaches the patient, preventing the collapse of the airway during sleep. This is why this therapy can be used at home in this type of patients, and its results are reflected in a reduction of daytime sleepiness, improving cognitive performance, decreasing sympathetic activation, blood pressure and mortality (Barbé et al., 2010; Bronc, 2005; Cano-Pumarega et al. 2011; Nogueira et al., 2013; Parra et al. 2015).

McMillan conducted several studies in 2014, which were designed to evaluate the efficacy of CPAP in older people and thus determined its cost-effectiveness. This technique reduces drowsiness in both the elderly and middle-aged populations by improving daytime surveillance, care, and thereby decreasing falls in the elderly.

If OSAS is not treated, the risk of physiological disorders such as cerebrovascular and cardiovascular disease increases. It can also be a cause of social dysfunction and poor quality of life. When an older person presents with any coronary event such as stroke, repeated falls or even a severe trauma due to a traffic accident, it would be appropriate to consider OSAS as part of the diagnosis to be differentiated (McMillan et al., 2014).

The masks used in the CPAP can have from one to four points of support, the latter being the most used in this type of population. The importance of choosing the right mask for the patient lies prominently in the discomfort and as a consequence in a high possibility of poor adherence to treatment (Mortimore, Whittle, & Douglas 1998).

The most frequent adherence of CPAP use is at least four hours a day, being its use at night (in 70%) (Martínez et al., 2018), without forgetting the importance of the number of nights that its use is necessary. It is estimated that patients who stop using CPAP and thus do not continue with the treatment are between 30% to 60% of those who are evaluated annually after initiating this therapy (Weaver et al., 1997).

There are several reasons why adherence to the treatment decreases or disappears. These have to do with the aging process and the problems related to this treatment, so as to establish a classification of the same (Real, Jiménez & Castro, 2016) such as:

- Doctor-patient relationship: the trust and motivation fostered by the multidisciplinary team is fundamental to the fulfillment of the treatment. The figure of the community nurse specialist related to OSAS and informal caregivers comes into play (Gómez, et al., 2015).
- The environmental factor is very important, as it directly influences treatment adherence. It has been observed that in chronic diseases such as OSAS there is less adherence. On the other hand, the severity of the disease, as well as receiving treatment at home, normally favors compliance with the treatment since the patient is in his habitual environment (De la Cuesta, 2005).
- It has been proven that when a treatment is short and easy to follow, adherence to it is increased, obtaining benefits in this type of patients.
- In prescribed treatments where several drugs are used over a long period of time and with drugs that require qualified personnel or that have great side effects, adherence is scarce.

These problems are usually related to the mask, since one of the main discomforts derived from the mask is the pressure exerted by the mask in the support areas, without forgetting irritation, skin abrasions and even allergic reactions or air leaks (Pépin et al., 1995; Vaca & Elizabeth 2019) This situation could be avoided if the IC of the patient with such treatment was offered prior health education and thus be able to prevent abrasions by indicating the use of Vaseline before and after using the mask; paying attention to air leaks, as well as a good placement of this and the various allergic reactions, in short, a good education of health (Eps) (Garcia, Sala, & Coscolla, 2009).

Oronasal dryness, congestion, runny nose, frequent sneezing and aerophagia also appear frequently in these patients, an issue that appears in up to 65% of patients (Pépin et al., 1995). Eye dryness and red eye should not be overlooked. All these discomforts are usually treated with saline solutions prior to sleeping and waking up, and it is even necessary to apply moisturizing ointments, which are carried out by the IC figure at home (Martínez & De la Cuesta, 2016).

Sometimes there is intolerance to air pressure and even difficulty breathing due to pressure and exhalation. We should not forget the above mentioned about the insomnia of the patient in relation to the sensation of drowning they feel when wearing the mask, as well as claustrophobia, and even the discomfort produced by its use. The discomfort caused by the noise of the CPAP itself is also one of the reasons for abandoning treatment (Martínez & De la Cuesta, 2016).

EpS is very important in this type of patients and therapies since the decrease in adherence of treatment is rarely due to a lack of information regarding the use of CPAP equipment, the mask and/or a poor awareness of the consequences of the disease and the benefits of using this treatment (Martínez & De la Cuesta, 2016). Non-adherence to treatment is usually related to lack of information regarding the use of the equipment or mask, a poor awareness of the disease or excessive IC fatigue (Molina, et al., 2005).

In this pathology, it is necessary to take into account the family and, above all, the person within the family nucleus who carries out the IC work. Dependence is defined in our country, according to Law 39/2006, of 28 December on the Promotion of Personal Autonomy, which informs us of the state of people who, due to their advanced age, suffer some illness or disability, all of this together with the lack or loss of physical, mental, intellectual or sensory autonomy, need to be cared for by other people to carry out basic activities of daily life, and even deals with the help that people with intellectual disability or mental illness should receive (García, et al., 2009).

The IC is being substituted by the hiring of services of personnel external to the family, falling massively on the female figure. This situation is largely due to the flexibility of schedules, ensuring the presence of the latter even in the home, going so far as to remain in the same domicile for twenty-four hours, at the same time that this situation for the family lowers costs with respect to proximity services within their community (Molina, et al., 2005).

Formal Care of the OSA Patient: Nurse Specialist

Formal carers are those professionals who dedicate themselves to the care of the dependent person receiving a salary for their work. One of the most important causes of dependency is dementia, a syndrome characterized by cognitive, functional, motor and behavioral deterioration of negative and irreversible evolution, not forgetting patients diagnosed with obstructive apnea syndrome (OSAS / OSAHS), a situation that causes great dependence for the basic daily activities, for these reasons the elderly need the permanent care of other people in order to survive (Martínez & De la Cuesta, 2016).

The infirmary for the attention of the elder counts on the formation of the specialist infirmary in Geriatrics (EIR-Geriatrics), which is inserted in this way with its own perspective in the integral care of the greater adult, for which it is necessary to strengthen during the formative period of these professionals (regulated formation and duration of two years in Teaching Units Nurses-UDE), the foundations that support the humanized care of the elderly and the technical-professional training of their formal and informal caregivers since these professionals are the link between hospital care and home care (Acker, 2011).

Nursing guides the planned care of human beings through an intentional process that encompasses aspects such as the promotion and prevention of disease, health-sickness process and even death. Taking care of people's health implies having a broad theoretical knowledge and support of phenomena related to health and illness, which is generated from the nursing discipline itself through its models and theories, as well as sciences related to the care of human beings such as medicine, psychology, among others (Gómez, et al., 2015).

The teaching of geriatrics and gerontology in undergraduate nursing schools and in continuous training within the training of specialist nurses, must be considered essential to respond adequately to the changes facing our country and particularly in relation to the increase of older adults and the increase in the quality of care given to this group of people, in addition to know the most accentuated pathologies in this age (Ruiz, 2013).

It should be taken into account that the preferences to be attended by professional caregivers are directly related to the level of training people have, so the culturally better trained people prefer to be attended by non-family caregivers. In these cases, the role of nursing becomes important in order to avoid the increase of possible future problems that dependent persons may suffer. According to the definition of the Advisory Committee for Nursing Training, a specialized nurse is a nurse who has complementary qualifications to those of a nurse responsible for general care, within the meaning of Directive 77/EEC, and is entitled to practice as a specialist with advanced knowledge in a given area of nursing care.

During the training period, a multipurpose professional profile must be acquired, linked to both primary and specialized care, by means of teaching and assistance activities closely linked to the practice of care and to the ordinary activity of health centers and services. Therefore, Eir-Geriatrics nursing is the professional who provides attention and nursing care to the elderly population, being able to teach, supervise, investigate, manage and lead the care for this group in complex situations, in which it also acts as an advisor at all levels of the social health system (Gómez, et al., 2015; Balboa, Pérez, & Sarasola, 2012).

It is important to point out that, in addition to working with some knowledge and skills, the humanist aspect must be taken into account in the relationship with the patient-client, seeking the improvement or cure of the disease, alleviating suffering, or in the latter case, collaborating with the patient in the process of death. Therefore, the nurse replaces the patient when he cannot take charge of his self-care and encourages and reinforces him when he can do it himself, but does not have the necessary strength or will (Bellido & Lendínez, 2010; Porcel, 2011; Rodríguez, et al., 2005), in addition to training informal caregivers as in the case of patients with sleep disorders.

The objective of nursing is well-being, for which it is necessary to take care of the person from the totality in its biopsychosocial dimension. There is no daily record to write down small details, nor can the impact of help and relief from the conversation with the family in the corridor be measured, however, they are always present (Gómez, 2014; Vargas, 2012).

Adaptation to aging is not an easy task for older adults and requires health professionals, both in the participation of their care and by their vocation to it, to transmit an attitude that transcribes values such as: respect for others, autonomy and compassion to provide humanized care to the older adult, thus favoring adherence to established treatments and that also extends to their direct group of formal and informal caregivers (Overbeek, 1984; Livi-Bacci, 2002).

The purpose of geronto-geriatric specialist nursing (Eir-Geriatrics), is to help the elderly and their caregivers to face the aging process, understanding it as a natural and adaptive process and intervening in maximizing their sources of power. In the case of the treatment of CPAP in patients with OSAS, this nurse provides technical and regulated IC training, an issue that prevents alterations and complications in the elderly patient (Gómez, et al., 2015).

Nursing professionals currently stand out for their attitudes, skills and values in the field of ethics, humanitarian attitude, sensitivity, respect and love for the elderly and interest in professional development based on continuous research, playing a fundamental role in education, research, advice and involvement in public policies (Moreno, Recio, Borrás, & Torns, 2016; INE, 2013).

In view of the above, the figure of the specialist nurse is essential, as from a biopsychosocial point of view and with continuous training that will help in the diagnosis of diseases such as OSA. Likewise, contributions to the training of IC and in the care of the elderly patient work to reduce the most common risks that appear at this stage of life.

MAIN FOCUS OF THE CHAPTER

To establish a relationship to prevent and treat pathologies such as OSAS through informal care and health professionals (doctor, nurse, nurse specialist), using continuous positive airway pressure (CPAP) devices as treatment.

FUTURE RESEARCH DIRECTIONS

Within the importance in primary health care and development that have in the socio-health context the care of people in situations of dependency, at home within their usual context to increase their health and welfare. One of the objectives to be developed is to create tools that facilitate early diagnosis in the syndrome of obstructive apnea in the elderly.

DISCUSSION

Studies carried out on the health of the elderly, such as those of (Cordero, 2013) report on the essential role of achieving active ageing, an issue that will boost a population of healthy elderly people with less burden of complications and, therefore, less chronicity in diseases (Vilardell, 2014). In this sense (García Lizana, 2013) is inclined to improve the pluripathology of the group of people in advanced age from each person, being that who potentiates its own care and controls its disease. On the other hand (Gluzmann, 2013), based on data from the Gallup World Survey, indicates the existence of a positive relationship between welfare and growth, therefore, the countries with higher rates of economic development are those that currently show an increase in welfare levels. However, there is a very strong relationship with the health of the elderly in relation to the place of residence and the health care network that exists in the area (Parra et al., 2015). Although, it is true that the most predominant chronic processes in the elderly are related to the cardiovascular system, in which the majority of cases have a great impact on the respiratory system (Nogueira et al., 2013). It is true that we find studies that agree that respiratory pathology can provoke OSAS (Moreno, 2015; Nogueira et al., 2013), an issue that implies the application of CPAP in most cases. On the other hand, several studies indicate that there is no significant improvement in the elderly patient with CPAP administered at the hospital level compared to home treatment (Gray et al. 2008; Megido & Franco 2014; Vital, Ladeira, & Atallah 2013).

According to the study by (Alcántara, Torres, Martínez, & García, 2014), home treatment involves collaboration by a multidisciplinary team, with a strong involvement of general nursing, as well as specialist nursing (Gómez et al., 2015) and more personalized care by the family, not forgetting the person who will act as the main informal caregiver.

CONCLUSION

Obstructive sleep apnea syndrome (OSAS / OSAHS) is a chronic pathology that appears in advanced ages, with general signs and symptoms difficult to associate with this pathology due to the multiple diseases that may occur in later life.

For this reason, health professionals must be trained, especially geriatric specialist nurses, to care for this disease in patients suffering from it and thus increase adherence to treatment (CPAP).

In order to achieve this, it will be very important to carry out the EpS both on the patient themself and on their IC, with the aim of preventing patients from abandoning treatment and increasing the quality of life in people who dedicate themselves to administering informal care.

In order to favor adherence to treatment, a line of research could be proposed that includes the importance of the nursing consultation in this type of pathology and the value of adequate initial information in the patient who begins the therapy in order to avoid the abandonment of it and, therefore, suffer repercussions on his or her health.

In addition, there should be a connection between the geriatric specialist nurse and the IC of this pathology, since it will be the best reference figure to guide the latter in the care of the dependent person and thus avoid abandonment in the therapeutic treatment and health problems in the caregiver themselves.

ACKNOWLEDGMENT

This research received no specific grant from any funding agency in the public, commercial, or not-for-profit sectors.

To thank the associated study HISAG-EP (Spain-Portugal) for the collaboration in the development of this research on obstructive sleep apnea.

REFERENCES

Acker, G. M. (2011). Burnout among mental health care providers. *Journal of Social Work, 24*(2), 112–119.

Alcántara Santaigo, Z. R., Torres Amengual, M., Martinez Fernandez, C. A., & García Jiménez, E. (2014). ¿Somos conscientes de nuestras creencias? Estudio piloto. *Paraninfo Digital.* Recuperado de: http://www.index-f.com/para/n20/pdf/381.pdf

Balboa, M., Pérez, M., & Sarasola, J. L. (2012). Propuestas saludables para el envejecimiento activo. *Revista de Educación Hekademos., 11*(5), 29–36.

Basheer, R., & Shiromani, P. J. (2001). Effets of prolonged wakefulness on c-fos and AP1 activity in Young and old rats. *Brain Research. Molecular Brain Research, 89*(1-2), 153–157. doi:10.1016/S0169-328X(01)00045-6 PMID:11311986

Bellido Vallejo, J. C., & Lendínez Cobo, J. F. (2010). *Proceso Enfermero desde el modelo de cuidados de Virginia Henderson y los Lenguajes NNN.* Ilustre Colegio Oficial de Enfermería de Jaén. España. Primera Edición. Disponible en: www. index-f. com/lascasas/documentos/lc0714.pdf

Bielicki, P., Byskniewicz, K., Kumor, M., Korczynski, P., & Chazan, R. (2006). Obstructive sleep apnoa syndrome in yourger and older age groups –differences and similarities. *Pneumonologia i Alergologia Polska, 74*(1), 56–58.

Bloom, H. G., Ahmed, I., Alessi, C. A., Ancoli-Israel, S., Buysse, D. J., Kryger, M. H., Phillips, B. A., Thorpy, M. J., Vitiello, M. V., & Zee, P. C. (2009). Evidence-based recommendations for the assessment and management of sleep disorders in older persons. *Journal of the American Geriatrics Society, 57*(5), 761–789. doi:10.1111/j.1532-5415.2009.02220.x PMID:19484833

Bronc, A. (2005). Documento consenso español sobre el síndrome de apneas-hipopneas del sueño. *Grupo Español de Sueño, 41*, 4.

Cano-Pumarega, I., Durán-Cantolla, J., Aizpuru, F., Miranda-Serrano, E., Rubio, R., Martínez-Null, C., de Miguel, J., Egea, C., Cancelo, L., Álvarez, A., Fernández-Bolaños, M., & Barbé, F. (2011). Obstructive Sleep Apnea and Systemic Hypertension: Longitudinal Study in the General Population: The Vitoria Sleep Cohort. *American Journal of Respiratory and Critical Care Medicine, 184*(11), 1299–1304. doi:10.1164/rccm.201101-0130OC PMID:21868499

Cantero, A. R. (2011). Control del riesgo cardiovascular en el anciano. *Revista Clínica Española, 211*, 2–7. doi:10.1016/S0014-2565(11)70002-9

Carreño, S. P., & Chaparro, L. (2016). Calidad de vida de los cuidadores de personas con enfermedad crónica. *Aquichan, 16*(4), 447–461. doi:10.5294/aqui.2016.16.4.4

Collop, N. A. (1997). The significance of sleep-disordered breathing and obstructive sleep apnea in the elderly. *Chest, 112*(4), 867–868. doi:10.1378/chest.112.4.867 PMID:9377944

Cordero del Castillo, P. (2013). *2012, Año Europeo del Envejecimiento Activo y la Solidaridad Intergeneracional.* Academic Press.

Crawford, E. (2013). Le sommeil physiologique et pathologique du sujet âge: impact sur la qualité du vieillissement et le vieillissement cognitif. Médecine humaine et pathologie. *Archives-Ouvertes: Université Jean Monnet – Saint-Etienne.*

Crepo, M., & López, M. (2007). *El apoyo a los cuidadores familiares mayores dependientes en el hogar: desarrollo del programa "cómo mantener su bienestar."* Recuperado en: https://www.imserso.es/InterPresent1/groups/imserso/documents/binario/apoyocuidadores.pdf

De la Cuesta, C. (2005). La artesanía del cuidado. Cuidar en la casa de un familiar con demencia avanzada. *Enfermeria Clinica, 15*(6), 335–342. doi:10.1016/S1130-8621(05)71140-2

Duffy, J. F., Zeitzer, J. M., Rimmer, D. W., Klerman, E. B., Dijk, D. J., & Czeisler, C. A. (2002). Peak of circadian melatonin rhythm occurs later within the sleep of older subjects. *American Journal of Physiology. Endocrinology and Metabolism, 282*(2), E297–E303. doi:10.1152/ajpendo.00268.2001 PMID:11788360

Eguía, V. M., & Cascante, J. A. (2007). Síndrome de apnea-hipopnea del sueño. Concepto, diagnóstico tratamiento médico. *Anales del Sistema Sanitario de Navarra, 30*(1), 53–74. doi:10.4321/S1137-66272007000200005 PMID:17491608

Falque-Madrid, L. (2014). La evidencia científica y el arte de envejecer. *Anales Venezolanos de Nutrición, 27*(1), 110–118.

Gabbay, I. E., & Lavie, P. (2012). Age- and gender-related characteristics of obstructive sleep apnea. *Sleep and Breathing, 16*(2), 453–460. doi:10.100711325-011-0523-z PMID:21499842

Ganga, H., Thangaraj, V., y Puppala, N. (2009). Obstructive Sleep Apnea in the ederly Population: Atypical Presentation and Diagnostic Challenges. *The Internet Journal of Internal Medicine, 8*(2).

García, D. A. R., & Martínez, E. G. (2015). El síndrome de apnea obstructiva del sueño en el anciano: características específicas. Investigación en Salud y Envejecimiento, 3, 77-84.

Garcia Oliva, M., Sala, E., & Coscolla Aisa, R. (2009). *La calidad de vida de las cuidadoras informales: bases para un sistema de valoración*. Recuperado en: http://www.segsocial.es/prdi00/groups/public/documents/binario/119780.pdf

Gluzmann, P. (2013). Bienestar Subjetivo y Crecimiento Económico: Analizando La Paradoja Del Crecimiento Infeliz En La Encuesta Mundial Gallup. *Económica, 59*, 231–258.

Gómez, S., Duque, T. C., & Sukkarieh, N. S. (2015). Otras unidades multiprofesionales en la formación sanitaria especializada desde el punto de vista de la enfermería. Principios de Educación Médica. Desde el grado hasta el desarrollo profesional. *Editorial médica Panamericana. S.A., 20*(6), 439-440.

Gómez Sánchez, A. (n.d.). Intervenciones de enfermería en el cuidador informal del adulto dependiente. *Nuberos Científica, 2*(11), 21-26. Recuperado de: http://nc.enfermeriacantabria.com/index.php/nc/article/view/35/33

González Castro, U., & Reyes, A. (2012). Algunos aspectos del proceso que viven los cuidadores primarios de un enfermo crónico-degenerativo. *Revista Electrónica de Psicología Iztacala, 15*(2), 636–661.

Grupo Español de sueño. (2005). Consenso Nacional sobre el síndrome de apneas-hipopneas del sueño. *Archivos de bronconeumología, 41*(4).

Inouye, K., Silva, E., Iost, S., & Yoshie, C. (2009). Perceived quality of life of elderly patients with dementia and family caregives: Evaluation and correlation. *Revista Latino-Americana, 17*(3), 35–41.

Instituto Nacional de Estadística. (2013). *Proyecciones de población a largo plazo.* Recuperado en: https://www.ine.es/jaxi/menu.do?type=pcaxis&path=%Ft20%Fp251&file=inebase&L=0

Jackson, C., & Wenger, N. (2011). Enfermedad cardiovascular en el anciano. *Revista Espanola de Cardiologia, 64*(8), 697–712.

Kendall, A. R., Lewy, A. J., & Sack, R. L. (2001). Effects of aging on the intrinsic circadian period of totally blind humans. *Journal of Biological Rhythms, 16*(1), 87–95. doi:10.1177/074873040101600110 PMID:11220783

Kleisiaris, C. F., Kritsotakis, E. I., Danil, Z., Tzanakis, N., Papaioannou, A., & Gourgoulianis, K. I. (2014). The prevalence of obstructive sleep apnea-hypopnea syndrome-related symptoms and their relation to airflow limitation in and elderly population receiving home care. *International Journal of Chronic Obstructive Pulmonary Disease*, *10*(9), 1111–1117. doi:10.2147/COPD.S67779 PMID:25336942

Lara, G., González-Pedraza, A., & Blanco, L. (2008). Perfil del cuidador: Sobrecarga y apoyo familiar e institucional del cuidador primario en el primer nivel de atención. *Revista de Especialidades Médico-Quirúrgicas*, *3*(1), 159–166.

Launois, S. H., Pepin, J. L., & Levy, P. (2007). Sleep apnea in the elderly: A especific entity? *Sleep Medicine Reviews*, *11*(2), 87–97. doi:10.1016/j.smrv.2006.08.005 PMID:17276106

Leiton-Espinoza, Z. E. (2016). El envejecimiento saludable y el bienestar: Un desafío y una oportunidad para enfermería. *Enfermería Universitaria*, *13*(3), 139–141. doi:10.1016/j.reu.2016.06.002

Livi-Bacci, M. (2002). *Historia mínima de la población mundial*. Ariel.

López-Dávalos, G., Domínguez-Guedea, M., & Ochoa, M. (2010). Validación de la Escala de Bienestar Subjetivo en cuidadores familiares de adultos mayores. *Revista Psicologia e Saúde*, *1*(1), 13–22.

López-Gil, M., Orueta, R., Gómez-Caro, S., Sánchez-Oropesa, A., Carmona, J., & Alonso-Moreno, F. (2009). El rol del cuidador de personas dependientes y sus repercusiones sobre su calidad de vida y su salud. *Revista Clínica Médica Familiar*, *2*(1), 332–339.

Martínez, L., Martín-Bejarano, L., Diéguez, Mª. D., Garrido, Mª. V., Romero, L., & Carrasco, Mª. A. (2018). Pincipales causas de la no adherencia al tratamiento con CPAP (Presión continua positiva de aire). *Hygia de enfermería: revista científica del colegio,* (98), 19–21.

Martínez, M., & De la Cuesta, C. (2016). La experiencia del cuidado de las mujeres cuidadoras con procesos crónicos de salud de familiares dependientes. *Atención primaria: Publicación oficial de la Sociedad Española de Familia y Comunitaria, 48*(2), 77-84.

Martínez-García, M. A., Durán-Cantolla, J., & Montserrat, J. M. (2010). El síndrome de apneas-hipopneas durante el sueño en edades avanzadas. *Archivos de Bronconeumologia*, *46*(9), 479–488. doi:10.1016/j.arbres.2010.05.003 PMID:20580480

McMillan, A., Bratton, D. J., Faria, R., Laskawiec-Szkonter, M., Griffin, S., Davies, R. J., Nunn, A. J., Stradling, J. R., Riha, R. L., & Morrell, M. J. (2014). Continuous Positive Airway Pressure in Older People with Obstructive Sleep Apnoea Syndrome (PREDICT): A 12-Month, Multicentre, Randomised Trial. *The Lancet. Respiratory Medicine*, *2*(10), 804–812. doi:10.1016/S2213-2600(14)70172-9 PMID:25172769

Megido, J. A., & Franco, Á. G. (2014). Ventilación Mecánica No Invasiva En El Tratamiento de La Insuficiencia Cardíaca Aguda. *Medicina Clínica*, *142*, 55–58. doi:10.1016/S0025-7753(14)70084-3

Molina-Linde, J., Iáñez, M., & Iáñez, B. (2005). El apoyo social como modulador de la carga del cuidador de enfermos de Alzheimer. *Revista Psicologia e Saúde*, *9*(1), 33–42.

Moreno, R. (2015). Terapias ventilatorias en el manejo del edema agudo de pulmón cardiogénico. *Revista Patología Respiratoria, 18*(1).

Moreno, S., Recio, C., Borrás, V., & Torns, T. (2016). Significados e imaginarios de los cuidados de larga duración en España. *Una aproximación cualitativa desde el discurso de las cuidadoras, 1*, 1-28.

Mortimore, I. L., Whittle, A. T., & Douglas, N. J. (1998). Comparison of Nose and Face Mask CPAP Therapy for Sleep Apnoea. *Thorax*, *53*(4), 290–292. doi:10.1136/thx.53.4.290 PMID:9741373

Naresh, M., & Punjabi, S. (2008). The Epidemiology of Adult Obstructive Sleep Apnea. *Proceedings of the American Thoracic Society*, *5*(2), 136–143. doi:10.1513/pats.200709-155MG PMID:18250205

Nogueira, F., Nigro, C., Cambursano, H., Borsini, E., Silio, J., & Ávila, J. (2013). Practical guidelines for the diagnosis and treament of obstructive sleep apnea síndrome. *Medicine*, *73*(4), 349–362. PMID:23924537

Onen, F., & Onen, H. (2010). Syndrome d'apnées obstructives du sommeil et troubles cognitifs chez les sujets âgés. *Psychologie & Neuropsychiatrie du Vieillissement*, *8*(3), 9–163. PMID:20739254

Ortiz, M. M., Aguilera, A., & Hernández, C. (2016). Analizando las patologías más prevalentes en la edad avanzada. In *Investigación en salud y envejecimiento* (pp. 129–133). ASUNIVEP.

Overbeek, J. (1984). *Historia de las teorías demográficas*. México: Fondo de Cultura Económica.

Parra, O., Sánchez-Armengol, A., Capote, F., Bonnin, M., Arboix, A., Campos-Rodríguez, F., & Macarrón, J. (2015). Efficacy of Continuous Positive Airway Pressure Treatment on 5-Year Survival in Patients with Ischaemic Stroke and Obstructive Sleep Apnea: A Randomized Controlled Trial. *Journal of Sleep Research*, *24*(1), 47–53. doi:10.1111/jsr.12181 PMID:25040553

Pépin, J. L., Leger, P., Veale, D., Langevin, B., Robert, D., & Lévy, P. (1995). Side Effects of Nasal Continuous Positive Airway Pressure in Sleep Apnea Syndrome: Study of 193 Patients in Two French Sleep Centers. *Chest*, *107*(2), 375–381. doi:10.1378/chest.107.2.375 PMID:7842764

Porcel, A. (2011). *Construcción y validación de un sistema de evaluación del nivel de dependencia para el cuidado de los pacientes hospitalizados*. Universidad de Granada.

Real, B. A., Jiménez, M. M., & Castro, E. M. (2016). Factores que predisponen al incumplimiento terapéutico en el anciano. In *Investigación en salud y envejecimiento* (pp. 111–115). ASUNIVEP.

Rodríguez, J. B., Carrión, M. R., Espina, M. A., Jiménez, J. P., Oliver, M. C., Péculo, J. A., & .... (2005). *Marco conceptual, proceso enfermero en EPES*. Empresa Pública de Emergencias Sanitarias.

Ruiz López, M. (2013). *Ni familiares ni profesionales: cuidadoras inmigrantes contratadas* (Tesis doctoral). Serie: Salud.

Salech, M. F., Jara, L. R., & Michea, A. L. (2012). Cambios fisiológicos asociados al envjecimiento. *Revista Médica Clínica Las Condes*, *23*(1), 19–29. doi:10.1016/S0716-8640(12)70269-9

Schubert, C., Cruickshanks, K., & Dalton, D., Klein, Klein, B., & Nondahl D. (2002). Prevalence of Sleep Problems and Quality of Life in an Older Population. *Sleep*, *25*(8), 48–52. PMID:12489896

Shiromani, J., Lu, J., Wagner, D., Thakkar, J., Greco, M. A., Basheer, R., & Thakkar, M. (2000). Compensatory sleep response to 12h wakefulness in Young and ol rats. *American Journal of Physiology. Regulatory, Integrative and Comparative Physiology*, *278*(1), 125–133. doi:10.1152/ajpregu.2000.278.1.R125 PMID:10644630

Sullivan, C. E., Berthon-Jones, M., Issa, F. G., & Eves, L. (1981). Reversal of obstructive sleep apnoea by continuous positive airway pressure applied through the nares. *Lancet*, *317*(8225), 862–865. doi:10.1016/S0140-6736(81)92140-1 PMID:6112294

Vaca, B., & Elizabeth, G. (2019). *Prevalencia y factores asociados a la Malnutrición en pacientes con Enfermedad Pulmonar Obstructiva Crónica*. Hospital José Carrasco Arteaga.

Vargas Escobar, L. M. (2012). Aporte de enfermería a la calidad de vida del cuidador familiar del paciente con alzheimer. *Aquichan*, *12*(1), 62–76. http://www.scielo.org.co/pdf/aqui/v12n1/v12n1a07.pdf

Vilardell, M. (2014). *Envejecer Bien*. Plataforma.

Vital, F. M. R., Ladeira, M. T., & Atallah, A. N. (2013). Non-Invasive Positive Pressure Ventilation (CPAP or Bilevel NPPV) for Cardiogenic Pulmonary Oedema. *Cochrane Database of Systematic Reviews*, (5), CD005351. doi:10.1002/14651858.CD005351.pub3 PMID:23728654

Weaver, T. E., Kribbs, N. B., Pack, A. I., Kline, L. R., Chugh, D. K., Maislin, G., Smith, P. L., Schwartz, A. R., Schubert, N. M., Gillen, K. A., & Dinges, D. F. (1997). Night-To-Night Variability in CPAP Use Over the First Three Months of Treatment. *Sleep*, *20*(4), 278–283. doi:10.1093leep/20.4.278 PMID:9231953

Wilkinson, T. M. A., Aris, E., Bourne, S., Clarke, S. C., Peeters, M., Pascal, T. G., Schoonbroodt, S., Tuck, A. C., Kim, V., Ostridge, K., Staples, K. J., Williams, N., Williams, A., Wootton, S., & Devaster, J.-M. (2017). A Prospective, Observational Cohort Study of the Seasonal Dynamics of Airway Pathogens in the Aetiology of Exacerbations in COPD. *Thorax*, *72*(10), 919–927. doi:10.1136/thoraxjnl-2016-209023 PMID:28432209

ADDITIONAL READING

Abellán, A., Esperanza, C., Castejón, P., & Pérez, J. (2011). Epidemiología de la discapacidad y la dependencia de la vejez en España. *Gaceta Sanitaria*, *25*(supl. 2), 5–11. doi:10.1016/j.gaceta.2011.07.010 PMID:22000866

Ayalon, L., Ancoli-Israel, S., & Drummond, S. P. (2010). Obstructive sleep apnea and age: A doublé insult to brain function? *American Journal Of Resperatory Critical Care Medicina*, *182*(3), 413–419. doi:10.1164/rccm.200912-1805OC PMID:20395556

Carliste, T., Carthy, E. R., Glasser, M., Drivas, P., McMillan, A., Cowie, M. R., Simonds, A. K., & Morrel, M. J. (2014). Upper airway factors that protect against obstructive sleep apnoea in healthy older males. *The European Respiratory Journal*, *44*(3), 685–693. doi:10.1183/09031936.00177213 PMID:24833768

Degache, F., Sforza, E., Dauphinot, V., Celle, S., Garcin, A., Collet, P., Pichot, V., & Roche, F. (2013). Relation of Central Fat Mass to Obstructive Sleep Apnea in the Elderly. *Sleep (Basel)*, *36*(4), 501–507. doi:10.5665leep.2532 PMID:23564997

Lara, G., González Pedraza, A., & Blanco, L. (2008). Perfil del cuidador: Sobrecarga y apoyo familiar e institucional del cuidador primario en el primer nivel de atención. *Revista de Especialidades Médico-Quirúrgicas*, *3*(1), 159–166.

Oliva, J., Vilaplana, C., & Osuna, R. (2011). El valor social de los cuidados informales provistos a personas mayores en situación de dependencia en España. *Gaceta Sanitaria*, *25*(Supl. 2), 100–107. doi:10.1016/j.gaceta.2011.09.005

KEY TERMS AND DEFINITIONS

Apnea: Transient suspension of breathing.

Cares: The action of caring (preserving, guarding, conserving, assisting). Care implies helping oneself or another living being, trying to increase their well-being and avoid suffering any harm. It is also possible to care for objects (such as a house) to prevent incidents such as damage and theft from occurring.

CPAP: Continuous positive airway pressure and is the treatment of choice in patients with moderate to severe symptomatic apnea. It is equipment used while you sleep that prevents the collapse of the airway.

Drowsiness: A state in which there is a feeling of tiredness, heaviness, sleep, dullness of the senses and clumsiness in the movements.

Mask: An object or piece of cloth or paper that is placed over the nose and mouth and fastened with a rubber band or headband to prevent or facilitate the inhalation of certain gases or substances.

Nursing: Body of knowledge required to obtain the title of nurse.

Pathology: Part of medicine that studies the anatomical and physiological disorders of diseased tissues and organs, as well as the symptoms and signs through which diseases manifest themselves and the causes that produce them.

SAOS: A frequent disease and carries certain risks due to possible secondary complications (traffic accidents, cardiovascular disease, etc.). It is easy to diagnose and generally responds positively to treatment.

Snoring: A rough, severe, hoarse noise produced by breathing while sleeping, due to the vibration of the veil of the palate.

Therapy: A set of means that are applied to cure or alleviate a person's illness.

Chapter 8
Non-Invasive Ventilation in Alveolar Obesity-Hypoventilation Syndrome

Rute Pires
Hospital do Espírito Santo de Évora, Portugal

ABSTRACT

Obesity is the main risk factor for several sleep breathing disorders, including obstructive sleep apnea syndrome (OSAS), either alone or associated with chronic obstructive pulmonary disease (COPD), and alveolar obesity-hypoventilation syndrome (AOHS). In several of these conditions, the indicated treatment includes the use of non-invasive ventilation during sleep, such as the use of continuous positive airway pressure (continuous positive airway pressure or CPAP) and two-level pressure (BIPAP, bi-level positive airway pressure). In this chapter, a brief review is made of what the most recent studies say regarding the treatment of SOHA with non-invasive ventilation (NIV), comparing different ventilation modes and/or treatments.

INTRODUCTION

Obesity is the main risk factor for several sleep respiratory systems, including Obstructive Sleep Apnea Syndrome (OSAS), either alone or associated with Chronic Obstructive Pulmonary Disease (COPD), and Alveolar Obesity-Hippoventilation Syndrome (AOHS). In several of these conditions, the indicated treatment includes the use of non-invasive form of ventilation during sleep, such as the use of Continous Positive Airway Pressure (CPAP) and Bi-level Positive Airway Pressure (BIPAP).

DOI: 10.4018/978-1-7998-3531-8.ch008

Copyright © 2020, IGI Global. Copying or distributing in print or electronic forms without written permission of IGI Global is prohibited.

This chapter briefly reviews what the most recent studies say about the treatment of AOHS with non-invasive ventilation (NIV), comparing different ventilatory modes and/or treatments.

ALVEOLAR OBESITY-HYPOVENTILATION SYNDROME: DEFINITION

Obesity is one of the biggest public health problems in the developed world and has therefore been dubbed the "global epidemic of the 21st century" (López-Jiménez et al., 2016). This metabolic disease, recognised by the World Health Organisation as a serious health, social and economic problem, is associated with high morbidity and mortality rates (Ojeda Castillejo et al., 2015).

In addition to a pathology in its own right, obesity is a risk factor for the development of other chronic diseases, since it leads to significant changes in the physiology of the respiratory system that can lead to a wide spectrum of clinical manifestations, ranging from secondary dyspnea and restrictive ventilatory defect to hypercapnic respiratory failure, characteristic of Hypoventilation-Alveolar Obesity Syndrome (AOHS) (Ojeda Castillejo et al., 2015).

The Obesity-Alveolar Hypoventilation Syndrome (AOHS), or Pickwick Syndrome, or Obesity Hypoventilation Syndrome, or Obesity Hypoventilation Syndrome (OHS), which consists of the lack of effectiveness of the respiratory system in maintaining adequate gas exchange (Silva, 2006), was first described in 1956 and, is currently known as a condition characterized by obesity, hypercapnia and respiratory alterations during sleep, namely episodes of apnea and hypoventilation, in the absence of any other cause/disease that explains respiratory failure (López-Jiménez et al., 2016).

In 1999, AOHS was defined by the American Academy of Medicine of SONO (AAMS) as the association of obesity (BMI - Body Mass Index > 30 Kg/m2), chronic daytime hypercapnia (PaCO2 > 45 mmHg) and sleep breathing disorders, excluding all other causes of alveolar hypoventilation, such as severe obstruction or restrictive pulmonary diseases, chest wall disorders or neuromuscular diseases (Orfanos et al., 2017). Individuals may have symptoms such as daytime drowsiness, fatigue or morning headaches (Jacqueline et al., 2018).

In addition, AOHS is characterized by mild hypoxemia in wakefulness, associated with extreme oxygen desaturations during REM (Rapid Eye Movement) sleep and concomitant acute and repeated increases in PaCO2. Its importance today is due, in most cases, to the increased prevalence of obesity and the discovery of obstructive sleep apnea and hypopnea syndrome (OSAS) as a determining factor of symptoms - individuals with AOHS are more severely affected by cardiovascular diseases, compared to obese eukápnic individuals, with a mortality rate of 23% versus 9% (Nowbar et al., 2004).

Obstructive Sleep Apnea/Hypopnea Syndrome (OSAS), more commonly known as Obstructive Sleep Apnea Syndrome (OSAS), is a condition characterized by repeated partial narrowing (hypopnea) or total collapse (apnea) of the upper airways during sleep, resulting from an imbalance between the mechanisms that maintain airway permeability and the forces that promote its closure, with consequent hypoxemia and hypercapnia, associated with sleep fragmentation, pronounced snoring and excessive daytime sleepiness due to frequent nocturnal awakenings (Esquinas, 2011).

AAMS defines OSAS as a respiratory disturbance index (RDI) greater than 15 events per hour, or an RDI between five and 14 that is simultaneously accompanied by daytime sleepiness, roncopathy, observed apneas or awakenings with fighting movements or with a feeling of asphyxiation. RDI is the number of respiratory effort related arousals (REBA) apneas, obstructive hypopneas and awakenings per hour of sleep. The respiratory disturbances observed are predominantly obstructive and/or hypopnea-type apneas. Obstructive apnea is defined as the interruption, during sleep, of the oro-nasal flow for a period of ten seconds or more. The absence of airflow is due to the total occlusion of the pharynx during sleep, by collapse of the soft palate and/or base of the tongue against the walls of the former, due to decreased muscle tone, despite the continuous respiratory impulse that maintains the thoracic-abdominal respiratory movements. Hypopnea, in turn, results from an incomplete obstruction of the pharynx during sleep and can be defined as a decrease in oro-nasal flow of at least 5% and for at least ten seconds, being generally associated with a decrease in arterial oxygen saturation of at least 4% of the waking value, followed by an awakening. Thus, OSAS is defined when the number of obstructive apneas and/or hypopneas is equal to or greater than five respiratory events per hour. In terms of severity, the most commonly used criterion is based on the number of apneas and hypopneas per hour of sleep (AHI - Hypopnea Apnea Index): OSAS is mild when there are five to 14 events per hour, moderate with 15 to 29 events per hour, and severe with more than 30 events per hour (Esquinas, 2011).

The AOHS currently has a high prevalence among the adult population, as well as contributing to the development of several cardiovascular diseases, such as systemic arterial hypertension, auricular fibrillation, atherosclerosis, heart failure, acute myocardial infarction, stroke, increasing morbidity and mortality of individuals who suffer from it (Esquinas, 2011).

EPIDEMIOLOGY

Despite all the efforts that have been made to stop this epidemic, the proportion of adults with obesity has been increasing in recent decades. In the United States, one third of the population is obese and the prevalence of extreme obesity (BMI > 40 kg/m2) has increased dramatically. So much so that from 1986 to 2005, the prevalence of extreme obesity increased five times, from one in 200 adults to one in 33 adults (Bobak, 2010). Similarly, the prevalence of individuals with BMI > 50 Kg/m2 increased ten times, from one in 2000 adults to one in 230 adults (Sturm, 2007).

In Europe, on the other hand, more than half of the population is overweight, and of this 30% are obese; in Portugal, there is the same upward trend, although most estimates are based on self-reporting, given the scarcity of surveys with anthropometric measurements (Vânia Gaio, Liliana Antunes, Marta Barreto, Ana Gil, Irina Kislaya, Sónia Namorado, Ana Paula Rodrigues, Ana Santos, Baltazar Nunes, 2018). Recently, the National Food and Physical Activity Survey (IAN-AF 2015-2016) reported a prevalence of overweight[1] of 31% in women and 41.8% in men; regarding the prevalence of obesity, it was estimated that it was 23.7% in women and 19.7% in men, based on a representative sample of the population aged between 18 and 64 years (n = 3445) (ISNA, with Physical Examination the National Health Survey State of Health, 2016).

Obesity is an epidemic that affects not only adults, but also behaves as a global phenomenon affecting children and adolescents (Skidmore & Yarnell, 2004). Thus, the prevalence of AOHS has also increased. Several studies report that the prevalence of this entity is around 9-20% in obese individuals with OSAS. Similarly, the prevalence is higher in the subgroup of individuals with OSAS with extreme obesity. In a meta-analysis that included 4250 individuals with obesity and OSAS (in the absence of Chronic Obstructive Pulmonary Disease - COPD), a prevalence of hypercapnia of 19% was reported (Kaw, Hernandez, Walker, Aboussouan, & Mokhlesi, 2009). Another study, conducted with adult individuals hospitalized with a BMI > 35 kg/m2, indicated that 31% of them had AOHS (Nowbar et al., 2004).

Thus, AOHS is still a condition that is underdiagnosed and sub-treated. Although the prevalence of AOHS tends to be higher in men, in OSAS the predominance over males is still unclear, since it is estimated that 93% of women and 82% of men with moderate or severe OSAS are not yet diagnosed (Nowbar et al., 2004; Schlosshan & Elliott, 2004). Similarly, the predominance according to ethnicity has not yet been defined. However, the prevalence of AOHS is expected to be higher in African-Americans than in other races, given the higher prevalence of obesity in this ethnic group (Mctigue et al., 2006).

Despite its high prevalence in obese individuals, AOHS is also underdiagnosed due to the reduced specificity of its symptoms. In fact, when studying hospitalised obese individuals, it was possible to conclude that one third of them had AOHS and did not know it (Jennum & Kjellberg, 2011). In addition, AOHS is considered by many authors simply as a progressive form of OSAS in some obese individuals. However, although respiratory disorders during sleep are a defining condition of AOHS, they are always associated with OSAS. The prevalence of AOHS in the general obese population is not yet precisely defined, however, studies conducted in hospitalized obese individuals showed a higher prevalence, also revealing an increase in mortality rates in this group (Ojeda Castillejo et al., 2015; Orfanos et al., 2017).

The mortality and morbidity of these individuals is high. Individuals hospitalized with AOHS showed a mortality rate of 23% in 18 months, compared to only 9% of obese individuals without hypoventilation, who also died in the same period (Esquinas, 2011). These results were mainly due to respiratory failure and progressive or pulmonary thromboembolism (Jacqueline et al., 2018).

Less is known about the repercussions of AOHS than those of OSAS, although pulmonary hypertension, hyperlipemia, diabetes mellitus and cerebrovascular disease seem to be the most common. In a study conducted by Pihtili et al., with 419 individuals, 72.5% had metabolic syndrome, which would make it the most prevalent comorbidity in AOHS (Pıhtılı, Bingöl, & Kıyan, 2017). In fact, the higher risk of hypoxia in obese individuals with AOHS may produce a higher risk of cardiovascular events and mortality compared to obese individuals without respiratory failure (López-Jiménez et al., 2016). The non-recognition of this pathology becomes worrying due to the great loss in the quality of life of individuals with it, associated comorbidities, and the risk of sudden death that contribute to the increase in mortality and morbidity in this group (Schlosshan & Elliott, 2004).

PHYSIOPATHOLOGY

A vicious relationship is established between OSAS and obesity, since, just as obesity plays a decisive role in the pathophysiology of apnea and hypopnea episodes, they also contribute to the development or maintenance of obesity, since sleep is not peaceful at night, and the individual will have excessive daytime sleepiness, which predisposes to obesity, as well as other factors already widely described, such as smoking, alcoholism and sedentary lifestyle (Bhushan, Ayub, Thompson, Abdullah, & Billings, 2016).

Although it has been known for some years, the pathogenesis of AOHS has not yet been fully explained, although the exact mechanism leading to hypoventilation in obesity is complex and probably multifactorial in which altered ventilatory mechanics, muscle dysfunction secondary to obesity and ventilation control play an important role (Ojeda Castillejo et al., 2015).

The compliance of the thoracic cavity and lung volumes, and in particular the functional residual capacity and the volume of the functional reserve, is reduced in obese individuals. As a consequence, there is the possibility of small airway collapse and the potential development of limitation to expiratory flow, which increases the rise in respiratory work, already substantially enhanced by obesity. In addition, there is the increase in upper airway resistance found during wakefulness in individuals with AOHS. Muscle strength is also decreased, as is endurance (Esquinas, 2011).

PaCO2 is determined by the balance between CO2 production and removal (minute ventilation and dead space ventilation fraction). Thus, ventilatory responsiveness to hypoxia and hypercapnia is mitigated in individuals with AOHS due to hypoventiation. Thus, several physiological differences were observed between individuals with AOHS and those with obesity and/or OSAS: increased upper airway resistance, excessive mechanical load imposed on the respiratory system due to excess weight, imbalance in ventilation-perfusion secondary to pulmonary edema or low lung volumes/atelectasis, change in central response to hypoxemia and hypercapnia, presence of respiratory disorders during sleep and altered neurohormonal responses (leptinorresistance) (Jacqueline et al., 2018).

The excessive burden on the respiratory system is characterized by (Jacqueline et al., 2018):

- Obstruction of the airways, as individuals with AOHS present greater airway resistance, both in the sitting and standing positions, when compared to individuals with eukarypnic OSAS with a similar degree of obesity;
- Mechanics of the respiratory system and respiratory muscles: in AOHS there is an increase in respiratory work to mobilize the excess weight of the thoracic cavity and abdomen during breathing, although it is not clear what the contribution of these changes is in the mechanics of breathing. Pulmonary capacity in individuals with AOHS is lower compared to obese individuals without AOHS, which explains why the former presents a three-fold increase in pulmonary resistance.

The mechanisms related to changes in ventilation control in individuals with AOHS are not fully known. However, there is evidence that substances such as leptin are involved. Leptin is a hormone secreted by fat tissue, which is related to the control of appetite and energy expenditure, since its function is to inhibit hunger and increase energy expenditure. It is believed that obesity is associated with leptin, leading to hyperleptinemia, so, high levels of leptin are found in individuals with AOHS. On the other hand, studies in animal models have shown that leptin is a powerful respiratory stimulant, helping its increase in the maintenance of ventilation in the face of increased respiratory work, so its absence or defect could cause hypoventilation.

DIAGNOSTIC

AOHS is defined, as already mentioned, as the presence of hypercapnia and diurnal hypoxemia (PaCO2 > 45 mmHg and PaO2 < 70 mmHg) in an obese individual accompanied by respiratory disorders during sleep, in the absence of any other cause of hypoventilation (Esquinas, 2011; Orfanos et al., 2017).

The diagnosis of OSAS (which is characterized by recurrent episodes of partial or total upper airway obstruction during sleep) is made through nocturnal polysomnography, which shows the rate of respiratory events per hour of sleep. Respiratory breaks during sleep, witnessed by family members are the most specific symptoms, although snoring is the main clinical sign, present in virtually all individuals. Other associated symptoms include, in turn, loss of quality of life, fatigue, nictury, sexual impotence, morning headache and insomnia (Esquinas, 2011).

Thus, clinical manifestations alone do not allow for discrimination between AOHS and OSAS, since there is a significant overlap between the two, which makes it essential to perform a polysomnography during the night, in order to detail the respiratory disorder associated with sleep and its consequent severity (Jacqueline et al., 2018).

Before proposing any therapy to the individual, the diagnosis should be correctly established, determining its severity. In fact, the assessment of the severity of the disease enables guiding of the treatment, identifying the individuals at higher risk of suffering complications resulting from it and providing a basis for determining the effectiveness of the subsequent treatment (Esquinas, 2011).

TREATMENT

One of the treatments used for AOHS is weight loss, as it improves the physiological abnormalities that may be involved in pathogenesis, helps to reverse respiratory failure, pulmonary hypertension and sleep disorders. Weight loss of at least 10 kg produces a significant improvement in vital lung capacity and maximum voluntary ventilation, as well as a significant reduction in daytime PaCO2. Although studies are limited, weight loss has been shown to increase the central ventilatory response measured by the diaphragmatic electromyogram response to carbon dioxide inhalation. In individuals with AOHS and OSAS concomitantly, weight reduction decreases the number of sleep-associated respiratory events (apneas and hypopneas), decreases the severity of desaturation associated with any residual apnea and leads to the resolution of daytime hypercapnia (Jacqueline et al., 2018; López-Jiménez et al., 2016).

Although weight loss seems to be the most ideal treatment for this syndrome, it tends to be slow and difficult to achieve and maintain, so it cannot be used initially as the only treatment. In addition, the ideal amount of weight loss and its long-term result have not yet been studied. In fact, most individuals find it difficult to achieve and maintain significant weight loss, so bariatric surgery would be another option, but it is associated with higher mortality and is generally rejected for that very reason (Jacqueline et al., 2018; López-Jiménez et al., 2016). In this sense, the consensus of the National Institutes of Health (NIH), in the United States, addressed the issue of surgical treatment for obesity and obesity with comorbidities: according to these guidelines, in individuals with BMI above 35 kg/m2 with presence of comorbidities, including AOHS, or individuals with BMI above 40 kg/m2, surgical treatment is recommended ("Gastrointestinal surgery for severe obesity: National Institutes of Health Consensus Development Conference," 1992). These recommendations are supported by studies that evaluated the effect of gastric surgery in individuals with AOHS and OSAS, where, although one of the groups presented a significantly higher operative mortality rate, surgery was associated with weight loss, considerable improvement in sleep apnea, pulmonary volumes, arterial gas analysis results, polycythemia and pulmonary hypertension (Sugerman, Baron, Fairman, & Evans, 1987).

However, changes in lifestyle and medical treatment should not be ruled out. In any case, the initial goal should be a weight reduction of at least 5%, for a period of six months to one year. Regardless of the approach used, a consultation with the psychologist may clearly contribute not only to initial weight loss, but also to a long-term commitment by the individual (Darío & Andrés, 2017).

Thus, and currently, there are no established guidelines for the treatment of AOHS, and few randomized clinical trials have been published. The available treatments can be divided into medical, surgical or specific treatment of alveolar sleep/hypoventilation respiratory disorders, through adequate ventilatory support depending on the clinical and gasometric conditions of each individual, although the ideal therapeutic approach should include all three (Ramírez-Molina, Gómez-de-Terreros, Barca-Durán, & Masa, 2017).

As previously mentioned, there are a variety of sleep-associated respiratory disorders (apneas, hypoventilation or both), which are found in AOHS; treatment that corrects specific sleep-associated respiratory disorders produces the resolution of chronic daytime hypercapnia. In individuals with AOHS, Continuous Positive Airway Pressure (CPAP) was for a long time the first-line treatment; this therapy provides continuous positive pressure during the respiratory cycle, which produces and maintains upper airway permeability, eliminating apneas/hypopneas and resurrecting daytime euchapnia. However, noninvasive ventilation (NIV) with the use of BiPAP (Bilevel Positive Pressure Airway), Positive Airway Pressure at two levels, is of great importance and has been imposing itself as the first method of choice in the treatment of this syndrome, as it allows the correction of hypercapnia. Several studies suggest that BiPAP suppresses respiratory events during the night, normalizes sleep structure and restores daytime vigil (Chouri-Pontarollo, Borel, Tamisier, Wuyam, Levy & Pépin, 2007; De Llano et al., 2005). Others, in turn, reported a significant reduction in morbidity and mortality, with a consequent improvement in the quality of life of individuals with AOHS (Budweiser, Riedl, Jörres, Heinemann & Pfeifer, 2007; Heinemann, Budweiser, Dobroschke & Pfeifer, 2007).

Several factors have been identified today, which may explain why some individuals with AOHS and OSAS are not adequately treated with CPAP. In some of them and despite the use of CPAP, airway permeability is not maintained; individuals may need higher inspiratory pressure peaks, which only volume ventilation can provide. Other individuals, on the other hand, may present both pathologies simultaneously, which requires noninvasive ventilatory support to increase ventilation (Sullivan & Ph, n.d.).

Bi-Level positive pressure ventilators, introduced in the late 1980s, have become by far the most commonly used ventilators in most chronic respiratory failure situations, such as Chronic Obstructive Pulmonary Disease (COPD) or AOHS. There are, however, considerable variations in the performance of Bi-Level positive pressure ventilators available. In addition, one of the limitations of Bi-Level Positive Pressure (BiPAP) ventilators is the lack of guarantee as to the volume made available to the individual, as a pre-established fixed Pressure Support (PS) is provided, and it is therefore not possible to determine the volume delivered for each breath (Area, Janssens, Derivaz, & Breitenstein, 2003; Donaldson et al., 2005; Strumpf et al., 1991).

In contrast, in AVAPS (Average Volume Assured Pressure Support) mode, recently available on certain hybrid ventilators (integrating pressure or volumetric ventilation modes), the inspiratory pressure varies automatically from breath to breath, to ensure a predefined volume, better adjusted to the individual's needs, at each moment. This new mode allows you to estimate the tidal volume with each breath, comparing it to the target tidal volume for each individual and responding by adjusting (either increasing or decreasing) the inspiratory positive airway pressure (IPAP) to maintain ventilation and reach the estimated target tidal volume. Its objectives are: to facilitate the adjustment process; to improve ventilatory efficiency and individual comfort; and to increase safety by ensuring an average tidal volume (Anne et al., 2005).

However, few studies were conducted in this area. In the study conducted by Janssens et al. (Janssens, Metzger, & Sforza, 2009), in order to assess the correction of night-time hypoventilation, as well as the quantity and quality of sleep with Bi-Level Fixed Support Pressure (BiPAP) versus AVAPS, We selected 12 individuals (8 males and 4 females) with AOHS (defined by the authors as BMI > 30 Kg/m2 and PaCO2 > 45 mmHg) treated with NIV at the Division of Pulmonary Diseases of the University Hospital of Geneva, from June 1 to March 20, 2007. As inclusion surgeries to select their sample, the authors defined: 1) stable clinical condition; 2) home treatment with a two-level pressure support ventilator for AOHS for at least 2 months; 3) initiation of NIV after at least one episode of acute respiratory failure. Exclusion criteria were: any unstable cardiac or respiratory clinical condition and/or lack of compliance defined by daily use of the ventilator for less than four hours.

The individuals were distributed into two groups in order to receive NIV according to the ST mode (spontaneous/timed)/BiPAP or AVAPS on the first night and then moved to the alternative ventilatory mode. A nocturnal polysomnography was performed in the Sleep Laboratory of the University Hospital of Geneva with transcutaneous capnography. The AVAPS mode requires an objective determination of the tidal volume (TV), and a range of IPAP values, allowing the ventilator to adapt to a certain support pressure to reach the estimated target volume for each individual (through a pneumotachograph embedded in the ventilator). The recommended target volume for obese individuals is 7 and 8 ml/Kg (or 8 and 12 ml/Kg ideal body weight). The maximum IPAP was initially set at 30 cm/H2O and then adjusted according to the tolerance and leakage presented, over a period of 30 minutes. The minimum IPAP value was set according to the usual IPAP value minus 3 cm/H2O. Definitions of Expiratory Positive Airway Pressure (EPAP), back-up respiration rate and the inspiration/expiration time ratio were not modified. The standard interface used was a face mask or, when not tolerated, a nasal mask. Where oxygen was required, its flow was identical for both measurements.

During the night recording performed at the Laboratory, a standard polysomnography (PSG) was performed; respiratory air flow was monitored through a nasal cannula connected to a pressure transducer; thoracic and abdominal respiratory movements were monitored with pressure gauges; arterial oxygen saturation (SpO2) aggravated by a pulse oximeter and a finger probe was continuously evaluated; recorded the minimum and average SpO2, percentage of total sleep time with SpO2 < 88% and the oxygen desaturation index (ODI) (transient desaturation defined as a decrease in SpO2 of 3%); and, measured continuously the positive pressure level at the mask and recorded during the night study. Transcutaneous measurements of carbon dioxide (CO2) were also taken. The following sleep parameters were monitored: total sleep time (TST); sleep efficiency; percentage of each sleep stage; wakefulness after the onset of sleep; and sleep latency. Sleep fragmentation indices included the number of awakenings (lasting > 20 seconds and > 2 minutes), sleep phases, sleep fragmentation index (defined as the number of awakenings > 20 seconds/total sleep time per hour) and microawakening index (> 1.5 seconds). A subjective assessment of sleep quality (latency and duration of sleep) and ventilation comfort (perception of ventilator-individual synchrony, airflow, leaks and ventilator noise) was also performed through a questionnaire.

According to the results of transcutaneous capnography and pulse oximetry, the use of AVAPS mode significantly improved transcutaneous control of nocturnal CO2 and increased tidal volume. Polysomnography data and subjective evaluation of sleep quality revealed that, objectively, individuals slept better with the ST/BiPAP mode: total sleep time and sleep phase 2 were longer and wakefulness after the onset of shorter sleep. Although the microawake index and sleep fragmentation index were not affected, the number of awakenings was lower. However, no statistically significant difference was found between NREM (Non-rapid Eye Movement) or REM (Rapid Eye Movement) sleep between the two modes of ventilation. Subjectively, the individuals classified the quality of sleep and continuity as worse with AVAPS: their sleep was perceived as lighter and they reported more awakenings. However, no statistically significant difference was reported in relation to sleep latency and/ or satisfaction between ventilation modes.

In fact, individuals complained of less comfortable general ventilation with the target volume through the AVAPS mode, with a more frequent perception of "too much delivered air" and increased number of leaks, leading to poorer sleep quality. However, since individuals were familiar with conventional NIV through the BiPAP mode, the introduction of the target volume through the AVAPS mode may have been perceived as less comfortable than in individuals without any kind of contact with NIV therapy, which may have influenced the results. In fact, the introduction of the target volume with the AVAPS mode is potentially useful to increase the effectiveness of bi-level positriva pressure ventilation, at the expense of correcting night-time hypoventilation in stable individuals with AOHS, at the expense of minor changes in sleep structure and fragmentation, and a slight decrease in individual comfort.

In another study, carried out by Murphy et al. (Murphy et al, (Murphy et al., 2012), in order to verify whether the pre-defined target volume through automatic adjustment of the PS, in the AVAPS mode, is more effective in reversing daytime hypercapnia than the fixed PS, in the BiPAP mode, in very obese individuals with chronic respiratory failure, the inclusion criteria used for the selection of participants were: BMI > 40 Kg/m2; stable daytime respiratory failure; absence of another identifiable cause of hypoventilation; relationship between forced expiratory volume in 1 second (FEV 1) for forced vital capacity (FVC) > 0.70; and CVC < 70% of predicted. The exclusion criterion considered was the inability to provide written informed consent.

Sixty-two individuals were randomly selected, 50 of whom consented to participate in the study, and four (two from each group) were subsequently removed during follow-up. The individuals were randomly selected for the two-level AVAPS or Fixed Pressure Support (PS) mode and submitted to initial evaluations of spirometry, arterial gasometry and anthropometry, including body composition measurements using the bioelectric impedance method. Health-related quality of life was also assessed through the severe respiratory failure questionnaire.

The results of the study showed that the AVAPS mode is as effective in reducing daytime hypercapnia as the fixed PS mode, results that contrast with the previous ones, which suggest that the AVAPS mode allows better night-time ventilatory control, although with an increase in sleep disorders. Thus, data suggest that in less obese individuals (as in the previous study) the BiPAP mode may be sufficient, while in more obese individuals with chronic respiratory failure, the AVAPS mode shows better results. In addition, the data from this study also showed that nocturnal ventilatory support not only improves daytime symptoms, but also increases the physical activity of individuals during the day, which is associated with weight loss in obese individuals, highlighting the potential to increase this effect by introducing a healthy lifestyle.

In order to understand the role of healthy lifestyle counseling in the treatment of individuals with AOHS, compared to treatment with NIV, Borel et al, 2012) developed a study with this objective, which included individuals aged between 20 and 75 years with a BMI of 30 kg/m2 and a PaCO2 of 45 mmHg, except for those with significant airway obstruction (FEV1/FVC 70%), scoliosis, heart failure or progressive neuromuscular disease, resulting in a total of 37 who met the inclusion criteria. All individuals were submitted to an initial evaluation with the study of sleep by polysomnography to characterize abnormal respiratory events during sleep, as well as to respiratory function tests (spirometry, plethysmography and SNIP - Nasal Inspiratory Pressure).

Subsequently, they were randomly assigned, through a computer program, to the control group that received lifestyle counseling and to the group that received NIV treatment during the one-month period. Those who received lifestyle counselling had a one-hour education session, where they were informed about the risks associated with obstructive sleep apnea and obesity (namely, information on harmful factors such as smoking, reduced physical activity and alcohol consumption). A specialist nurse provided them with dietary counselling, in addition to being encouraged to change their lifestyle with regard to increased daily physical activity. The other group, in turn, initiated NIV with two pressure levels (BiPAP - Bilevel Positive Pressure Airway): inspiratory pressure 18 ± 2 cm/H2O and expiratory pressure 11 ± 2 cm/H2O (with a mean support pressure of 8 ± 2 cm/H2O), with a back-up respiratory rate of 13 ± 2 cycles/minute, with none of the individuals receiving additional oxygen. In one month, the mean use of NIV at night was 5.6 ± 2.2 h/night. At the end of this period, all individuals repeated the initial tests.

Compared to lifestyle counseling, NIV treatment was more effective in reducing daytime PaCO2 and blood bicarbonate values, with the consequent increase in total daytime pulmonary capacity, which can be explained by improved lung compliance related to the resolution of collapsed alveolar spaces during NIV. In other words, the application of NIV during sleep was associated with an improvement in all nocturnal oxygenation indices (pulse oximetry oxygen saturation during sleep and apnea-hypopnea index), which was not observed in the control group (who underwent lifestyle counselling), although this difference was not statistically significant after only one month of intervention. These results can be explained by the fact that this study included individuals who were in the mild spectrum of the disease, with ventilatory response values at the lower limit of normality and, perhaps, by the treatment time (one month) that can be considered insufficient. In terms of metabolic parameters (glucose metabolism and lipid profile), no statistically significant changes were observed, although in the control group there was a significant improvement in BMI, without any change in the NIV group, which may be due to the higher prevalence of type 2 diabetes in the group submitted to NIV. Although there was no difference in the groups in relation to subjective sleepiness, there was a great improvement in the general clinical level. Compared to the control group that underwent lifestyle counseling, NIV improved sleep quality by suppressing abnormal respiratory events and reducing sleep fragmentation, with a significant shift to deeper and more stable sleep.

In the last two decades, growing evidence in the literature has confirmed the role of NIV as a first-line therapy for certain forms of acute respiratory failure (ARF). In addition, it was used in individuals with more severe clinical situations and with proven efficacy, such as in restrictive lung diseases, AOHS and weaning from invasive mechanical ventilation. However, the efficacy of NIV depends not only on the careful selection of individuals, but also on their early identification. In the review prepared by Cavalleri et al. (Cavalleri, Barbagelata, Scudeletti, & Nicolini, 2018) three critical periods were defined to detect NIV failure: 1) immediate failure (in minutes to < 1 hour), due for example to a weak cough reflex that leads to inefficient clearance of excessive secretions or hypercapnic encephalopathy due to low adherence by confusion/agitation; 2) early failure (from 1 to 48 hours) due to severe respiratory acidosis, low level of consciousness, higher age and higher hypoxemia; and, 3) late failure (after 48 hours), which occurs after a good initial response to NIV. The latter is more frequent in individuals who, at the time of admission, had functional limitations assessed by a score correlated with daily life activities, higher number of comorbidities, lower ph at the beginning of the study and basic cause of ARF, such as Pneumonia. Obese individuals thus need a longer NIV therapy than non-obese individuals, especially at night, when apneas or hypoventilation worsen.

However, and despite the increasing use of BiPAP today, the superiority of NIV over CPAP has not yet been proven. In fact, around 26 to 50% of individuals with AOHS are diagnosed in an acute setting and, in most cases, treated with NIV, which continues to be their usual mode of ventilation for the rest of their lives. Once stability is achieved, the question arises as to whether NIV should be changed to CPAP; recent studies have assessed the possibility of starting treatment with non-invasive ventilation and, as soon as the individual stabilizes, begin maintenance with CPAP. Thus, and with the aim of testing the feasibility and effect of a standardized protocol, alternating individuals with AOHS, from NIV to CPAP, Orfanos et al, 2017) developed a study in which they hypotentatized that there would be no difference in efficacy after changing NIV to CPAP, as well as in daytime and night-time alveolar gas exchange, transcutaneous nocturnal saturation, but also on sleepiness, sleep quality and quality of life (Epworth Sleepiness Scale (EsS), Pittsburg Sleep Quality Index (PSQI), Severe Respiratory Insuficiency Questionnaire (SRI).

We then recruited individuals over 18 years of age (between February 2015 and February 2016), with AOHS and who had been using NIV for more than two months, from the Pneumology Wards of the University Hospital and the Military Hospital in Marseille, France. To be included in the study, individuals had to be clinically stable for a period of four weeks before inclusion in the study (without prior hospitalisation or emergency hospitalisation); individuals with hypercapnia secondary to other causes, interstitial pneumonia, neuromuscular or chest wall diseases, severe hypothyroidism or congenital central hypoventilation syndrome and individuals unable to give their consent were excluded.

Subsequently, several clinical information were collected, namely the history of the diagnosis of AOHS, the occurrence of acute exacerbations, the NIV configurations in use (brand, mode, respiratory rate, positive expiratory airway pressure, positive inspiratory airway pressure and interfaces used) and the quality of life, daytime sleepiness and quality of sleep were assessed. Finally, a gasometry analysis was performed during the consultation and the individual at home, during a night with NIV, was submitted to night-time pulse oximetry with a pulse oximeter and transcutaneous nocturnal capnometry, with the respective preparation of a report. After all these procedures, the individuals were removed from NIV for a period of seven nights and at the end of the week were submitted to pulmonary function tests (PFTs) according to the guidelines of the American Thoracic Society and European Respiratory Society, and a polygraph at night in spontaneous breathing. In this phase, individuals with obstructive ventilatory disorder or mild sleep apneas continued their treatment with NIV; the rest were changed to CPAP and adjustments were made such as constant pressure, EPAP 2 cmH2O above the EPAP of the previous NIV to compensate for the absence of IPAP in CPAP. After more than one month with CPAP, the SRI, ESS and PSQI questionnaires were reassessed and the same analysis was performed under the conditions described above. During one night with CPAP at home, the individuals were submitted to night-time oximetry, transcutaneous nocturnal capnometry, mean compliance report, median loss and mean AHI index of the last month spent with CPAP were extracted (Orfanos et al., 2017).

There were no significant differences after the change to CPAP, in mean AHI, diurnal and nocturnal, gas exchange and compliance. The only significant difference was in ESS, which was lower after the change to CPAP. At the end of the study and after a self-administration questionnaire, the effective preference of individuals for a mode of ventilation was determined. Twelve of them (80%) reported preferring CPAP over NIV and wanting to continue treatment with CPAP. Two (13%) did not have any preference and only one wished to discontinue CPAP and return to NIV, although there were no objective criteria for deterioration during treatment with CPAP. In other words, the efficiency in gas exchange, sleep quality and quality of life is maintained once the change has been made. These results, however, need to be confirmed by a larger assessment, which could also assess the clinical consequences of this change in the long term, namely the cardiovascular consequences (Orfanos et al., 2017).

CONCLUSION

Alveolar obesity-hypoventilation syndrome (AOHS) is defined by the presence of chronic alveolar hypoventilation, and therefore chronic hypercapnia (PaCO2 > 45 mmHg) accompanied by equivalent degree of hypoxemia (PaO2 low), in obese individuals (with BMI > 30 Kg/m2), without any other respiratory disease that justifies it. This syndrome is of great importance because of the risk it adds to disease conditions and the poor quality of life of the obese. The differential diagnosis is mainly made with Chronic Obstructive Pulmonary Disease (COPD) and Obstructive Sleep Apnea Syndrome (OSAS).

The therapeutic approach is therefore based on hypoxemia control, sleep and wakefulness. This control is achieved through Continuous Positive Airway Pressure (CPAP) or Non Invasive Ventilation (NIV) with the use of Positive Airway Pressure at two levels (inspiratory and expiratory) (BiPAP, Bilevel Positive Pressure Airway), both applied during the night, during sleep. This last ventilatory mode, BiPAP is indicated whenever the individual maintains sustained hypoxemia after correction of sleep apneas with CPAP. However, the effective treatment of Alveolar Obesity-Hip Ventilation Syndrome also implies an action on obesity and, as such, a real change in lifestyle. Although CPAP is considered the first-line treatment in AOHS, it is certain that NIV increasingly occupies a prominent place, since most individuals besides hypercapnia also have hypoxemia.

However, there is still much to study and find out about this subject. It would be important to carry out studies that included stable and unstable individuals, in order to effectively understand whether or not there are significant differences between the different ventilatory modes in the treatment of AOHS, simultaneously including other variables such as lifestyle counseling, since, although NIV alone improves ventilation, it is not sufficient for all the chronic consequences of AOHS, such as cardiovascular and metabolic parameters.

REFERENCES

Anne, B., Didier, T., Jean-paul, J., Jean-bernard, M., Samir, J., & Philippe, J. (2005). laboratory and animal investigations Performance Characteristics of 10 Home Mechanical Ventilators in. *Chest*, *127*(5), 1784–1792. doi:10.1378/chest.127.5.1784 PMID:15888859

Area, G. L., Janssens, J., Derivaz, S., & Breitenstein, E. (2003). *Changing Patterns in Long-term Noninvasive Ventilation: A 7-Year Prospective Study in the*. doi:10.1378/chest.123.1.67

Bhushan, B., Ayub, B., Thompson, D. M., Abdullah, F., & Billings, K. R. (2016). *Impact of Short Sleep on Metabolic Variables in Obese Children With Obstructive Sleep Apnea*. doi:10.1002/lary.26420

Bobak, M., Bobrova, N., West, R., Malyutina, D., & Malyutina, S. (2010). Gender differences in drinking practices in middle aged and older Russians. *Alcohol and Alcoholism (Oxford, Oxfordshire)*, *45*(6), 573–580. doi:10.1093/alcalc/agq069 PMID:21075855

Borel, J., Tamisier, R., Gonzalez-bermejo, J., Baguet, J., Pharmd, D. M., Arnol, N., ... Pépin, J. (2012). Noninvasive Ventilation in Mild Obesity. *Chest*, *141*(3), 692–702. doi:10.1378/chest.10-2531 PMID:21885724

Cavalleri, M. A., Barbagelata, E., Scudeletti, M., & Nicolini, A. (2018). Effectiveness of non-invasive ventilation in acute respiratory failure of obese patients: A brief narrative review. *Italian Journal of Medicine*, *12*(1), 5–9. doi:10.4081/itjm.2018.916

Darío, I., & Andrés, E. (2017). *Tratamiento médico-quirúrgico de la obesidad en el síndrome de apnea-hipopnea obstructiva del sueño (SAHOS)*. Academic Press.

De Llano, L. A. P., Golpe, R., Piquer, M. O., Racamonde, A. V., Caruncho, M. V., Muinelos, O. C., & Carra, C. A. (2005). Short-term and long-term effects of nasal intermittent positive pressure ventilation in patients with obesity-hypoventilation syndrome. *Chest*, *128*(2), 587–594. doi:10.1378/chest.128.2.587 PMID:16100142

Donaldson, G. C., Ambrosino, N., Escarabill, J., Farre, R., Fauroux, B., Robert, D., ... Wedzicha, J. A. (2005). *Patterns of home mechanical ventilation use in Europe: results from the Eurovent survey*. doi:10.1183/09031936.05.00066704

Esquinas, A. M. (2011). *Princípios de Ventilação Mecânica Não Invasiva: do Hospital ao Domicílio*. GASINMédica.

Gaio, Antunes, Barreto, Gil, Kislaya, Namorado, Rodrigues, Santos, & Nunes. (2018). Prevalência de excesso de peso e de obesidade em Portugal: resultados do primeiro Inquérito Nacional de Saúde com Exame Físico (INSEF 2015). *Boletim Epidemiológico Observações*, *22*(7), 29–33.

Gastrointestinal surgery for severe obesity. (2018). *National Institutes of Health Consensus Development Conference*.

Jacqueline, S., Espinoza, N., Alexandra, K., Lozano, A., Geovanny, C., & Rivera, A. (n.d.). *S índrome de hipoventilación del obeso : revisión de la literatura*. Academic Press.

Janssens, J., Metzger, M., & Sforza, E. (2009). Impact of volume targeting on efficacy of bi-level non-invasive ventilation and. *Respiratory Medicine*, *103*(2), 165–172. doi:10.1016/j.rmed.2008.03.013 PMID:18579368

Jennum, P., & Kjellberg, J. (2011). *Health, social and economical consequences of sleep-disordered breathing : a controlled national study*. doi:10.1136/thx.2010.143958

Kaw, R., Hernandez, A. V., Walker, E., Aboussouan, L., & Mokhlesi, B. (2009). Determinants of Hypercapnia in Obese Patients With Obstructive Sleep Apnea A Systematic Review and Metaanalysis of Cohort. *Chest*, *136*(3), 787–796. doi:10.1378/chest.09-0615 PMID:19567489

López-Jiménez, M. J., Masa, J. F., Corral, J., Terán, J., Ordaz, E., Troncoso, M. F., ... Cancelo, L. (2016). Mid- and Long-Term Efficacy of Non-Invasive Ventilation in Obesity Hypoventilation Syndrome: The Pickwick's Study. *Archivos de Bronconeumologia*, *52*(3), 158–165. doi:10.1016/j.arbr.2016.01.012 PMID:26656679

Mctigue, K., Larson, J. C., Burke, G., Kotchen, J., Lewis, C. E., & Stefanick, M. L. (2006). Article. *Mortality and Cardiac and Vascular Outcomes in Extremely Obese Women*, *296*(1), 79–86.

Murphy, P. B., Davidson, C., Hind, M. D., Simonds, A., Williams, A. J., Hopkinson, N. S., ... Hart, N. (2012). *Volume targeted versus pressure support non-invasive ventilation in patients with super obesity and chronic respiratory failure : a randomised controlled trial*. doi:10.1136/thoraxjnl-2011-201081

Nowbar, S., Burkart, K. M., Gonzales, R., Fedorowicz, A., Gozansky, W. S., Gaudio, J. C., Taylor, M. R. G., & Zwillich, C. W. (2004). Obesity-Associated hypoventilation in hospitalized patients: Prevalence, effects, and outcome. *The American Journal of Medicine*, *116*(1), 1–7. doi:10.1016/j.amjmed.2003.08.022 PMID:14706658

Ojeda Castillejo, E., de Lucas Ramos, P., López Martin, S., Resano Barrios, P., Rodríguez Rodríguez, P., Morán Caicedo, L., Bellón Cano, J. M., & Rodriguez Gonzalez-Moro, J. M. (2015). Noninvasive Mechanical Ventilation in Patients with Obesity Hypoventilation Syndrome. Long-term Outcome and Prognostic Factors. *Archivos de Bronconeumologia*, *51*(2), 61–68. doi:10.1016/j.arbr.2014.06.016 PMID:24703500

Orfanos, S., Jaffuel, D., Perrin, C., Molinari, N., Chanez, P., & Palot, A. (2017). Switch of noninvasive ventilation (NIV) to continuous positive airway pressure (CPAP) in patients with obesity hypoventilation syndrome: A pilot study. *BMC Pulmonary Medicine*, *17*(1), 1–11. doi:10.118612890-017-0391-9 PMID:28288605

Pıhtılı, A., Bingöl, Z., & Kıyan, E. (2017). *The Predictors of Obesity Hypoventilation Syndrome in Obstructive Sleep Apnea*. doi:10.4274/balkanmedj.2015.1797

Ramírez-Molina, V. R., Gómez-de-Terreros, F. J., Barca-Durán, J., & Masa, J. F. (2017). Non-invasive Positive Airway Pressure in Obesity Hypoventilation Syndrome and Chronic Obstructive Pulmonary Disease: Present and Future Perspectives. *COPD*, *14*(4), 418–428. doi:10.1080/15412555.2017.1317730 PMID:28485989

Schlosshan, D., & Elliott, M. W. (2004). Sleep·3: Clinical presentation and diagnosis of the obstructive sleep apnoea hypopnoea syndrome. *Thorax*, *59*(4), 347–352. doi:10.1136/thx.2003.007179 PMID:15047962

Silva, G. A. (2006). *Obesidade-Hipoventilação Alveolar*. Ribeirão Preto: Medicina.

Skidmore, P. M. L., & Yarnell, J. W. G. (2004). *Commentary The obesity epidemic : prospects for prevention*. doi:10.1093/qjmed/hch136

Strumpf, D. A., Millman, R. P., Carlisle, C. C., Grattan, L. M., Ryan, S. M., Erickson, A. D., & Hill, N. S. (1991). *Nocturnal Positive-Pressure Ventilation via Nasal Mask in Patients with Severe Chronic Obstructive Pulmonary Disease*. Academic Press.

Sturm, R. Ã. (2007). *Increases in morbid obesity in the USA*. doi:10.1016/j.puhe.2007.01.006

Sugerman, H. J., Baron, P. L., Fairman, R. P., & Evans, C. R. (1987). *Hemodynamic Dysfunction in Obesity Hypoventilation Syndrome and the Effiects of Treatment with Surgically Induced Weight Loss*. Academic Press.

Sullivan, C. E., & Ph, D. (n.d.). *Effects of Short-term NIPPY in the Treatment of Patients With Severe Obstructive Sleep Apnea and Hypercapnia.* doi:10.1378/chest.105.2.434

ENDNOTE

1 The prevalence of overweight and obesity is based on the calculation of the Body Mass Index (BMI), with a BMI of 25 or more and less than 30 kg/m2 being considered as an indicator of overweight and a BMI of 30 kg/m2 or more as an indicator of obesity.

Section 3

Coadjuvants of Non-Invasive Ventilation

Chapter 9
Ambulatory Oxygen Therapy From Narrative-Based Medicine:
The Importance of Patient Experience in Care Plans

Carmen Cipriano-Crespo
University of Castilla-La Mancha, Spain

David Conde-Caballero
https://orcid.org/0000-0002-5967-4371
University of Extremadura, Spain

Pablo Sánchez-García
University of Extremadura, Spain

Lorenzo Mariano-Juárez
University of Extremadura, Spain

ABSTRACT

Oxygen therapy consists on administering oxygen at a higher concentration than that found in the air in order to treat problems due to respiratory failure. When the oxygen therapy treatment is not necessary to administer in the hospital, within a hospital admission, it can be prescribed for the patient to receive at home, referred to as continuous home oxygen therapy. This type of therapy has great advantages for patients and their families because it allows them to stay together longer. But there are also important difficulties to be taken into account that have to do with the handling of the devices that are used for the administration of oxygen, as well as the compliance or not of the time prescribed by the health professional.

DOI: 10.4018/978-1-7998-3531-8.ch009

Copyright © 2020, IGI Global. Copying or distributing in print or electronic forms without written permission of IGI Global is prohibited.

INTRODUCTION: AMBULATORY OXYGEN THERAPY: CONCEPTS, USES AND INDICATIONS

Oxygen therapy is a therapeutic technique that allows the controlled administration of oxygen at high concentrations (Ortega *et al.*, 2014). Since its introduction in the 1960s (De la campa, 2014), it has been routinely used in the treatment of, among others, Chronic Obstructive Pulmonary Disease (COPD)[1], a condition that is one of the most common causes of hospital admission (Masclans, Pérez-Terán & Roca, 2015). In addition, it has also been used in many other situations where ventilation/perfusion is compromised, such as left heart failure, diffuse interstitial lung disease, pulmonary hypertension, and dyspnea secondary to neoplastic disease, hepato-pulmonary syndrome or patients with exclusive hypoxemia during physical activity, among others. (Codinardo *et al.*, 2016). The goal is always to treat and/or prevent the manifestations of hipoxia[2], and thereby reduce respiratory and myocardial work, while increasing tolerance to exercise and Activities of Daily Living (ADL) (Salcedo *et al.*, 2001).

Although the use is to a greater extent in the hospital, it can also be prescribed in the patient's own home on an outpatient basis, especially in a supplementary manner when the person in question is unable to perform normal physical exercise and/or daily activities (Bradley & O'Neill, 2007), something known as Continuous Home Oxygen Therapy (OCD) (González-Moro, Navarrete, Michavila & Lobato, 2016). The scientific literature has described, in detail, the benefits for people who use oxygen therapy at home. The time spent in the hospital is less, the social and family disadvantages of being in an institution for so long are less when staying in their natural environment surrounded by their people at any time, without the obligations and schedules that the institution establishes for the patient and his/her companions. All of these factors clearly improve the quality of life of the patient and his/her loved ones. In this sense, the Spanish Society of Pneumology and Thoracic Surgery (SEPAR) establishes a series of indications that are necessary to be able to establish the oxygen therapy in the home, such as obtaining a stabilized situation for the patient, to receive the correct medical treatment, to give up the habit of smoking, and of course, to have the patient's willingness to collaborate (SEPAR,2014).

When the time comes to start using OCD, the patient is forced to completely change his/her life habits, especially when it is often necessary that the therapy be applied at least 15 hours a day, including the hours of sleep, following the evidence provided by classical studies such as the Nocturnal Oxygen Therapy Trial or the British Medical Research Council, which demonstrated increased survival in patients with oxygen therapy, a survival that was greater the more hours of oxygen they received (Party, 1981; NOTT, 1980). A fact with which health professionals are often inflexible (Alonso & Sobradillo, 2004), forcing the person to spend a good part of the day at home or, in some cases, to use some kind of portable device[3] which the patient must carry if he/she intends to go outdoors (Ruiz *et al.*, 2014).

Beyond the impact in the field of physiology, the irruption of disease and treatment in the body, this work seeks to study the impact it has on life, identity, the patient's self and even relatives. Illness and outpatient treatment also lead to a complex universe of meanings determined by their new way of living, which the oxygen therapy patient faces on a daily basis. In spite of the obviousness of this statement, most of the approaches that science has made to these experiences have been carried out from the biological paradigms that prevail in *Evidence-Based Medicine* (EBM). These approaches tend to underestimate the importance of experiential worlds that connect patients with their own feelings about what they are experiencing and the way everything has changed in their own existence, sometimes conceptualizing them as "side effects" over which the clinician can do little. As a result, today the most that a healthcare professional who wishes to improve a patient's care plans through scientific literature can choose is to consult research that has been mainly concerned with analysing aspects such as the improvement in oxygen saturation levels, the quantification of changes that occur in dyspnoea processes or the physiopathology of pulmonary hypertension, among others. To cite just a few recent examples in this regard, Branson described, in 2018, the physiological impact of oxygen therapy and the use of oxygen during the exacerbation of symptoms, while Zappia *et al.* spoke, in 2013, of the advantages of using this type of therapy in pediatric patients in order to reduce healthcare costs, something they spun through the fact that it involves improving the physical health of patients as measured by increasing levels of oxygen saturation. However, these studies do not pretend to know how people who require oxygen therapy live and to analyze the type of important modifications that occur in their personal and family life.

A very dense line of biomedical literature, however, has handled these approaches from the works that conceptualize and evaluate "quality of life". This concept is defined in biomedical research as "a desired state of personal well-being that is multidimensional, and that is experienced when a person's needs are met and there is opportunity for improvement in the most important life areas" (Verdugo *et al.*, 2012). It is also defined by Ardila in 2013 as "a state of general satisfaction, derived from the realisation of the person's potentialities. It has subjective and objective aspects. It is a subjective sensation of physical, psychological and social well-being. It includes, as subjective aspects, intimacy, emotional expression, perceived security, personal productivity and objective health. Objective aspects include material well-being, harmonious relations with the physical and social environment and with the community, and objectively perceived health".

In a study by Collado *et al.* (2017) COPD patients have a lower "quality of life" due to the symptoms they have from the disease, as well as reduced ability to perform activities of daily living and the medications they take.

In most cases, these are attempts to quantify areas of much denser and more complex significance, blurring much richer intersubjective spaces. In a certain way, concepts or categories such as mobility, identity, mental health, perspectives on the future... try to be collected in the most usual questionnaires. For example, the GENCAT scale that evaluates the "quality of life" of adult users in an objective way (Verdugo *et al.,* 2007). As does the FUMAT scale, an objective evaluation of the "quality of life" of users of social services, which evaluates emotional, physical and material well-being, interpersonal relations, social inclusion, personal development, self-determination and people's rights (Gómez *et al,* 2008). However, these attempts to turn the worlds of meaning into scales and numbers always involve losses.

BACKGROUND: A DIFFERENT PROPOSAL. THE NARRATIVE BASED MEDICINE

The personal and subjective world of people who receive oxygen therapy in their own homes, which means getting sick and the patient's experience itself, has therefore been, in function of the underlined, cornered in the concerns of medical science. A fact that undoubtedly distances us from the possibility of creating holistic care plans and therefore quality, by reducing more and more the interest and contributions that come from the experience of the afflicted and the narrative that carries.

Faced with this, what we have proposed, in our research, has been just the opposite, having been interested in approaching just those experiences of patients from the possibilities offered by the approach of *Narrative Based Medicine* (NBM). This is a paradigm that emerged in the mid-1990s around a reconsideration of what was excluded from positivism (Evans & Sweeney, 1998) and is based on an attempt to improve that oligopoly of quantitative approaches in which clinical trials usually prevail over the subject's own experience (Mariano Juárez, Rodríguez Martín & Conde, 2013; Greenhalgh & Hurwitz, 1999). The aim is to rescue the narrative by shortening the distance between "knowing" about the disease and "understanding" the experience (Greenhalgh & Hurwitz, 1998; Charón, 2001; 2002; 2006), in order to offer each person what they really need at each moment. In contrast to the predominance of clinical observation of the *Evidence-Based Medicine* (EBM) model, active listening by the clinician is proposed here; in contrast to the centrality of the physical sign, the importance of the subjective symptom; in contrast to the merely biological, the significant world of biography (Greenhalgh & Hurwitz, 1998). What interests us in this paradigm, is the phenomenological way in which the patient perceives his/her health and his/her illness (Márquez Romero, 2010), something that professionals can only approach through a narrative (Gefael, 2009)[4] which makes it possible, in the words of Cano (2013) or Kleinman (1998), on the one hand, to give meaning to the experience of suffering in a way that is outside the domain of the voice of biomedicine (Hydén, 1997), and on the other, to allow the patient to create his/her own self-referential explanatory model with a logical-temporal order that allows him/her to resignify his/her life (p.368).

Along with all this, also under the focus of Narrative Based Medicine (NBM) arises the possibility of its use as a therapeutic tool, since according to Cortés, Uribe and Vásquez (2005). "Narratives by themselves are therapeutic, since the fact of telling the story allows the patient to free him/herself from them, to exteriorize it, which generates a vision of him/herself as someone capable of making choices and making choices in relation to the problems linked to the malaise" (p.190). As Mariano Juárez (2012) affirms, when narrative is understood as an act that allows a person to construct a narrative of what he or she is living, the patient is allowed to show his or her world of experience and affliction, but it also offers professionals who are in contact with him or her individual information about the biography, something that is otherwise difficult to access, avoiding, according to Martínez-Hernáez (2008), possible errors in the medical act derived from the almost systematic disauthorization of the narratives of the sick and the skepticism with which doctors receive such narratives (p.239)[5].

From this approach to care plans, as stated by Mariano Juárez and Cipriano (2013), the accounts of patients' experiences would then be considered as "evidence". The objective would be to build a bridge between clinical studies and the medical art of applying knowledge to an individual case, in such a way that the EBM and the NBM should be understood in complementary terms (Kalitzkus and Matthiessen, 2009), something for which it is essential that this epistemology be incorporated into the curricula of healthcare professionals. In this way, says Rosas Jiménez (2017), future healthcare professionals could acquire, strengthen and explore the narrative capacities they possess, a fact that would undoubtedly be of great help in improving clinical practice in healthcare.

Methodology

Based on these postulates, our research has approached the experience of eight OCD patients from a narrative perspective. It is carried out from this approach because it is considered that knowing the experiences of affected people who receive oxygen treatment at home can improve the relationship between patients and professionals, in addition to being able to help make the person comply more strictly with the treatment.

In the study conducted by Banfi *et al.* (2018) on narrative writing by physicians treating patients who require this type of treatment, it is shown that this reflective writing helps to establish empathetic relationships between physician and patient and will therefore improve the "quality of life" of the patient.

The perception among doctors and patients is sometimes not the same, the asymmetrical relationships that occur between the two, causes patients not to comply as they should with the doctor's prescription on the time and mode of receiving oxygen. In research by Fioretti, *et al.* (2016) the concordance is greater between physicians and patients with more severe COPD compared to those with moderate diseases, something that can be attributed to an increased risk of hospitalization, greater intensity of COPD symptoms, and better doctor-patient communication.

Stories of experiences of patients with domiciliary oxygen therapy have been taken for the accomplishment of this study by means of *YouTube* videos.

Blogs have also been consulted from people who receive this type of therapy for different illnesses that cause respiratory difficulties that are so important that they affect the activities of daily life, in order to know how and in what way they experience everything that happens to them from the obligation to receive oxygen therapy.

It has also been tracked in databases of individual patient experiences of their disease such as *DIPEx*.

The empirical materials on which we have based the research that gave rise to this text have come from ethnographic research (Velasco & Díaz de Rada, 1997; Reeves, Kuper & Hodges, 2008), something that has undoubtedly allowed us to attend to the narratives of each informant to the point of placing them at the very heart of our work. In this way, we have managed, through the stories and in accordance with the NBM, to give a unique value to each individual experience: the uniqueness of each case (Ugarte, 2012). In this sense, we consider it essential to know what it meant for each of these people to spend most of the day connected to a device that at the end of the day is the ballast that separates them from a previous life, but it is also the ballast that unites them with the world and allows them to continue with life. An experience that in our opinion can only be accessed through individualized interviews, enabling the amplification of the verbalization of a wealth of emotions and feelings.

MAIN FOCUS OF THE CHAPTER

"Living Plugged In": Stories as First-Rate Evidence

The empirical evidence from our fieldwork has highlighted the fact that the use of oxygen therapy has a significant impact on the life of the person using it, as well as that of their own family. The obligation to be at home in order to be able to comply with the medical prescription often entails a good number of problems that affect very different levels. Sometimes, the time that the patient can be without oxygen is very little, and therefore is forced to choose the activities he/she can partake in, very well. Work problems then arise, since many have to give up the work they have done until then. Their personal competence is diminished, while their purchasing power is diminished. The personal and social spheres are also affected most of the time. Many times, patients are impelled to change their habits when performing the activities of daily living, so that sitting to shower, shave or brush teeth will be the usual way to do it from the arrival of oxygen therapy. Something as everyday as eating, for example, also becomes a *via crucis*, since sometimes, some devices such as those of the Venturi® type, prevent ingesting anything[6]. Or sleep, since most of the time patients end up sleeping alone, in a separate room, as a result of the discomfort caused by the devices and their functioning: "You sleep with the oxygen bottle and wake up next to it, what I have is not a life," says Albano.

Sometimes even intimacy is lost, as they often require the help of other people to be able to perform any activity of daily life, something that strongly affects their feelings of personal competence (Vinaccia & Quiceno, 2011). Routines are similarly forced to change, and sometimes there is a change of interests for activities they could do before, but not now. They can no longer, for example, engage in intense physical exercise; they can no longer continue their leisure activities [7] … without a doubt, all of this can make it easier, in the words of Rio *et al.* (2007), for people to isolate themselves and decide not to explore new interests, thus building isolated lives in their own homes, confined in their own world of anguish and grief[8].

Manuel, a 65-year-old COPD patient, recounts that he can no longer live without the machine, that everything is "hooked" on it, and explicitly acknowledges, sadly, that "without it he can no longer live". Manuel tells us how from the moment he started the treatment, all his life and that of his family has changed, having to adapt radically to a new situation he had never imagined. At home, he must have oxygen for a large part of the day, and he openly acknowledges that this problem has affected his social relationships, since "I can't stay away from home for long"[9]. A similar story can be found in Albano, a 60-year-old patient with COPD and Pulmonary Emphysema, who counts as the oxygen cylinder that must be used "occupies and weighs a lot", in a way that forces him to spend most of the day confined to his own home.

A new difficulty arises in many patients in relation to the amount of preparations they have to face before going to a particular place outside their usual abodes. The spontaneity for them is over. Now it is not like before, since they must make an exhaustive study of the place where they want to go. The story of Emilio and his wife shows it clearly. He must remain connected to the machine 24 hours a day, at home he has a static device, but he has also recently been prescribed a portable one to be able to go out into the street. Even so, they do not do it as often as they would like, since they are always very aware of where they are going, whether or not there is, for example, an elevator to avoid fatigue. Checking that everything meets the requirements Emilio needs is exhausting, and often leads to feelings of frustration that play against him.

For those who have greater mobility the thing is not much better. Patients who can go out on the street with a portable device often feel the social stigma, the prying eyes of those who don't understand the different ones, something that, in the words of some of our informants, "deeply marks them" and makes them feel ashamed to be looked at as "weird bugs"[10]. Views that often go from being "compassionate" about what a person may be living through, to imagining the discomfort of living like this... to becoming inquisitive, views that all too often allow themselves to make value judgments about why they think patients must carry a machine in order to live, such as tobacco abuse. Gazes, anxieties and fears that contribute to the fact that every day outings to the outside are less frequent, often limited to going to closed places, with people that as they really understand the situation they're going through, where they don't feel judged.

Antonio, also 65 years old and suffering from COPD, reflects on another aspect of no less importance, which is the symbiosis that seems to be generated in this type of treatment between the person and the machine. Those unbreakable anchors that we highlighted earlier:

Being hooked means that the machine is part of your life, and vice versa [...] there is a clear dependence and I have to learn to accept that now it is something obligatory and necessary in my daily life. The machine is a very important part of my life, the most...

Emilio, 55 years old, tells us about the afflictions, the feelings, the generous emotional costs that are generated when one becomes aware that with the arrival of oxygen therapy everything has changed forever: desires, self-esteem... everything, so that on occasion he has come to think that "he is no longer alive":

At first, I had no clear awareness that the disease was so bad, as it progresses it is when you realize you are losing. Your mind is not aware of the reality, of what you are going to live from then on, it is fundamental not to abandon yourself because you feel that desire...

Around all these situations described in many of our informants, there appear to be strong feelings of nostalgia for a world that used to be and no longer is. They constantly compare what was possible before, and it no longer is... and of course, one longs for, one suffers. León, 65 years old, with Pulmonary Emphysema, has been "stuck to the machine" for two years. For him, his greatest wishes are that the past be the future: "I would love to breathe for myself again, as I did before, but I know that it is impossible because this is not cured ...". Emotional losses that increase the barriers that must be overcome, to face daily life. Emilio, for example, talks about how, thanks to the difficulties of his illness and his treatment, he has realized that he has lost the possibility of doing things that he used to do unconsciously:

You know... I used to go for a walk, talk without having to take a breath... I try not to hold on to anything, when you have to lose something, then you lose it and that's it, but it's been hard for me to accept the changes that COPD has caused me. Before, I used to climb two floors in nothing and now maybe it will take me ten minutes. Possibly you become more sensitive to the things you lack than when you were not aware that you had those things and now they are no longer ...

If before we talked about the fear of people's glazes, of what people will say, many other types of fears can also be added to complete an atmosphere that sometimes becomes unbreathable, giving the paradox that what allows breathing, now suffocates. Thus, many of the patients manifest a deep distress caused by the fear of drowning when unable to breathe due to the presence of dyspnea (Costa *et al.*, 2016).

Others talk about the fear they feel when they don't know how to use the different devices that are part of the therapy in the right way[11]. In this sense, it is also common for patients to live with some anguish during the first moments, when many of them feel overwhelmed by the large amount of technical information they must assimilate and with which in many cases they are not accustomed to deal. [12] The way in which they receive information is decisive here, since it depends on whether their anxiety decreases or increases. A point confirmed by a study carried out by Clèries *et al.* (2016), who evidence that the type of information provided by doctors and nurses and how it was transmitted to them is the main reason for concern among new patients undergoing oxygen therapy[13].

CONCLUSION AND PROPOSALS

The narratives of the patients included in this text tell us about the impact of the disease, but above all about the treatment in their lives. They are windows to the "quality of life" they experience, to their losses, in the form of first-person accounts. They are not subjective elements without value, but spaces for the construction of intersubjective experiences that form part of the evidences that Medicine must face. Oxygen therapy used during most of the day substantially modifies their lives, in different ways, affecting the emotional contexts, mental health, and the definitions of person. A world of coexistence with the disease and its physiopathology opens up for them, but also a world of feelings, afflictions and subjectivities. However, while the former are good, collected in protocols, graphs and clinical histories, patients' worlds of experience often go unnoticed, and consequently swell the exclusive privacy reserves, with no possibility of them being incorporated into their own care plans as a result.

What we have tried to demonstrate in this text are the possibilities that the MBN presents in this sense, based on the conviction that the only way to achieve holistic care plans that attend to the physical, psychic, social and spiritual spheres is through the use of the EBM and the NBM in complementary terms, while at the same time we would manage to limit the rates of abandonment of treatment that are so high in this type of patients. It is therefore necessary to take into account the patient's narratives in relation to the treatment, since only by knowing their experiences of the process, will we be able to understand it and thus help and care for them in a situation as complex as the one they have had to live in. Along with the stories, our experience has shown the importance of the ethnographic method to get closer to the daily reality lived by this type of patient, in order to know and better understand the emotional impact of the pathology.

In addition, we are convinced that it is fundamental for the researcher to enter the field or circle in which the informant who uses oxygen therapy lives, that is, in his/her own home, since it is essential to take into account the context in which the patient develops, in order to see how he/she can influence the process that he/she is experiencing. This must be considered in order to be able to develop it in the future.

Through all the empirical materials generated through the survey relationships and participant observation we have described, this research has sought to produce evidence from the necessary reflected reflexivity (Bourdieu, Passeron & Chamboredon, 1968) and the NBM paradigm. A fact that has been particularly necessary in the analysis of some speeches loaded with a special emotiveness and social sense, that will allow us in a not too distant future to know better the universe of afflictions and needs associated to this type of therapeutic reality.

ACKNOWLEDGMENT

This work was supported by the 4IE project (0045-4IE-4-P) funded by the Interreg V-A España-Portugal (POCTEP) 2014-2020 program.

REFERENCES

Allué, M. (2002). *Temporarily valid: an ethnography on the environment of disability* (PhD thesis). Universitat Rovira i Virgili.

Alonso, J., & Sobradillo, V. (2004). Continuous home oxygen therapy: A good treatment if it is done well. *Anales de Medicina Interna (Madrid, Spain)*, *21*, 5–7.

Álvarez-Sala, J., Cimas, E., Masa, J., Miravitlles, M., Molina, J., Naberan, K. . . . of Pneumology, E. (2001). Recommendations for the care of patients with chronic obstructive pulmonary disease. *Bronchopneumology Archives, 37*(7), 269 278.

Ancochea, J., Badiola, C., Duran-Tauleria, E., Rio, F. G., Miravitlles, M., Muñoz, L., ... Soriano, J. (2009). EPI-SCAN study: Summary of the protocol of a study to estimate the prevalence of COPD in people aged 40 to 80 in Spain. *Bronchopneumology Archives*, *45*(1), 41–47. doi:10.1016/j.arbres.2008.06.001

Ardila, R. (2003). Quality of life: An inclusive definition. *Revista Latinoamericana de Psicología*, *35*(2), 161–164.

Banfi, P., Cappuccio, A., Latella, M. E., Reale, L., Muscianisi, E., & Marini, M. G. (2018). Narrative medicine to improve the management and quality of life of patients with COPD: The first experience applying parallel chart in Italy. *International Journal of Chronic Obstructive Pulmonary Disease*, *13*, 287–297. doi:10.2147/COPD.S148685 PMID:29391786

Boticario, C., & Angosto, M. C. (2010). Hypoxia and cancer. *Annals of the Royal National Academy of Pharmacy*, *76*(3).

Bourdieu, P., Passeron, J. C., & Chamboredon, J.-C. (1968). *Le Métier de sociologue*. Mouton, Bordas.

Bradley, J. & O'Neill, B. (2007). Short-term ambulatory oxygen for chronic obstructive pulmonary disease. *Cochrane Library Plus, 4*.

Cano, W. (2013). Evidence and narratives in health care: An anthropological perspective. *The Journal of Pain and the Survival of Illness in Patients with Pain, 11*, 357.

Charon, R. (2001). Narrative medicine: A model for empathy, reflection, profession, and trust. *Journal of the American Medical Association, 286*(15), 1897–1902. doi:10.1001/jama.286.15.1897 PMID:11597295

Charon, R. (2005). Narrative medicine: Attention, representation, affiliation. *Narrative, 13*(3), 261–270. doi:10.1353/nar.2005.0017

Charon, R. (2008). *Narrative medicine: Honoring the stories of illness*. Oxford University Press.

Clèries, X., Solà, M., Chiner, E., & Escarrabill, J. (2016). Approach to the experience of the patient and their caregivers in home oxygen therapy. *Bronchopneumology Archives, 52*(3), 131–137. doi:10.1016/j.arbr.2016.01.005

Codinardo, C., Cáneva, J. O., Montiel, G., Uribe Echevarría, M. E., Lisanti, R., Larrateguy, L., ... Torres, R. (2016). Recommendations on the use of oxygen therapy in special situations. *American Journal of Respiratory Medicine, 16*(2), 150–162.

Collado-Mateo, D., Adsuar, J. C., Olivares, P. R. & García-Gordillo, M. Á. (2017). Health-related quality of life in Chilean patients with chronic obstructive pulmonary disease. *Medical Journal of Chile, 145*(2), 147-155.

Cortés Duque, C., Uribe, C. A., & Vásquez, R. (2005). Clinical ethnography and disease narratives of patients with obsessive-compulsive disorder. *Colombian Journal of Psychiatry, 34*(2).

Costa, X., Gómez-Batiste, X., Pla, M., Martínez-Muñoz, M., Blay, C., & Vila, L. (2016). Living with advanced chronic obstructive pulmonary disease: The impact of dyspnoea on patients and caregivers. *Primary Care, 48*(10), 665–673. PMID:27288085

De la Campa. (2014). Actualización en oxigenoterapia. *Revista de Patología Respiratoria, 17*(1).

Evans, M., & Sweeney, K. (1998). The human side of medicine. *Occasional Paper (Royal College of General Practitioners)*, 76. PMID:9707989

Fioretti, C., Mazzocco, K., Riva, S., Oliveri, S., Masiero, M., & Pravettoni, G. (2016). Research studies on patients' illness experience using the Narrative Medicine approach: A systematic review. *BMJ Open, 6*(7), e011220. doi:10.1136/bmjopen-2016-011220 PMID:27417197

Fontanella, L., Rigon, L. A., Serena, P. & Munarin, F. (2010). Rischio clinico per le persone che utilizzano a domicilio ossigenoterapia e ventilazione meccanica: indagine di prevalenza. *SCENARIO: Official Italian Journal of ANIARTI, 27*(4).

Gefael, C. V. (2009). Patients bleed stories: A narrative approach to decrease clinical misunderstandings. *North Mental Health*, *8*(34), 9.

Gómez, L., Verdugo, M., Arias, B., & Navas, P. (2008). Evaluation of the quality of life in elderly and disabled people: The Fumat Scale. *Intervención Psicosocial*, *17*(2), 189–199.

Greenhalgh, T., & Hurwitz, B. (1998). *Narrative Based Medicine Dialogue and discourse in clinical practice*. PhilPapers.

Kalitzkus, V., & Matthiessen, P. (2009). Narrative-based medicine: Potential, pitfalls, and practice. *The Permanente Journal*, *13*(1), 80. doi:10.7812/TPP/08-043 PMID:21373252

Kleinman, A. (1988). *Suffering, healing and the human condition.* New York: Basic Book Publication.

Mariano Juárez, L. (2012). *Definitions of evidence between signs and words. From Medical Anthropology to Narrative-Based Medicine. In Medicine and narratives. From theory to practice*. Editorial Círculo Rojo.

Mariano Juárez, L., Rodríguez Martín, B., & Conde, D. (2013). Narrative-based care: Redefining the hierarchy of evidence. *Nursing Index*, *22*(1-2), 55–59.

Márquez Romero, M. (2010). From the narratives of madness: I'm not mad! Why am I here? Approach to the narratives of illness in a mental health unit. *Periphery: Journal of Research and Training in Anthropology,* (12).

Masana, L. (2013). Between doctors and anthropologists. Attentive and committed listening to the narrated experience of chronic disease. In Evidence and narratives in health care: an anthropological perspective. Tarragona: Publicacions URV.

Masclans, J., Pérez-Terán, P., & Roca, O. (2015). Role of high flow oxygen therapy in acute respiratory failure. *Intensive Medicine*, *39*(8), 505–515. doi:10.1016/j.medin.2015.05.009 PMID:26429697

NOTT. (1980). Continuous or nocturnal oxygen therapy in hypoxemic chronic obstructive lung disease. *Annals of Internal Medicine*, *93*(3), 391–398. doi:10.7326/0003-4819-93-3-391 PMID:6776858

Ortega, F., Lobato, S. D., Iturri, J. B. G., Rio, F. G., Rous, R. G., Velez, F. M., ... Camarasa, J. T. (2014). Continuous home oxygen therapy. *Archives of Bronchopneumology, 50*(5), 185-200.

Paredes, M. L., De la Cruz, O. A., Aznar, I. C., Carrasco, M. M., de Agüero, M. B. G., Ruiz, E. (2009). Fundamentals of oxygen therapy in acute and chronic situations: indications, methods, controls and follow-up. *Annals of Pediatrics Peneumology.*

Party, M. W. (1981). Long-term domiciliary oxygen therapy in chronic hypoxic cor pulmonale complicating chronic bronchitis. *Lancet, 1*, 681–685. PMID:6110912

Reeves, S., Kuper, A., & Hodges, B. D. (2008). Qualitative research methodologies: Ethnography. *BMJ (Clinical Research Ed.), 337*(3), a1020. doi:10.1136/bmj.a1020 PMID:18687725

Río, F. G., Clau, L. B., Macario, C. C., Celli, B. R., Sanglás, J. E., Mangado, N. G., ... Romero, F. U. (2007). Respiratory pathology and airplane flights. *Bronchopneumology Archives, 43*(2), 101–125.

Rosas Jiménez, C. A. (2017). Narrative medicine: The patient as "text", object and subject of compassion. *Bioethical Act, 23*(2), 351–359.

Ruiz, F. O., Lobato, S. D., Iturri, J. B. G., Rio, F. G., Rous, R. G., Velez, F. M., . . . Camarasa, J. T. (2014). Continuous home oxygen therapy. *Archives of Bronchopneumology, 50*(5), 185-200.

Salcedo Posadas, A., Neira Rodrıguez, M., Beltrán Bengoechea, B., Albi Rodrıguez, S., & Sequeiros González, A. O. (2001). *Diagnostic and therapeutic protocols at pediatrıa.* Spanish Association of Pediatrıa.

Ugarte, I. (2012). Narrative evidence and quality of care in the National Health System. In *Medicine and Narratives. From theory to practice*. Editorial Círculo Rojo.

Velasco, H., & Díaz de Rada, A. (1997). *The logic of Ethnographic Research.* Trotta.

Verdugo, M. A., Canal, R., Jenaro, M. C., Badía, M., & Aguado-Díaz, A. L. (2012). *Application of the paradigm quality of life to the intervention with people with disabilities from a holistic perspective.* INICO.

Verdugo, M. A., Gómez, L., & Arias, B. (2007). The integral scale of quality of life: Development and preliminary study of its psychometric properties. *Zero Century, 38*(4), 37–56.

Villaescusa, C., Pinares, M., & Pieras, E. (2014). *Oxygen management systems. SEPAR procedures manual.* Oxygen Therapy Systems.

Vinaccia, S. & Quiceno, J. M. (2011). Health-related quality of life and psychological factors: a study from chronic obstructive pulmonary disease-EPOC. *Psychological Therapy, 29*(1), 65-75.

Zappia, T., Peter, S., Hall, G., Vine, J., Martin, A., Munns, A., Shields, L., & Verheggenn, M. (2013). Home oxygen therapy for infants and young children with acute bronchiolitis and other lower respiratory tract infections: The HiTHOx program. *Issues in Comprehensive Pediatric Nursing*, *36*(4), 309–318. doi:10.3109/01460862.2013.834397 PMID:24083944

KEY TERMS AND DEFINITIONS

Ambulatory: That which does not require the patient to be admitted to a hospital.

Complementarity: Set of characteristics that make one thing complement another.

Narrative-Based Medicine: The NBM proposes a redefinition of the *ethos* of medical practice by placing the patient's experience as first-order evidence.

Oxygen-Therapy: Medical treatment of certain diseases based on the application of oxygen inhalations.

Quality Of Life: Is a concept that alludes to various levels of generalization through society, community, to the physical and mental aspect, therefore, the meaning of quality of life is a complex and with definitions from sociology, political science, medicine, development studies, etc.

Impact: Impression or intense effect produced in a person by an action or event.

ENDNOTES

1 COPD is a permanent and progressive disorder characterised by decreased airway flow, which may be partially reversible and may improve somewhat with treatment (Álvarez-Sala *et al.*, 2001). Smoking is associated with the main cause of the disease. COPD has a very high prevalence in Spain, specifically 10.2% of the population (15.1% in men and 5.7% in women) between 40 and 80 years of age. The estimate of deaths in our country from this disease is more than 18,000 people a year, becoming the third cause of death (Ancochea *et al.*, 2009).

2 We speak of hypoxia when we refer to the state of deficiency of oxygen in the blood, cells and tissues of the organism, with possible compromise of their function (Boticario & Angosto, 2010).

3 In the market it is possible to find several portable sources: those of continuous flow and of flow on demand. In addition, depending on the volume of gas to be supplied there are two types of devices, high and low flow (Masclans *et al.*,

2015). Regardless of the way it is administered, the goal is always the same, to improve the patient's hypoxia situation.

4 A positioning that undoubtedly demands a redefinition of the doctor/patient relationships prevailing in contemporary biomedical systems, since, as Ugarte (2012) states, what really happens is that the patient is seen as someone who simply benefits but is not seen as a person with sufficient capacity to take charge of his or her health, illness and/or rehabilitation process. A clear example of this is lived in daily medical consultations. The professional in a white coat, sitting behind the table, writes without often raising his gaze from the keyboard, emitting a judgment based on a series of questions that have to do with symptoms only, without even being attentive to the tone of voice in which this is narrated. The judgment is not only clinical, sometimes they also question the personal characteristics of the patient who narrates, and writes in the medical history terms such as, "perfectionist", "anxious", "fearful", which will end up stigmatizing them even more in every contact I have with healthcare professionals.

5 This doctor's deauthorization of patients is common in clinical practice. The following is an example of this, narrated by Allué (2002): At a conference of intensive care physicians and nurses who were invited years ago to tell about their experience in the Intensive Care Unit, a physician refuted his arguments about suffering and treatment on the grounds that the patient's perception in such circumstances can never be objective and, therefore, was not meaningful. She still thinks, and this was made known to her at the time, that she disavowed her only because he was a doctor and she was one of the many patients who passed through this unit at a specific time.

6 A situation that is solved, in the words of Paredes *et al.* (2009), by using adapted oxygen cannulae in meals.

7 For example, most patients who receive ambulatory oxygen therapy are discouraged from flying because of the risks of pressure in the airplane and because of the hypoxia problems that occur normally in the rest of the passengers, something that increases even more in those with respiratory failure.

8 For example, patients who live on a fourth floor without an elevator must exert a great deal of physical effort that leads to a great deal of respiratory fatigue that they cannot withstand. Therefore, they end up restricting considerably their exits to the outside, and with it they reduce their social relations. But not only theirs, but they also indirectly produce a decrease in the relationships of their relatives, since, in most cases, they do not want to go out and leave them alone at home.

9 And not only the presence of the "machine" influences. The dyspnea that accompanies respiratory pathologies, for example, is also a reason for a decrease in social relations (Costa *et al.*, 2016). Thus, breathing problems cause significant difficulties in speaking, so that patients who suffer from it need to make many stops in the thread of a conversation making it difficult, and making other talkers lose interest in what they say or get tired of the conversation. A fact that can provocate, in some cases, avoidance of the person to whom this happens, something that they perceive clearly and, consequently, they stop participating more and more in gatherings and group meetings.

10 A study by Lynes, O'Brien & Shaw (2018) explores the perception of a group of patients receiving oxygen therapy, finding that in many cases people felt shame and stigma, which limited their lifestyles and eventually affected their body image.

11 To a certain extent this is a fear not without a certain basis, since it is true that there is risk when using the devices. Studies such as that of Fontanella, Rigon, Serena and Munarin, (2010), for example, have provided evidence on the dangers that can involve the use of oxygen therapy at home.

12 In this sense, in order for people to obtain success in the use of oxygen therapy, it is essential, according to González-Moro et al. (2016), a great coordination at the time of giving the correct information on the part of the doctor and/or nurse and the commercial house in charge of the supply.

13 On many occasions, although the way in which health education has been done has been the right way, other fears may appear. For example, the points of support of the masks, the nasal glasses, etc...can cause discomfort and even ulcers in the person, for which the prevention by means of cushions and/or pressure changes is important (Villaescusa, Pinares & Pieras, 2014). The appearance of these discomforts may lead to rejection of this type of treatment or failure to comply adequately with the prescription.

Chapter 10
Outpatient Oxygen Therapy, Illness Experience, and Mental Health:
Contributions in the Occupational Area

Pablo Sánchez-García
University of Extremadura, Spain

David Conde-Caballero
https://orcid.org/0000-0002-5967-4371
University of Extremadura, Spain

Carmen Cipriano-Crespo
https://orcid.org/0000-0002-0584-8030
University of Castilla-La Mancha, Spain

Lorenzo Mariano-Juárez
University of Extremadura, Spain

ABSTRACT

This chapter is a literary review based on the experience of patients with ambulatory oxygen therapy treatment that analysed the way in which this treatment influences patients from an occupational point of view. The relationship of these pathologies and treatments with mental health, especially with depression, anxiety, and stress, is also addressed, with an interest in the treatment of possible functional limitations from the intervention of the discipline of occupational therapy. Oxygen therapy allows patients to continue in their performance contexts, although it can generate new limitations and deficiencies derived from episodes of anxiety and mood disorders, causing greater occupational disfunction. A function-dysfunction process that can be approached from occupational therapy with the aim of minimizing the impact both physical and psychological, enhancing the autonomy and independence of these patients.

DOI: 10.4018/978-1-7998-3531-8.ch010

Copyright © 2020, IGI Global. Copying or distributing in print or electronic forms without written permission of IGI Global is prohibited.

INTRODUCTION

Oxygen-Therapy is considered one of the most relevant and important therapeutic instruments for patients with chronic respiratory diseases (Ortega *et al.*, 2014). It has been nearly 240 years since Chaussier first used oxygen on patients with dysnea and cyanotic newborns. History advances through several milestones: in 1887 Dr. Holzapple used it to treat a young man suffering from pneumonia, generating oxygen from potassium chlorate and manganese dioxide. At the end of the nineteenth century was discovered the process to produce liquid air by compression and cooling, being able to isolate oxygen by fractional distillation of liquid air. During the 20th century, beneficial effects were demonstrated for some of the most common consequences of respiratory diseases (reduction of polycythemia, reduction in the number and days of hospitalization...). In the eighties of the last century, the selection criteria basis of patients who would benefit from the use of continuous home oxygen therapy was established (Ortega *et al.*, 2014).

Oxygen-Therapy is defined as the beneficial use of oxygen for therapeutic purposes (Jarillo, 2004). It is considered a specific intervention for the treatment of acute and chronic respiratory failure caused by different respiratory diseases (Paredes, Cruz & Aznar, 2009). This therapeutic use of oxygen consists of administering it in concentrations higher than the environmental ones, in order to treat or prevent complications resulting from hypoxia (López Riolobos *et al.*, 2014). In acute hypoxemia its use is unquestionable as in chronic (Neves & Lobão, 2012). Hypoxemia is defined as the lowering of oxygen blood pressure as well as the deficit of hemoglobin saturation in arterial blood. It is also considered as the lack of tissue oxygen (Jarillo, 2004). Many other sources consider oxygen therapy as the most recommended treatment in ventilation/perfusion deficit (Rodríguez Ibagué *et al.*, 2008).

The use of oxygen, once linked to technological innovation and use in professionalized spaces, is now also used in family home environments. The so-called ambulatory Oxygen-Therapy changes the traditional sense of movement, being the treatment and not the person who moves: this therapeutic practice is incorporated into the daily life of people with chronic respiratory pathologies that require oxygen treatment. This implies a series of advantages, but also drawbacks that must be taken into account. Ambulatory Oxygen-Therapy is considered an effective treatment in people with severe respiratory failure due to the results it offers in improving the quality of life of these people and reducing mortality in this type of patient (Olmedo & Sierra, 2004). As we pointed out above, this therapeutic proposal has been applied since the beginning of the 20th century; however, it was in the 1980s that the papers that established the basis for the criteria for selecting patients who would benefit from continuous administration of supplemental oxygen were published, based on two controlled clinical studies in patients with chronic obstructive pulmonary disease. This ambulatory Oxygen-Therapy is characterized by the fact that it allows the patient to receive supplemental oxygen during exercise and activities of daily living (Codinardo *et al.*,2018). This treatment aims to facilitate and enhance the functionality of the patient in their day to day, whether in the family, work, school, etc. to improve their quality of life (Díaz Lobato, García González, & Mayoralas, 2015). The relationship of Oxygen-Therapy with quality of life is a central issue in the available literature, highlighting the following elements that impact the maintenance or recovery of certain levels.

BACKGROUND

The use and indications of ambulatory Oxygen-Therapy differ according to the pathologies to be treated. Among respiratory pathologies, it stands out mainly in Chronic Obstructive Pulmonary Disease (COPD), where Oxygen-Therapy is considered fundamental in its treatment. Oxygen-Therapy is also used in cardiovascular alterations and disorders of the nervous system that interfere with respiratory function: tachycardia, Cor Pulmonale, arterial hypotension, alteration of the state of consciousness, alteration of the pulmonary function, hypoventilation by depression of the Central Nervous System (CNS), toxicity by drugs, etc. Regarding other respiratory alterations like asthma, atelectasis, cardiogenic pulmonary edema, pulmonary thrombus embolism, adult respiratory distress syndrome, pulmonary fibrosis… are worth to be mentioned (Rodríguez Ibagué *et al.*, 2008).

Chronic Obstructive Pulmonary Disease (COPD) is characterized by a specific symptomatology in which persistent respiratory signs and chronic limitation to airflow, caused by alterations in the airway, produced by significant exposure to harmful elements, among which tobacco smoke stands out as the main risk factor. COPD is a major health problem due to its high prevalence worldwide. It entails a significant economic cost, including the direct costs of hospitalization and other health care. It also includes indirect costs due to sick leave of patients or even family members who must remain for care (López & Cob, 2018). European data from recent years show a prevalence between 2.1% and 26.1%, varying from country to country. In Spain, it is estimated that 10% of the population between the ages of 40 and 80 suffers from this disease. The Madrid Community's 2013/2017 COPD Strategic Plan estimates around 300,000 patients diagnosed with COPD. Spain originates between 10%-12% of Primary Care consultations, 35-40% of pneumology consultations, and 7% in terms of hospital admissions. It causes an annual expense of 3,000 million euros just in treatments to the Spanish Government. (*Consejería de Sanidad de Madrid*, 2013). Mortality data tends to account for 6% of deaths worldwide. According to the latest study of the global burden of disease carried out in 2015, it is estimated to be the fifth cause of premature death in the country (*Sociedad Española de Neumología y Cirugía torácica*, 2018).

COPD can be understood as a broader disorder and not just a disease of the respiratory system. It is associated with other chronic diseases, comorbidities such as high blood pressure, left ventricular failure, ischaemic heart disease and arrhythmias (Gabriel *et al.*, 2014). It is a disease with a high morbidity and mortality which is a public health problem of great magnitude. The main symptoms are breathlessness, coughing and expectoration. Its clinical presentation is very heterogeneous (Miravitlles, *et al.*, 2017a).

On patients with COPD, the aim is to reduce symptoms, minimise severity, control the disease, reduce risk and improve the prognosis of the disease. For this, treatment is essential: vaccination, bronchodilators, corticosteroids, mucolytics, antibiotics and ambulatory oxygen therapy. (Cueva Chenche, 2018). The long-term effectiveness of home oxygen therapy has been widely documented (López & Cob, 2018). The benefits are: decrease in mortality and reduction of pulmonary arterial hypertension, polyglobulia, nocturnal arrhythmias, dyspnea and neuropsychiatric symptoms (Hernández Hernández, 2016).

To indicate and prescribe ambulatory Oxygen-Therapy, a series of aspects must be taken into account depending on the particularities of each patient (Ortega *et al.*, 2014). It should be founded on data obtained by arterial blood gases in a stable patient receiving optimal pharmacological treatment. On certain occasions, a provisional indication can be made after a respiratory exacerbation. Oxygen-Therapy is dispensed through different sources that must be taken into account in the impact they may have on the daily activity of patients in their contexts (Martínez Muñiz *et al.*, 2017). Some examples are:

- High pressure cylinders are economical but complicated to handle and require continuous spare parts.
- An oxygen concentrator is more manageable and displaceable but requires electricity and is noisy.
- Liquid oxygen allows wandering, but is economically expensive.

As far as equipment is concerned, nasal goggles are usually used which offer comfort, allow eating, communication and expectoration and are quite stable during the state of sleep. They provide a variable concentration of oxygen. The effect of Oxygen-Therapy depends on the hours of use. No benefits have been demonstrated with less than 12 hours a day, for which a minimum duration of 15-18 hours is recommended, which should include hours of sleep (Hernández Hernández, 2016).

The impact of different respiratory pathologies as well as the prescription and use of Oxygen-Therapy in the daily work of these patients and their families make their lives very limited functionally. It is already complicated to accept and live with a constraining pathology, but even more complicated is to bear the use of Oxygen-Therapy for a large number of hours daily. It has been pointed out on numerous occasions how the disease is an event that floods people's lives, sometimes altering the patient's world until it completely collapses. Disease is something that occurs not in the body, but in the world of the patient (Cedano, 2013). This sort of pathology is a good example of this metaphor, to which is added the process of invasion and demolition implied by the therapeutic proposal: it is as beneficial as it is hoarding the times, the spaces and the movements of the patients. Both factors -disease and treatment- mean that these people's day-to-day life lacks occupational functionality (Martínez Muñiz *et al.*, 2017). It may be noted that one of the major limitations suffered by these people is the loss of mobility:

Modern Oxygen-Therapy requires an assessment of the patient's mobility profile, the mobility allowed by the available oxygen sources, the appropriate selection of patient and oxygen source. The search for the ideal oxygen equipment, to improve the regulation and information systems of therapies, to advance in the education of patients and to promote research.

On the other hand, the characteristics of the therapeutic context, the irruption in the life of the patients may imply a series of impacts in the psychological sphere and the mental health that influence the mood, appearing other underlying complications such as anxiety, stress and depression. As usual, we must remember that the irruption of disease in life implies that it affects not only the body, but also social and family relations, the life built: it has repercussions not only on patients but also on their main carers, spouses and children fundamentally. In the words of López & Cob (2018):

The costs from the clinical and psychological point of view start from its main symptom, dyspnea. This symptom is present from the early stages of the disease and is aggravated as the disease progresses, making difficult speech, wandering and necessitating the use of portable oxygen delivery devices in advanced stages. All this has a series of psychosocial effects that gradually appear as the disease progresses, generating behaviors of self-isolation, self-marginalization and avoidance of social contacts, as well as feelings of shame, anger and disappointment that increase the psychological impact and influence a negative view of life in general. The repercussions in health if an adequate treatment or necessary self-care is not carried out are reflected in a significant worsening, an increase in the number of hospital admissions, the acceleration of the progress of the disease and the decrease in the quality of life of the person who suffers it and his or her environment.

In short, we can understand that Oxygen-Therapy is vital for these patients, they need to integrate it into their daily lives to survive, but it is paradoxical that in turn limits the occupational functionality of these people. It would be unfair to blame only Oxygen-Therapy since the pathological respiratory process itself is a large part of that limitation of functional capabilities. Oxygen-Therapy makes it easier to continue living, but its impact is significant from the point of view of the personal autonomy and independence of these people. The emotional world is altered, with an impact on evaluation processes, contributing to stigmatization, feelings of shame or depression (Martinez Rivera *et al.*, 2016). Thus, there is a double need for attention on the part of medical professionals: they need to attend to the person suffering from the disease as well as the impact of the therapeutic proposal of ambulatory Oxygen-Therapy. Let us enter the world of experience of those who live with the feeling that the air is not enough. Knowing the reality of the patient and those around him, is the beginning to find the most appropriate solutions (Dueñas-Espín *et al.*, 2016).

LIVING WHEN THERE'S NO AIR: IMPACT ON MENTAL HEALTH

The functional impact on the lives of patients suffering from respiratory diseases is substantial, especially in terms of quality of life. The category "Quality of Life" is proposed in the biomedical literature to address a set of subjective experiences. Generally speaking, "Quality of Life" refers to the set of conditions that contribute to making life pleasant and valuable or to the degree of happiness or satisfaction enjoyed by an individual, especially in relation to health and its domains" (Antonio, Fernández-Fidalgo, & Cieza, 2010). "Quality of Life" has been defined as a popular term that expresses a global sense of well-being, including aspects of happiness and satisfaction with life as a whole. (Fernández Mayoralas & Rojo Pérez, 2005). WHO (World Health Organization) defines "Quality of Life" as "individual's perception of their position in lifein the context of the culture and value systems in which they live and in relation to their goals, expectations, standards and concerns". It is a concept that is influenced by the physical health of the subject, his psychological state, his level of independence, his social relations, as well as the relationship with his environment (Huerta *et al.*, 2017). Despite referring to intersubjective spaces, "Quality of Life" has been measured in positivist terms through different scales and questionnaires: GENCAT, QLS, WHOQOL, WHOQOL-BREF, SEIQoL-DW, FUMAT, The Quality of Life scale of Sharlock & Keith, EuroQol-5D; European Quality of Life-5 Dimensions, etc. (Leland *et al.*, 2017).

The impact on "Quality of Life" derives mainly from dyspnea, the most limiting symptom that appears at the onset of the disease and is progressively aggravated. (Escarrabill, 2003). It causes problems in speech and walking, causing psychosocial limitations of self-isolation and avoidance of social contacts, as well as feelings of shame, anger or disappointment (Balbo, Acosta, & Kevorkof, 2012). Dyspnea becomes a symptom of difficult control, without an "effective" treatment, only palliated by Oxygen-Therapy and the administration of different drugs (Costa *et al.*, 2016).

We can trace this impact in the stories of the patients that show a shortening of the social life spaces, but also speak of impacts in intimate areas, such as sexual relations, the construction of the couple's affections or with family members (Gabriel *et al.*, 2014). In these narratives one can appreciate feelings of hopelessness, fear, helplessness, undervaluation, anger, indignation, feeling of slavery and humiliation. (Muñoz-Cobos *et al.*, 2015):

One day she said she would send everything to hell, but it's normal goes with a cable (note: the oxygen tube). I also see it... is as if it was always with a chain... she feels very attached to this machine. As if she were humiliated [...] I can't wash, I need her (his wife). Now, to shave, I do it myself. I usually do the dressing myself, but according to what, for example, if I have to bend down, then she helps me. Now she's almost taken it as a rule to help me all the time. When I get up she is always there. As a rule almost always...

Concern and suffering are sensations that invade these patients and their closest relatives (Muñoz-Cobos *et al.*, 2015):

What worries me is that there will come a time when he will be completely dependent and that he will become aware of this dependency. This is what most... because he will suffer.

Isolation and stigma are also clear exponents of the terrible consequences of this disease in everyday life (Muñoz-Cobos *et al.*, 2015):

No, I don't like going out on the street in places. I know a lot of people. And I don't like it because I have to talk to everyone, give explanations to everyone...

And as a consequence, the avoidance appears when faced with habitual situations in their daily life (Muñoz-Cobos *et al.*, 2015):

I am not one of those who go to mass every week but when I can I do go. Now I've also given up a lot because of the machine. I'm embarrassed to go to mass and have to carry oxygen. They are my hobbies, because people have to do without what others do...

The impact of the disease also carries risks for mental health: mood disorders, anxiety disorders and stress are the main exponents, with all the consequences that lie of these mental disorders (Rosalía,2016):

What affects me the most is the part about anxiety... I get nervous, I'm constantly buzzing my mind. It's very difficult for others to see how you are for everyday life... I'm getting afraid to go out into the street... the clash you have with society... friends don't understand that you're pushing yourself away... that impotence you feel, that anxiety that you'd want to do things but you can't... I'm getting kind of autistic or very weird, but let's just say I'm fine on my own...

So now it is necessary to add new limiting problems referred by psychiatric pathology in many cases misdiagnosed (Montserrat-Capdevila *et al.*, 2018). Even different studies show how anxiety itself directly influences the COPD clinic (Miravitlles *et al.*, 2017b) and "Quality of Life". Anxiety and depression are commonly found together in patients with COPD (Rubio *et al.*, 2009) and also in patients with other diseases that require Oxygen-Therapy as a treatment. These pathologies interfere daily with their social relationships, leisure activities, work, sleep, etc. The emotional changes experienced by these people often lead to a substantial decrease in professional activities and leisure possibilities, with the consequent repercussion on the personal sphere and on the family itself (Miravitlles *et al.*, 2017b). These circumstances substantially limit the performance of their Daily Living Activities. In addition, they have an important impact on the course of the disease itself (Rubio *et al.*, 2009).

Evidence shows poorer perception of "Quality of Life" by COPD patients and home Oxygen-Therapy compared to non-users (Betancourt-Peña & Tonguino-Rosero, 2016) but in addressing the underlying mental health problems we must do so not only from a negative perspective of the usefulness of Oxygen-Therapy (Ivziku *et al.,* 2018). Other studies argue that patients who receive home oxygen experience an improvement in their "Quality of Life" that is reflected in the decrease in the level of distress and the disappearance of depressive symptoms (Bello *et al.*, 2002). Studies show this controversial relationship between the role of anxiety and depression in the functioning of COPD patients (Dueñas-Espín *et al.*, 2016). Depression is considered an important comorbidity associated with the prognosis of these patients (Martinez Rivera *et al.*, 2016). Although there are studies that maintain that the relationship between COPD and comorbidity of mental disorders is evident, they offer weaknesses, because few studies investigate such a relationship (Rapsey *et al.*, 2015). Problems in the field of mental health are aggravated when there is an infra-diagnostic process and a consequent inattention or a misguided therapeutic itinerary (Rubio *et al.*, 2009):

Symptoms of anxiety and depression are common in patients with chronic obstructive pulmonary disease (COPD), but they are poorly diagnosed and there is little published data on this association. Their prevalence varies considerably from study to study, but is likely to be higher than currently known. Only one-third of these patients receive adequate treatment. Some drugs, behavioural treatment and care by a multidisciplinary team may improve the treatment of these disorders in these patients...

Anxiety, stress and depression are the primary mental health problems with significant impact on patients and their families (Fritzsche *et al.*, 2011) which can be seen in higher health costs and the number of hospitalizations or other health resources If these psychiatric pathologies are not properly treated, their repercussion is important in COPD itself and in the general health of the patient, even with the increase in mortality (Rubio *et al.,* 2009; Pelgrim *et al.,* 2019; Schuler *et al.,* 2018; Coventry *et al.,* 2014) or with the exacerbation of other mental health conditions (Jørgensen *et al.*, 2018).

Regarding the treatment of mental health pathologies that arise in people suffering from respiratory problems such as COPD, the prescription of anxiolytics and antidepressants is routine, not always with the monitoring and protocol of normative prescription. Symptoms of depression and anxiety are often not recognized and therefore are not treated or not treated correctly (Pommer *et al.,* 2012). It is necessary to know the cost and medical and pharmacological care of these comorbidities (Dalal *et al.*, 2011) and he impact of psychiatric medication on the "Quality of Life" of these patients (Usmani *et al.,* 2011). The pharmacology and other therapies used for these cases are diverse and their benefit and utility is not palpable in all patients equally, so it is necessary to design individualized plans (Weatherspoon, Weatherspoon, & Abbott, 2015).

In addition to pharmacological treatment, it is essential that the patient learns to identify situations of emotional complications and stress, by controlling the pulse, breathing, sweating, restlessness, and so on. "Breathing exercises and relaxation techniques and knowledge of your own process will reduce anxiety and help you consume less energy" (Hernández Hernández, 2016). Cognitive-Behavioral Therapy becomes another real possibility (Fritzsche *et al.*, 2011). Other therapeutic modalities have not been shown to be effective in reducing the psychiatric clinic associated with COPD, such as interpersonal psychotherapy, self-management, supportive therapies and self-help groups (Cafarella *et al.,* 2012).

In the analysis of the impact on the "Quality of Life" suffered by these patients we cannot ignore the main caregivers or informal caregivers, who suffer a significant burden both physically and psychologically (Ivziku *et al.*, 2018). Typically, informal carers form an integrated community support system in family, neighbors, friends, institutions, etc. who provide essential care and attention such as support in basic and instrumental activities of daily living, without the help of qualified professionals (Gatti *et al.*, 2018). The tasks of the informal carer affect their daily life and that of their families, causing significant stress, overload of care. The caregiver is forced to give up part of his own life, and become involved in continuous tasks of care and attention to the different needs of these patients (Strang *et al,* 2018). This implies that their quality of life is diminished, leading in many cases to psychological and emotional problems due to overloading, to exhaustion and claudication (Cedano, 2013). In addition, in most cases the situation leads to palliative care, leading to increased wear and tear on non-formal caregivers (Scheerens *et al.*, 2018). Detecting these symptoms is vitally important, as they are related to disease progression, treatment and rehabilitation procedures, and their relationship to the care provided by caregivers and family members (Tselebis *et al.*, 2016).

Depression and anxiety are two different disorders, but many times they go together (Yohannes & Alexopoulos, 2014). Bittner points out that having an anxiety disorder is an important risk factor for developing a major depressive disorder in the future. Spanish studies show data to support comorbidity between anxiety and depression (Agudelo, Buela-Casal, & Mental, 2007). Its negative influence on the evolution of other pathologies is emphasized, having been demonstrated that depressive patients have a higher mortality than the general population. On the other hand, it generates a greater functional disability than the rest of the chronic medical illnesses (Montserrat-Capdevila *et al.,* 2018).

Regarding anxiety, like depression, it acts as a stressor stimulus that can affect patients physically and emotionally. Each person responds to emotional disturbances differently. According to different authors, anxiety is defined as "irrational, unreal and disproportionate fear or worry, and daily life becomes a constant worry. It ends up dominating the individual's life, negatively affecting their normal functioning in different areas of their life, such as social activities, work or interpersonal relationships" (Hernan Silva, 2014). Validated tools exist to measure anxiety and stress in COPD, an example of which is the DASS-21 scale that offers acceptable results in its measurements (Yohannes, Dryden, & Hanania, 2018). Studies show that stressful situations aggravate anxiety and depression in COPD and it is necessary to avoid these stressful triggers, psychological intervention is considered necessary in many cases of these patients and their caregivers (Yu *et al.,* 2018). And even though the literature on the treatment of anxiety and depression in COPD patients is not very extensive, we believe that their therapeutic approach should be directed towards a more multidisciplinary approach and individualized care (Tselebis *et al.*, 2016). Promising findings have been noted regarding pulmonary rehabilitation, smoking cessation, psychological therapy and antidepressant medication to reduce anxiety and depressive symptoms in COPD patients (Yohannes & Alexopoulos, 2014).

The therapeutic effects of oxygen therapy are evident, but its high cost, together with the psychological problems such as anxiety, depression and stress suffered by both patients and their families and caregivers, requires meticulous control in the use of home oxygen. (OCD, 2015). The choice of oxygen administration is fundamental when it comes to improving the "Quality of Life" of these patients and their carers (Rodríguez Ibagué *et al.*, 2008). How to administer Oxygen-Therapy affects the process of occupational functionality of these people, and therefore in their daily work in the different areas that integrate and define the human being as an occupational individual, through propositive and significant activities. Occupational Therapy, as a discipline, can work in a clear way in respiratory rehabilitation and in the treatment of chronic diseases such as COPD. Its contribution allows minimizing the impact and functional limitations offered by the pathology clinic itself, the comorbidity of psychiatric diseases and the needs arising from the use of oxygen therapy as a treatment for these people. In other words, the occupational therapist's intervention affects the burden that these patients and their caregivers carry in terms of quality of life, health, daily activities, sleep, physical activity, exacerbations and prognosis (Miravitlles & Ribera, 2017).

NEEDS AND PROPOSALS FROM OCCUPATIONAL THERAPY

Multidisciplinary intervention is where Occupational Therapy takes on a relevant role, specifically in rehabilitation and in minimising the impact of COPD on "Quality of Life" (Bonsaksen, Fagermoen, & Lerdal, 2016). Some studies show how Occupational Therapy contributes to the prognosis of these COPD patients, including the reduction of exacerbations and hospital admission. Today there are programs with a great therapeutic specificity, as is the case of a specific rehabilitation program of Occupational Therapy aimed at preventing desaturation and activation of the sympathetic nerve during daily occupations in COPD patients (Maekura *et al.*, 2015). Proposals from Occupational Therapy contribute decisively to the development of COPD and adjacent psychiatric comorbidity (Petersen & Larsen, 2011). Respiratory rehabilitation from Occupational Therapy minimizes symptomatology, facilitates capacity and tolerance to physical effort, reduces hospitalizations and improves "Quality of Life" (Lorenzi *et al.*, 2004). In other respiratory pathologies it has also shown benefits, although the degree of evidence is lower (Papp *et al.*, 2017).

The fundamental components of rehabilitation are muscular training, education and respiratory physiotherapy, and it is also recommended to consider Occupational Therapy, psychosocial support and nutritional intervention (Güell Rous *et al.*, 2014), because the sequels in functionality are more than evident from an occupational point of view, that is, from the restriction of human activity in all areas of day-to-day daily life (Papp *et al.*, 2017).

One of the main lines of therapeutic intervention from Occupational Therapy is to try to return to the patient the ability to perform the activities of daily living (ADL), through conservation techniques or energy saving that seek to reduce respiratory limitation and extreme lack of activity as a result of the clinic caused by anxiety, depression and stress: abulia, apathy, anhedonia, social isolation, emotional lability, and so on. The aim is to interrupt the vicious circle that causes dyspnea with the reduction of activity and social isolation (Corhay *et al.*, 2014) and foster the ability to cope with day-to-day life in different occupational contexts (Gunnarsson *et al.*, 2018). The training of the activities of daily life ADLs, means that patients perceive how to perform work effectively and carry out an energy efficiency of movement, so that day-to-day tasks such as clothing, housework, personal grooming, leisure activities, shopping, etc. are performed functionally without a limiting energy cost and awakening the lack of initiative caused by low mood and anxiety (Leibold *et al.*, 2014).

The disease appears with significant changes, from a physical, psychic and social perspective. The activities and different tasks are progressively reduced, even reaching, in some cases, the total loss of functioning and incapacity to carry out the activities of daily life, such as eating, dressing, grooming, cooking, walking, shopping, maintaining social relations, etc. (Roll, 2015). The focus of the intervention must be aimed at improving the patient's "Quality of life" and occupational context, contributing to obtaining optimum results based on quality, specific and correctly focused intervention programmes (Leland *et al.*, 2015).

These rehabilitation programmes include a wide range of elements (McCarthy *et al.*, 2015) where to direct the intervention in order to achieve certain therapeutically proposed objectives from the Occupational Therapy and with the significant, propositive and functional activity as a vehicle with an adequate process of previous evaluation that sustains the practice centered in the client (Asaba *et al.*, 2017). Several studies show that rehabilitation programs through exercises with different levels of intensity, reduce stress, anxiety and depression, also improving the physical and functional fitness of patients (Godoy, 2007). In this context, incorporating intervention programs from Occupational Therapy acquires a relevant value for the daily life of patients and their families (Inzunza *et al.*, 2016). Of particular interest are pulmonary rehabilitation programs aimed at reducing anxiety and depressive symptoms (Tselebis *et al.*, 2016) which have an impact on the daily life of patients, leading to activity limitations and restrictions on social participation. The realization of daily occupations is fundamental to give sense and identity to the human being, who needs to be occupied daily and to adapt to different environments where to carry out those occupations, to be competent and to obtain achievements. The nature of the human being highlights, let us remember, as an occupational being (Sainburg *et al.*, 2017).

All human beings, regardless of their cultural origin, need to interact with the environment in order to achieve a functional homeostasis. This is manifested through participation in activities and occupations that are propositive, meaningful and symbolic for people (Kielhofner, 2004). Occupational Therapy proposes a work from a holistic perspective of the person. Occupational performance is important taking into account the values and needs of each person, and their participation in meaningful occupations (Willard *et al.*, 2005). The aim is to improve the "Quality of Life", maximising as far as possible the different occupational areas in the different environments or contexts (Ribeiro & Oliveira, 2005), that is, to evaluate the skills and functionalities that are impaired and that affect the different occupational areas of the person and how they can impact the performance of activities in different contexts through roles, habits and routines of patients (Da Silva *et al.*, 2011).

Interventions from Occupational Therapy with specific programs in mental health must be based on techniques and procedures recognized in the discipline and supported by scientific evidence (Pablos & Lozano, 2012). These programmes should promote the empowerment of patients with occupational dysfunction and enhance self-esteem, competence and self-confidence (Maceiras *et al.*, 2016). A specific intervention protocol in Occupational Therapy for patients with COPD and comorbidity of anxiety and depression is proposed below. This program must be based on the specific phases that any treatment applied with an Occupational Therapy program must include (Escobar, Ruiz, & Muela, 2013). The programme includes the points displayed in Figure 1.

Figure 1. Specific intervention protocol in occupational therapy for patients with COPD and comorbidity of anxiety

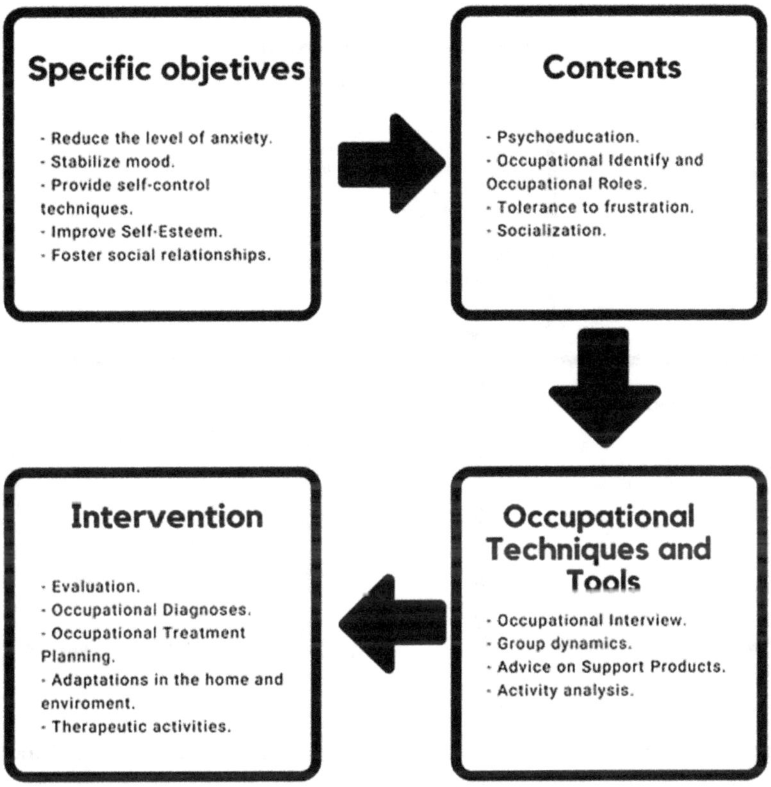

Rehabilitation programs from Occupational Therapy in patients with respiratory diseases and psychopathological clinic focuses on a process of evaluation and occupational intervention aimed at the elements that make up a person's occupation (occupational areas, occupational skills and occupational environments) in order to prevent occupational dysfunction and improve their "Quality of Life", minimizing the loss of functionality and trying to achieve the greatest possible autonomy and independence in their daily work. Figure 2 shows these elements in further detail.

Figure 2. The interaction of the three sets of elements makes it easier for the person to have an occupational function and to be autonomous and independent occupationally (AOTA)

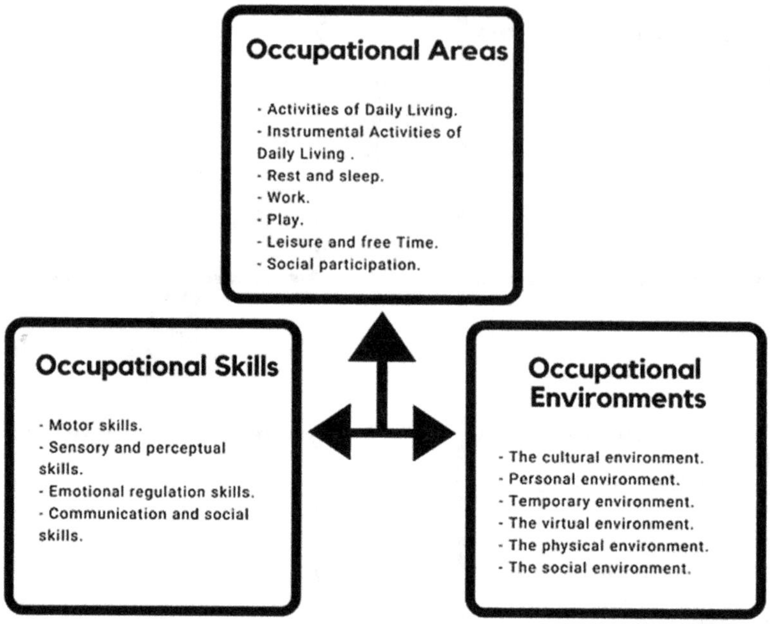

Occupational areas are the set of occupations that make a person functional in different areas of his life (Santos Del Riego, 2005). Occupational or performance skills make it possible for the person as an occupational being to participate in different occupational areas and to perform meaningful and purposeful occupations. It would be the abilities and capacities of the person that make it possible for them to carry out habits, roles, tasks, activities and occupations (Fernández & Sánchez, 2017). The contexts and environments would be the physical and external environment that surrounds the person and where the day-to-day occupations are carried out. That is to say, the conditions that are found around the person (Mercado, 2010). The interaction of the three sets of elements makes it easier for the person to have an occupational function and to be autonomous and independent occupationally.

In relation to COPD patients and anxiety and depression comorbid clinic (Rapsey *et al.*, 2015), it should be pointed out that they have alterations in their occupational capacities and skills: motor, emotional, social and communication skills that make them unable to carry out tasks and activities in the different areas of occupation: Activities of Daily Living (ADLs), leisure, social participation, rest and sleep, etc. and at the same time they show dependence to handle themselves in the different occupational contexts: physical, cultural, social, etc. (Arbillaga-Etxarri *et al.*,

2017).They show respiratory, motor, psychic, social and even cognitive alterations that impede an adequate adaptation to the environment. (Yu *et al.*, 2018). It is considered necessary functional treatments from Occupational Therapy beyond vital oxygen: energy conservation techniques, psychoeducation, mobilization techniques, relaxation, group dynamics, adaptations and elimination of architectural barriers, use and advice on support products, cognitive stimulation, etc. focused and applied with activities previously analyzed for a therapeutic application. (Macarena Inzunza *et al.*, 2016).

CONCLUSION

COPD and other pathologies requiring ambulatory oxygen therapy have been explained in the literature from purely biological approaches. However, the need to live hooked to machines, which are an essential part of the treatment, also leads to a loss that can be seen in the different functional areas of the human being. Psychosocial alterations arise, exemplified in mood alterations, anxiety, stress, sleep alterations, isolation, loss of confidence and control of their lives, etc. This interferes in the occupational functioning of these people. Self-care, leisure, rest, work environment and social participation are reduced... Lives that are biologically maintained by oxygen, but paradoxically truncated by their necessity. Feelings of rage, incomprehension, denial, social isolation, emotional lability, etc. arise, which limit the Activities of Daily Life both Basic and Instrumental: food, hygiene, cleanliness, clothing, transfers, household tasks, shopping, decision making, etc.

Health Professionals are faced here with the need to pay attention to the biological needs of the disease as well as to the social and cultural needs of the illness, the consequences of a treatment that invades daily life. A multidisciplinary therapeutic approach is needed, where Occupational Therapy can play an important role in improving the quality of life of these people and their families through the implementation of functional programs focused on minimizing the loss of autonomy and dependence on third parties. To do this, we need to deepen the knowledge of the experience of relatives and patients, considering the accounts of those as evidence at the level of oxygen saturation levels. Mental health is at stake.

ACKNOWLEDGMENT

This work was supported by the 4IE project (0045-4IE-4-P) funded by the Interreg V-A España-Portugal (POCTEP) 2014-2020 program.

REFERENCES

Agudelo, D., Buela-Casal, G., & Mental, C. (2007). Ansiedad y depresión: el problema de la diferenciación a través de los síntomas. *Medigraphic.Com*. Retrieved from https://www.medigraphic.com/cgi-bin/new/resumen.cgi?IDARTICULO=16113

Antonio, J., Fernández-Fidalgo, M., & Cieza, A. (2010). Los conceptos de calidad de vida, salud y bienestar analizados desde la perspectiva de la Clasificación Internacional del Funcionamiento (CIF). In *Revista española de salud pública. Revista Española de Salud Pública* (Vol. 84). Ministerio de Sanidad y Consumo. Retrieved from http://scielo.isciii.es/scielo.php?script=sci_arttext&pid=S1135-57272010000200005

Arbillaga-Etxarri, A., Gimeno-Santos, E., Barberan-Garcia, A., Benet, M., Borrell, E., Dadvand, P., Foraster, M., Marín, A., Monteagudo, M., Rodriguez-Roisin, R., Vall-Casas, P., Vilaró, J., & Garcia-Aymerich, J. (2017). Socio-environmental correlates of physical activity in patients with chronic obstructive pulmonary disease (COPD). *Thorax*, *72*(9), 796–802. doi:10.1136/thoraxjnl-2016-209209 PMID:28250201

Asaba, E., Nakamura, M., Asaba, A., & Kottorp, A. (2017). Integrating Occupational Therapy Specific Assessments in Practice: Exploring Practitioner Experiences. *Occupational Therapy International*, *7602805*, 1–8. Advance online publication. doi:10.1155/2017/7602805 PMID:29333112

Balbo, N. A., Acosta, M. A., & Kevorkof, G. V. (2012). *Calidad de vida en pacientes EPOC con oxigenoterapia crónica domicialiaria* (Vol. 69). Retrieved from http://www.revista2.fcm.unc.edu.ar/2012.69.2/Epoc/EPOC.pdf

Bello, S., Naranjo, C., Hinrichsen, J., & Morales, M. (2002). Oxigenoterapia domiciliaria a largo plazo, necesidad apremiante en enfermos con insuficiencia respiratoria crónica. *Revista Chilena de Enfermedades Respiratorias*, *18*(3), 175–181. doi:10.4067/S0717-73482002000300007

Betancourt-Peña, J., & Tonguino-Rosero, S. (2016). Impacto de la oxigenoterapia domiciliaria en la capacidad funcional de pacientes con enfermedad pulmonar obstructiva crónica. *Rehabilitacion*, *50*(1), 13–18. doi:10.1016/j.rh.2015.10.001

Bonsaksen, T., Fagermoen, M. S., & Lerdal, A. (2016). Trajectories of physical and mental health among persons with morbid obesity and persons with COPD: A longitudinal comparative study. *Journal of Multidisciplinary Healthcare*, *9*, 191. doi:10.2147/JMDH.S102630 PMID:27175082

Cafarella, P. A., Effing, T. W., Usmani, Z.-A., & Frith, P. A. (2012). Treatments for anxiety and depression in patients with chronic obstructive pulmonary disease: A literature review. *Respirology (Carlton, Vic.)*, *17*(4), 627–638. doi:10.1111/j.1440-1843.2012.02148.x PMID:22309179

Cedano, S. (2013). Qualidade de vida e sobrecarga dos cuidadores de portadores de Doença Pulmonar Obstrutiva Crônica em oxigenoterapia. *Revistas.Usp.Br*. Retrieved from https://www.revistas.usp.br/rlae/article/view/75996

Codinardo, C., Cáneva, J., Gil, B., & Echevarría, M. (2018). Recomendaciones sobre el uso de oxigenoterapia ambulatoria. *Vitalaire.Com.Ar*. Retrieved from https://www.vitalaire.com.ar/sites/vitalaire_ar/files/2018/09/19/recomendaciones_sobre_el_uso_de_oxigenoterapia_ambulatoria.pdf

Consejería de Sanidad de Madrid. (2013). *Plan Estratégico en EPOC de la Comunidad de Madrid 2013/2017*. Retrieved from http://www.madrid.org/es/transparencia/sites/default/files/plan/document/307_158_planepocmadrid_1abr13_lowres_0.pdf

Corhay, J.-L., Dang, D. N., Van Cauwenberge, H., & Louis, R. (2014). Pulmonary rehabilitation and COPD: Providing patients a good environment for optimizing therapy. *International Journal of Chronic Obstructive Pulmonary Disease*, *9*, 27–39. doi:10.2147/COPD.S52012 PMID:24368884

Costa, X., Gómez-Batiste, X., Pla, M., Martínez-Muñoz, M., Blay, C., & Vila, L. (2016). Vivir con la enfermedad pulmonar obstructiva crónica avanzada: El impacto de la disnea en los pacientes y cuidadores. *Atencion Primaria*, *48*(10), 665–673. doi:10.1016/j.aprim.2016.02.008 PMID:27288085

Coventry, P., Panagioti, M., Scott, C., & Blakemore, A. (2014). Overview of the prevalence, impact, and management of depression and anxiety in chronic obstructive pulmonary disease. *International Journal of Chronic Obstructive Pulmonary Disease*, *9*, 1289. doi:10.2147/COPD.S72073 PMID:25419126

Cueva Chenche, M. E. (2018). *Enfermedad pulmonar obstructiva crónica (EPOC): método diagnóstico de elección y tratamiento indicado usado con mayor frecuencia para evitar agudizaciones*. Retrieved from http://repositorio.utmachala.edu.ec/handle/48000/12585

Da Silva, L., Fierro Jordán, N., Guitérrez Monclus, P., & Rodriguez, O. (2011). Ciencia de la ocupación y Terapia Ocupacional: Sus relaciones y aplicaciones a la práctica clínica. *Revista Chilena de Terapia Ocupacional*, *11*(1), 79. doi:10.5354/0719-5346.2011.17084

Dalal, A. A., Shah, M., Lunacsek, O., & Hanania, N. A. (2011). Clinical and Economic Burden of Depression/Anxiety in Chronic Obstructive Pulmonary Disease Patients within a Managed Care Population. *COPD*, *8*(4), 293–299. doi:10.3109/15412555.2011.586659 PMID:21827298

De Pablos, C. M., & Lozano, S. G. (2012). *Funciones del Terapeuta Ocupacional en el ámbito de la Salud Mental.* Retrieved from www.revistatog.com

Díaz Lobato, S., García González, J. L., & Mayoralas Alises, S. (2015). Controversias en oxigenoterapia continua domiciliaria. *Archivos de Bronconeumologia*, *51*(1), 31–37. doi:10.1016/j.arbres.2014.05.002 PMID:24976235

Dueñas-Espín, I., Demeyer, H., Gimeno-Santos, E., Polkey, M., Hopkinson, N., Rabinovich, R., Dobbels, F., Karlsson, N., Troosters, T., & Garcia-Aymerich, J. (2016). Depression symptoms reduce physical activity in COPD patients: A prospective multicenter study. *International Journal of Chronic Obstructive Pulmonary Disease*, *11*, 1287. doi:10.2147/COPD.S101459 PMID:27354787

Escarrabill, J. (2003). *Enfermedad pulmonar obstructiva crónica (EPOC): visión global y continuidad de cuidados*. Retrieved from www.coldcopd.org

Escobar, J. C., Ruiz, C. C., & Muela, P. G. (2013). *Protocolo de intervención desde Terapia Ocupacional.* Retrieved from www.madridsalud.es

Fernández, V., & Sánchez, M. (2017). *Roles a través de la ocupación, justificación bajo el modelo de atención centrada en la persona.* Retrieved from https://dialnet.unirioja.es/servlet/articulo?codigo=5915166

Fernández Mayoralas, G., & Rojo Pérez, F. (2005). *Calidad de vida y salud: planteamientos conceptuales y métodos de investigación.* Retrieved from https://www.raco.cat/index.php/Territoris/article/viewFile/117017/147939

Fritzsche, A., Clamor, A., & von Leupoldt, A. (2011). Effects of medical and psychological treatment of depression in patients with COPD – A review. *Respiratory Medicine*, *105*(10), 1422–1433. doi:10.1016/j.rmed.2011.05.014 PMID:21680167

Gabriel, R., Figueiredo, D., Jácome, C., Cruz, J., & Marques, A. (2014). Day-to-day living with severe chronic obstructive pulmonary disease: Towards a family-based approach to the illness impacts. *Psychology & Health*, *29*(8), 967–983. doi:10.1080/08870446.2014.902458 PMID:24617821

Gatti, V., Banfi, P., Centanni, S., D'Antonio, S., Giustini, S., Piraino, A., Zibellini, M., & Marini, M. G. (2018). Enlightening chronic obstructive pulmonary disease through patients' and caregivers' narratives. *International Journal of Chronic Obstructive Pulmonary Disease, 13*, 3095–3105. doi:10.2147/COPD.S172214 PMID:30323580

Godoy. (2007). El efecto del ejercicio sobre los niveles de ansiedad, depresión y autoconcepto de pacientes con dolencia pulmonar obstructiva crónica. *Rpd-Online. Com*. Retrieved from https://www.rpd-online.com/article/view/158

Güell Rous, M. R., Díaz Lobato, S., Rodríguez Trigo, G., Morante Vélez, F., San Miguel, M., Cejudo, P., Ortega Ruiz, F., Muñoz, A., Galdiz Iturri, J. B., García, A., & Servera, E. (2014). Rehabilitación respiratoria. *Archivos de Bronconeumologia, 50*(8), 332–344. doi:10.1016/j.arbres.2014.02.014 PMID:24845559

Gunnarsson, A., Wagman, P., Hedin, K., & Håkansson, C. (2018). Treatment of depression and/or anxiety - outcomes of a randomised controlled trial of the tree theme method® versus regular occupational therapy. *BMC Psychology, 6*(1), 25. doi:10.118640359-018-0237-0 PMID:29792226

Hernan Silva, I. (2014). DSM-5 Nueva clasificación de los trastornos mentales. *Revista Chilena de Neuro-psiquiatría, 52*. www.sonepsyn.cl

Hernández Hernández, J. (2016). *Enfermedad Pulmonar Obstructiva Crónica (EPOC) en pacientes ambulatorios*. Retrieved from https://www.semg.es/doc/documentos_SEMG/consenso_epoc_cyl.pdf

Huerta, J. A. L., Romo, R. A. G., & Tayabas, J. M. T. (2017). Propiedades Psicométricas de la Versión en Español de la Escala de Calidad de Vida WHO QoL BREF en una Muestra de Adultos Mexicanos. *Revista Iberoamericana de Diagnóstico y Evaluación-e Avaliação Psicológica, 2*(44), 105–115. doi:10.21865/RIDEP44.2.09

Inzunza, M., Moreno, C., & Vallejos, M. J. (2016). Nuevas estrategias de intervención desde Terapia Ocupacional para personas con Enfermedad Pulomar Obstructiva Crónica (EPOC). *Revista Chilena de Terapia Ocupacional, 16*(2), 77–91. Retrieved from https://revistas.uchile.cl/index.php/RTO/article/view/44753

Ivziku, D., Clari, M., Piredda, M., De Marinis, M. G., & Matarese, M. (2018). Anxiety, depression and quality of life in chronic obstructive pulmonary disease patients and caregivers: An actor–partner interdependence model analysis. *Quality of Life Research: An International Journal of Quality of Life Aspects of Treatment, Care and Rehabilitation*. Advance online publication. doi:10.100711136-018-2024-z PMID:30341578

Jarillo Quijada, A. (2004). *Oxigenoterapia*. Retrieved from http://himfg.com.mx/descargas/documentos/planeacion/guiasclinicasHIM/oxigenotrepia.pdf

Jørgensen, M., Mainz, J., Lange, P., & Paaske Johnsen, S. (2018). Quality of care and clinical outcomes of chronic obstructive pulmonary disease in patients with schizophrenia. A Danish nationwide study. *International Journal for Quality in Health Care*, *30*(5), 351–357. doi:10.1093/intqhc/mzy014 PMID:29432585

Kielhofner, G. (2004). *Terapia ocupacional : modelo de ocupación humana : teoría y aplicación*. Médica Panamericana.

Leibold, M., Holm, M. B., Raina, K. D., Reynolds, C. F. III, & Rogers, J. C. (2014). Activities and adaptation in late-life depression: A qualitative study. *The American Journal of Occupational Therapy : Official Publication of the American Occupational Therapy Association*, *68*(5), 570–577. doi:10.5014/ajot.2014.011130 PMID:25184470

Leland, N. E., Crum, K., Phipps, S., Roberts, P., & Gage, B. (2015). Advancing the value and quality of occupational therapy in health service delivery. *The American Journal of Occupational Therapy*, *69*(1), 1-7. . doi:10.5014/ajot.2015.691001

Leland, N. E., Fogelberg, D. J., Halle, A. D., & Mroz, T. M. (2017). Occupational Therapy and Management of Multiple Chronic Conditions in the Context of Health Care Reform. *The American Journal of Occupational Therapy*, *71*(1), 6. . doi:10.5014/ajot.2017.711001

López, S. H., & Cob, L. H. (2018). *Proyecto de educación para la salud para personas con EPOC*. Retrieved from https://repositorio.uam.es/handle/10486/684884

López Riolobos, C., García del Castillo, E., Gómez Punter, R. M., & Fernandes de Vasconcelos, G. M. (2014). Indicaciones de la oxigenoterapia domiciliaria. Regulación y seguimiento clínico. *Medicine - Programa de Formación Médica Continuada Acreditado*, *11*(63), 3777–3781. doi:10.1016/S0304-5412(14)70843-1

Lorenzi, C. M., Cilione, C., Rizzardi, R., Furino, V., Bellantone, T., Lugli, D., & Clini, E. (2004). Occupational Therapy and Pulmonary Rehabilitation of Disabled COPD Patients. *Respiration*, *71*(3), 246–251. doi:10.1159/000077422 PMID:15133344

Maceiras, M., Juan, F., Navarro, M., Ramón, C., & García, R. (2016). *Proyecto Editorial Terapia Ocupacional*. Retrieved from http://www.sintesis.com

Maekura, R., Hiraga, T., Miki, K., Kitada, S., Miki, M., Yoshimura, K., Yamamoto, H., Kawabe, T., & Mori, M. (2015). Personalized pulmonary rehabilitation and occupational therapy based on cardiopulmonary exercise testing for patients with advanced chronic obstructive pulmonary disease. *International Journal of Chronic Obstructive Pulmonary Disease*, *10*, 1787–1800. doi:10.2147/COPD.S86455 PMID:26366071

Martínez Muñiz, F. B., Esperanza Barrios, A., Pérez Labour, R. A., & Rodríguez González-Moro, J. M. (2017). Tratamiento de la insuficiencia respiratoria crónica. Oxigenoterapia. *Medicine - Programa de Formación Médica Continuada Acreditado*, *12*(46), 2755–2765. . doi:10.1016/j.med.2017.12.003

Martinez Rivera, C., Costan Galicia, J., Alcázar Navarrete, B., Garcia-Polo, C., Ruiz Iturriaga, L. A., Herrejón, A., Ros Lucas, J. A., García-Sidro, P., Tirado-Conde, G., López-Campos, J. L., Mayoralas Alises, S., de Miguel-Díez, J., Esquinas, C., & Miravitlles, M. (2016). Factors Associated with Depression in COPD: A Multicenter Study. *Lung*, *194*(3), 335–343. doi:10.100700408-016-9862-7 PMID:26932809

McCarthy, B., Casey, D., Devane, D., Murphy, K., Murphy, E., & Lacasse, Y. (2015). Pulmonary rehabilitation for chronic obstructive pulmonary disease. *Cochrane Database of Systematic Reviews*, (2), CD003793. doi:10.1002/14651858.CD003793.pub3 PMID:25705944

Mercado, R. (2010). *Los entornos y contextos dentro del proceso de valoración. Evaluación e intervención en Terapia Ocupacional* (Vol. 7). Retrieved from www.revistatog.com

Miravitlles, M., Izquierdo, J. L., Esquinas, C., Pérez, M., Calle, M., López-Campos, J. L., Rodríguez González-Moro, J. M., Casanova, C., Esteban, C., & de Lucas, P. (2017). The variability of respiratory symptoms and associated factors in COPD. *Respiratory Medicine*, *129*, 165–172. doi:10.1016/j.rmed.2017.06.017 PMID:28732827

Miravitlles, M., & Ribera, A. (2017). Understanding the impact of symptoms on the burden of COPD. *Respiratory Research*, *18*(1), 67. doi:10.118612931-017-0548-3 PMID:28431503

Miravitlles, M., Soler-Cataluña, J. J., Cataluña, C., Calle, M., Molina, J., Almagro, P., ... Ancocheã, J. (2017). Guía española de la enfermedad pulmonar obstructiva crónica (GesEPOC) 2017. Tratamiento farmacológico en fase estable. *Archivos de Bronconeumologia*, *53*(6), 324–335. doi:10.1016/j.arbres.2017.03.018 PMID:28477954

Montserrat-Capdevila, J., Godoy, P., Marsal, J. R., Ortega, M., Pifarré, J., Alsedà, M., Castañ, M. T., & Barbé, F. (2018). Mental disorders in chronic obstructive pulmonary diseases. *Perspectives in Psychiatric Care*, *54*(3), 398–404. doi:10.1111/ppc.12274 PMID:29577318

Moruno Miralles, P., & Talavera Valverde, M. A. (2012). *Terapia ocupacional en salud mental*. Elsevier Masson.

Muñoz-Cobos, F., Acero-Guasch, N., Cuenca-del-Moral, R., Barnestein-Fonseca, P., Leiva-Fernández, F., & García-Ruiz, A. (2015). Cómo vivir con EPOC: Percepción de los pacientes. *Anales de Psicología*, *32*(1), 18. doi:10.6018/analesps.32.1.186211

Neves, J. T., & Lobão, M. J. (2012). Estudo multicêntrico de oxigenoterapia – uma auditoria nacional aos procedimentos de oxigenoterapia em enfermarias de medicina interna. *Revista Portuguesa de Pneumologia*, *18*(2), 80–85. doi:10.1016/j.rppneu.2012.01.001 PMID:22280829

OCD. (2015). *Indicación y empleo de la oxigenoterapia continua domiciliaria*. Retrieved from https://www.fisiorespiracion.es/indicacion_y_empleo_de_la_oxigenoterapia_continua_domiciliaria.pdf

Olmedo, P., & Sierra, A. (2004). Oxigenoterapia domiciliaria. *Neumosur.Net*. Retrieved from http://www.neumosur.net/files/EB02-20 ocd.pdf

Ortega Ruiz, F., Díaz Lobato, S., Galdiz Iturri, J. B., García Rio, F., Güell Rous, R., Morante Velez, F., ... Tàrrega Camarasa, J. (2014). Oxigenoterapia continua domiciliaria. *Archivos de Bronconeumologia*, *50*(5), 185–200. doi:10.1016/J.ARBRES.2013.11.025 PMID:24461631

Papp, M. E., Wändell, P. E., Lindfors, P., & Nygren-Bonnier, M. (2017). Effects of yogic exercises on functional capacity, lung function and quality of life in participants with obstructive pulmonary disease: A randomized controlled study. *European Journal of Physical and Rehabilitation Medicine*, *53*(3), 447–461. doi:10.23736/S1973-9087.16.04374-4 PMID:27830924

Paredes, M. C., & Aznar, I. (2009). *Fundamentos de la oxigenoterapia en situaciones agudas y crónicas: indicaciones, métodos, controles y seguimiento*. Elsevier. Retrieved from https://www.sciencedirect.com/science/article/pii/S1695403309003294

Pelgrim, C. E., Peterson, J. D., Gosker, H. R., Schols, A. M. W. J., van Helvoort, A., Garssen, J., Folkerts, G., & Kraneveld, A. D. (2019). Psychological co-morbidities in COPD: Targeting systemic inflammation, a benefit for both? *European Journal of Pharmacology*, *842*, 99–110. doi:10.1016/j.ejphar.2018.10.001 PMID:30336140

Petersen, A., & Larsen, S. (2011). Occupational therapy intervention for patients with COPD rehabilitation at home. *International Journal of Integrated Care, 11*(Suppl). Retrieved from https://www.ncbi.nlm.nih.gov/pmc/articles/PMC3184825

Rapsey, C. M., Lim, C. C. W., Al-Hamzawi, A., Alonso, J., Bruffaerts, R., Caldas-de-Almeida, J. M., Florescu, S., de Girolamo, G., Hu, C., Kessler, R. C., Kovess-Masfety, V., Levinson, D., Medina-Mora, M. E., Murphy, S., Ono, Y., Piazza, M., Posada-Villa, J., ten Have, M., Wojtyniak, B., & Scott, K. M. (2015). Associations between DSM-IV mental disorders and subsequent COPD diagnosis. *Journal of Psychosomatic Research, 79*(5), 333–339. doi:10.1016/j.jpsychores.2015.08.005 PMID:26526305

Ribeiro, M. B. S., & de Oliveira, L. R. (2005). *Interface: Comunicacao, saude, educacao. Interface - Comunicação, Saúde, Educação* (Vol. 9). Fundacao UNI. Retrieved from https://www.scielosp.org/scielo.php?pid=S1414-32832005000200023&script=sci_arttext&tlng=en

Rodríguez Ibagué, L.-F., Díaz Castillo, L. Á., Martinez-Santa, J., Rodríguez Ibagué, L. F., Díaz Castillo, L. Á., & Martínez Santa, J. (2008). Oxigenoterapia. *Instname:Universidad Del Rosario*. Retrieved from http://repository.urosario.edu.co/handle/10336/3696

Roll, S. C. (2015). Role of sonographic imaging in occupational therapy practice. *The American Journal of Occupational Therapy, 69*(3), 1-8. . doi:10.5014/ajot.2015.015941

Rosalía. (2016). *La ansiedad de la EPOC*. Retrieved February 1, 2019, from https://www.tucuentasmucho.com/cuidarse/ansiedad-en-epoc/

Rubio, M. C., Hermosa, J. L. R., & Nebreda, M. J. G. (2009). Ansiedad y EPOC. *Archivos de Bronconeumologia, 45*(SUPPL.5), 51–53. doi:10.1016/S0300-2896(09)72865-0 PMID:20116751

Sainburg, R. L., Liew, S.-L., Frey, S. H., & Clark, F. (2017). Promoting Translational Research Among Movement Science, Occupational Science, and Occupational Therapy. *Journal of Motor Behavior, 49*(1), 1–7. doi:10.1080/00222895.2016.1271299 PMID:28166469

Santos Del Riego, S. (2005). *El ser humano como ser ocupacional* (Vol. 39). Retrieved from https://ruc.udc.es/dspace/bitstream/handle/2183/16961/SantosRiego_SerHumano.pdf?sequence=3

Scheerens, C., Deliens, L., Van Belle, S., Joos, G., Pype, P., & Chambaere, K. (2018). A palliative end-stage COPD patient does not exist: A qualitative study of barriers to and facilitators for early integration of palliative home care for end-stage COPD. *NPJ Primary Care Respiratory Medicine*, *28*(1), 23. doi:10.103841533-018-0091-9 PMID:29925846

Schuler, M., Strohmayer, M., Mühlig, S., Schwaighofer, B., Wittmann, M., Faller, H., & Schultz, K. (2018). Assessment of depression before and after inpatient rehabilitation in COPD patients: Psychometric properties of the German version of the Patient Health Questionnaire (PHQ-9/PHQ-2). *Journal of Affective Disorders*, *232*, 268–275. doi:10.1016/j.jad.2018.02.037 PMID:29499510

Sociedad Española de Neumología y Cirugía torácica. (2018). Retrieved from https://www.separ.es/sites/default/files/SEPAR_NP_muertes_anuales_EPOC.pdf

Strang, S., Osmanovic, M., Hallberg, C., & Strang, P. (2018). Family Caregivers' Heavy and Overloaded Burden in Advanced Chronic Obstructive Pulmonary Disease. *Journal of Palliative Medicine*, *21*(12), 1768–1772. doi:10.1089/jpm.2018.0010 PMID:30118371

Tselebis, A., Pachi, A., Ilias, I., Kosmas, E., Bratis, D., Moussas, G., & Tzanakis, N. (2016). Strategies to improve anxiety and depression in patients with COPD: A mental health perspective. *Neuropsychiatric Disease and Treatment*, *12*, 297–328. doi:10.2147/NDT.S79354 PMID:26929625

Usmani, Z. A., Carson, K. V., Cheng, J. N., Esterman, A. J., & Smith, B. J. (2011). Pharmacological interventions for the treatment of anxiety disorders in chronic obstructive pulmonary disease. *Cochrane Database of Systematic Reviews*, (11), CD008483. doi:10.1002/14651858.CD008483.pub2 PMID:22071851

Weatherspoon, D., Weatherspoon, C. A., & Abbott, B. (2015). Pharmacology Update on Chronic Obstructive Pulmonary Disease, Rheumatoid Arthritis, and Major Depression. *The Nursing Clinics of North America*, *50*(4), 761–770. doi:10.1016/j.cnur.2015.07.006 PMID:26596663

Willard, H. S., Spackman, C. S., Crepeau, E. B., Cohn, E. S., & Schell, B. A. B. (2005). *Terapia ocupacional*. Médica Panamericana.

Yohannes, A. M., & Alexopoulos, G. S. (2014). Depression and anxiety in patients with COPD. *European Respiratory Review : An Official Journal of the European Respiratory Society*, *23*(133), 345–349. doi:10.1183/09059180.00007813 PMID:25176970

Yohannes, A. M., Dryden, S., & Hanania, N. A. (2018). The Validity and Responsiveness of the Depression, Anxiety and Stress Scale (DASS-21) in Chronic Obstructive Pulmonary Disease. *Chest*. Advance online publication. doi:10.1016/j.chest.2018.12.010 PMID:30594559

Yu, T., Frei, A., ter Riet, G., & Puhan, M. A. (2018). Impact of Stressful Life Events on Patients with Chronic Obstructive Pulmonary Disease. *Respiration*, *95*(2), 73–79. doi:10.1159/000481714 PMID:29156451

KEY TERMS AND DEFINITIONS

Ambulatory: Does not require the patient to be admitted to a hospital.

Anxiety: The emotions present in anxiety disorders range from simple nervousness to episodes of terror or panic. An anxiety disorder is diagnosed when a person has an extreme response (for example, a lot of fear) to a situation.

Depression: A psychiatric and psychological diagnosis describing a mood disorder, transient or permanent, characterized by feelings of dejection, unhappiness, and guilt.

Identity: A set of traits or characteristics of a person or thing that allow it to be distinguished from others in a set.

Mental Health: In general terms, the state of balance between a person and his socio-cultural environment that guarantees his labor, intellectual and relationship participation to achieve a welfare and quality of life.

Occupational Therapy: Occupational therapy, and its professionals, occupational therapists, help people throughout their lives to participate in the activities and tasks they want and need to perform through the therapeutic use of daily activities.

Oxygen-Therapy: Medical treatment of certain diseases based on the application of oxygen inhalations.

Quality of Life: A concept that alludes to various levels of generalization through society, community, to the physical and mental aspect, therefore, the meaning of quality of life is a complex and with definitions from sociology, political science, medicine, development studies, etc.

Chapter 11
Inhalotherapy in Noninvasive Ventilation

Mónica Helena Correia Pereira
Lisbon North University Hospital Center, Portugal

João Miguel Bettencourt Sena Carvalho
Lisbon North University Hospital Center, Portugal

Paula Maria Gonçalves Pinto
Lisbon North University Hospital Center, Portugal & Faculty of Medicine of Lisbon, University of Lisbon, Portugal

Maria do Carmo Oliveira Cordeiro
Independent Researcher, Portugal

ABSTRACT

The use of non-invasive ventilation (NIV) has markedly increased over the last decades, and NIV has now become an important alternative to invasive ventilation and has gained popularity particularly as treatment option for patients with obstructive sleep apnea, chronic obstructive pulmonary disease (COPD), and acute respiratory failure. The most prominent forms of NIV are noninvasive positive pressure ventilation (NPPV) and the recently introduced high-flow nasal cannula (HFNC) therapy. Many patients who received NIV may also benefit from the administration of pharmaceutical aerosols, typically bronchodilators, which are best delivered without interrupting respiratory support. For example, nowadays, the use of NIV is considered the standard of care for some forms of acute respiratory failure such as COPD exacerbation and acute cardiogenic pulmonary edema. Patients with COPD exacerbation also benefit from inhaled bronchodilator therapy.

DOI: 10.4018/978-1-7998-3531-8.ch011

Copyright © 2020, IGI Global. Copying or distributing in print or electronic forms without written permission of IGI Global is prohibited.

INHALOTHERAPY IN NONINVASIVE VENTILATION

The use of non-invasive ventilation (NIV) has markedly increased over the last decades, and NIV has now become an important alternative to invasive ventilation and have gained popularity particularly as treatment option for patients with obstructive sleep apnea, chronic obstructive pulmonary disease (COPD) and acute respiratory failure. The most prominent forms of NIV are noninvasive positive pressure ventilation (NPPV) and recently introduced high-flow nasal cannula (HFNC) therapy.

Many patients who received NIV may also benefit from the administration of pharmaceutical aerosols, typically bronchodilators, which are best delivered without interrupting respiratory support.

For example, nowadays, the use of NIV is considered standard of care for some forms of acute respiratory failure such as COPD exacerbation and acute cardiogenic pulmonary edema. Patients with COPD exacerbation also benefit from inhaled bronchodilator therapy.

Throughout the history of medicine, the use of aerosols has played a prominent role in the treatment of respiratory diseases that is perpetuated to the present. Currently the inhalation route is widely accepted by the international scientific community as being the recommended way to administer drugs in the treatment of pathologies of the airways and lungs (acute or chronic) (Walenga, Longest, Kaviratna, & Hindle, 2017).

An aerosol is a colloid system in which liquid or solid particles, especially the suspension of a drug, can be administered by nebulization.

Aerosoltherapy or inhalotherapy is defined as the therapeutic modality consisting of the administration of drugs in therapeutic dose in the form of respirable particles ($<5\mu m$ of diameter) within a short period of time, by inhalation. It is used for the treatment of acute or chronic bronchopulmonary disease.

Inhalotherapy has some specificities that need to be taken into account in order to ensure better efficacy and results from its use (Fink & Dhand, 2000).

Bronchodilators, corticosteroids and antibiotics can be administered by inhalation. Bronchodilators are the most frequently used and they can improve ventilatory parameters and gas exchange. They relax airway smooth muscles, reversing airway obstruction and preventing bronchoconstriction. Patients with COPD or asthma, for example, routinely receive treatment with inhaled bronchodilators. In patients with exacerbation of COPD or severe asthma, emergency treatment with bronchodilators is recommended. In patients with COPD the treatment with bronchodilators is the key of the therapy, and they are able to relieve symptoms, improve quality of life, improve lung function and prevent exacerbations (Beeh, et al. 2017; Yang et al., 2017).

Inhalotherapy

Nowadays, inhalotherapy is currently recognized as the route of choice in the pharmacological treatment of respiratory diseases and has contributed to improve the quality of life of respiratory patients, especially those with COPD and asthma.

Several advantages have been pointed out in the use of inhalotherapy, but the main ones are the possibility of obtaining a faster action in the therapeutic efficacy, with lower doses and minor side effects. Compared to oral and systemic road, inhalation has a faster therapeutic action because of direct deposition of the drug in the lung (Price, Østrem, Thomas, & Welte, 2017).

There are many groups of drugs available to administration in the form of aerosol, like bronchodilators of short action (beta-2 agonists), anticholinergics, non-steroidal anti-inflammatory drugs, antibiotics and mucolytics (Calzetta, Rogliani, Matera, & Cazzola, 2016).

The term aerosol defines a stable suspension of small particles, solid or liquid, dispersed in a gas (Fink & Dhand, 2000; Walenga, Longest, Kaviratna, & Hindle, 2017).

This type of therapy has deposition of the drug in lower airways as the main goal. According to many studies there is a significant variability between the prescribed drug fraction, the fraction generated by the inhaler, the fraction inhaled by the patient and the deposited fraction that is the amount of drug reaching the lower airways (Boer et al., 2017).

The administered dose of the drug is therefore much lower than that actually deposited in the lung, since the fraction of active product deposited is conditioned by factors such as particle diameter, ventilatory pattern and anatomic characteristics of the airways. There are other factors that influence the drug deposition in the lung like patient age and underlying diseases (Walenga et al., 2017).

The lung is a complex organ with multiple divisions of the airway structures, since the trachea, bronchi and their branches, end in the alveoli. So the anatomical characteristics of the lung influence the particles deposition. Aerosol particles travel along the branched airway system along with air, on which a system of dynamic forces acts. These forces include the inspired air drag force and inertial forces. Thus at the level of the upper airways whose function is the filtration and humidification of the air, the particles deposit by impaction. In bronchi of smaller caliber, the articles deposit by sedimentation. In the more distal portions of the airways, the particles deposit by sedimentation or by Brownian diffusion. Then in patients with respiratory disease the deposition along the respiratory tract will be different because of anatomical and physiological modifications. The presence of obstructive processes, diseases with pulmonary parenchyma alterations and ventilatory mechanics influence the deposition of the inhaled drug at the level of the airways. In situations where there is bronchial obstruction, the aerosol is deposited in the airways where the inspiratory flow encounters less resistance, being thus distributed heterogeneously and depositing more in the airways of greater caliber. In patients with COPD, the particles deposition will be preferably more proximal in consequence of the airway flow limitation. This is a limitation of this therapy so that the drug could not reach the ideal deposition site. The same situation could occur in diseases with changes in ventilatory mechanics or emphysema (Borghardt, Kloft & Sharma, 2018)-

The diameter of the inhaled particles and their granulometric distribution are factors that also contribute to the correct deposition of the drug. The particle size is not constant along the airways and can decrease its diameter, as in aerosols pressurized by evaporation of the propellant. Relative to particle size, particles with a size more than 10 μm deposit themselves mainly in the mouth and oropharynx, particles with a size between 5 to 10μm, deposit in the zone of transition between oropharynx and lower airways. Finally particles with less than 5μm can go to the lung and reach the alveoli, these being suitable for therapeutic aerosols (Fink & Dhand, 2000; Walenga et al., 2017).

The deposition of aerosol particles in the airways occurs by three main mechanisms (Deng et al., 2019; Miguel, 2017):

- Impact by inertia: This mechanism occurs mainly in particles of size greater than 5 μm in the upper airways, main bronchi and their bifurcations.
- Gravitational sedimentation: This mechanism favors the deposition of particles with a diameter between 1 and 5μm in the most distal airways. This mechanism is directly proportional to the particle size and inversely proportional to its velocity. It is favored by a slow inhalation.
- Brownian diffusion: It is the mechanism of deposition of particles with a diameter less than 1μm that acquire erratic movements along the bronchial tree.

Administration of drugs by inhalation can be performed through different inhalation devices. Nowadays there are many different devices available in the market, each one with their advantages and disadvantages with different clinical indications.

The inhalation devices are generally grouped into different categories according to the system of use for dispersion of the drug (Bosnic-Anticevich et al., 2017; Levy et al., 2016). These main groups are:

- Metered Dose Inhaler (MDI) or Pressurized Metered Dose Inhaler (pMDI);
- Dry Power Inhalers (DPI);
- Nebulization systems: pneumatic, ultrasonic and electronic;
- Inhaler with nebuliser solution.

The main difference between these categories is the way the aerosol is produced. Different devices condition different patterns of deposition along the airway and, in particular, in the lung.

During NIV, the most commonly used devices are pMDI. pMDI are the most prescript devices over the world and the most used in the hospital context.

The pMDI comprises several components, each of which is important to the success of the whole device. pMDI are constituted of a canister containing the pharmacologically active product, an antioxidant, a surfactant, the propellant gas, the solvent and the shaker, which together will constitute a final product which will be inhaled by the user. One of the most crucial components of a MDI is its propellant. The propellant provides the force to generate the aerosol cloud and is also the medium in which the active component must be suspended or dissolved. In 2009, the FDA banned the use of inhalers that use chlorofluorocarbons (CFC) as propellants, and now use hydrofluoroalkane (HFA). Use of hydrofluoroalkane (HFA) MDIs may diminish oropharyngeal deposition as they tend to deliver a greater proportion of the actuated dose to the airways in the lungs and less to the oropharynx compared with chlorofluorocarbon (CFC) MDIs. Another way to address this problem is to add a spacer device or valved holding chamber (VHC), which can decrease the oral deposition of medicine.

On activation, the metered-dose inhaler releases a fixed dose of medication in aerosol form. MDIs can be formulated as solutions, suspensions, or co-suspensions, with solutions typically having a finer aerosol particle size compared with suspensions.

There are some particularities to the good and correct use of pMDI, to optimize their effectiveness. It is consensual in the literature and fundamental, before each use: heating and shaking of the canister for correct suspension and dissolution of the drug, as well as acquisition of the ideal pressure inside the packaging for generation of the aerosol. It is also essential the synchronization with the beginning of inspiration.

Inhalation continues to be the route of choice in ventilated patients requiring the administration of pressurized inhalers in the ventilator respiratory circuit through a self-adaptive system. The inhaler device is adapted to the ventilator circuit and the principles of the recommended inhalation technique are followed: agitation of pMDI prior to administration and synchronization with the onset of inspiration.

Inhalotherapy and Ventilation

The administration of inhaled medications to mechanically ventilated patients requires special attention because of the propensity for deposition of the medication on ventilator tubing.

The use of inhaled drugs has some advantages like having a rapid onset of action, allowing selective treatment of the lung and being able to deliver high drug concentrations to the airway. They have few systemic adverse effects which is a positive point.

There are some studies that demonstrated that the beneficial effects of inhaled drugs are smaller in patients within ventilation therapy than those breathing spontaneously. It may be explained because of a substantial drug loss caused by the turbulent flow produced by ventilation (Fink & Dhand, 2000).

In general, there is evidence that there is an advantage in the use of metered dose inhalers (MDIs) because they are more economical and have a lower risk of nosocomial pneumonia. Nebulizers and MDIs have similar effects on lung function, both types resulting in equivalent changes in FEV_1.

In patients with NIV necessity, the inhaled drugs most commonly used are bronchodilators, like beta adrenergic agonists, anticholinergics and corticosteroids. Again, the inhaled administration is the preferred route of administration because of direct lung delivery, lower dose needed, rapid onset of action and reduced systemic absorption, thus reducing adverse effects.

There are some studies that tried to prove the efficiency of inhalotherapy during NIV. Currently, in daily practice, for bronchodilator administration in patients on NIV, the mask is removed and the drug is delivered, or the device is connected to the mask to the ventilator circuit. The concern is that patients might decompensate when NIV is discontinued. There is evidence available to support the concept that aerosols can be delivered effectively during NIV without discontinuation for inhaled therapy administration (Walenga, et al., 2017).

The use of an interface during NIV can be actually a problem, because there is some evidence that aerosol deposition in the mask and nasal cavity significantly reduces lung drug deposition, possibly reducing drug efficacy. For increase efficacy, the mask should be well secured because leaks can significantly reduce drug delivery.

França et al. (2006), compared pulmonary radioaerosol deposition during jet nebulization with NIV versus spontaneous breathing to measure lung deposition by scintigraphy. These authors concluded that although there was an increase in the total volume associated with an higher inspiratory flow during NIV, this didn´t result in an increase in lung deposition.

Maccari et al. (2014) tried to determine the effect of spontaneous breathing and NIV on lung technetium-99m deposition in subjects with normal lung. This study suggested that in individuals with normal lungs, aerosol delivery is not reduced during CPAP or NIV.

When aerosol is administered during NIV there is a concern to avoid leak of aerosol into the eyes of the patient.

Factors That Influence Inhaled Drug Delivery During Ventilation

Many factors influence the efficacy of the inhaled treatment and the aerosol deposition in the lower airways, generally based on the pharmacological properties of the drug and on lung drug deposition. Such factors include:

- Drug-related properties (physical and chemical properties);
- Characteristics of the aerosol generator;
- Position of the aerosol generator in the ventilatory circuit;
- Ventilator settings;
- Ventilation mode;
- Heating and humidification of the inhaled air;
- Characteristics of the endotracheal tube;
- Anatomy of the airways,
- Presence of respiratory secretions.

Generally, for better drug delivery, aerosol particles must be small enough to penetrate through the upper airway but large enough to avoid being eliminated by the expiratory flow. More efficiency of pulmonary deposition during NIV is achieved with devices that can produce aerosols with mass of less than 2μm.

Heating and humidification of the inhaled air prevent damage to the airway mucosa and prevent bronchospasm. However, an elevated humidification seems to increase the particles dimension of the drug, decreasing its lung deposition, and increase particle impaction in the ventilator circuit. But more studies are necessary to prove this. On the other hand, humidification improves the comfort of the patent during NIV and reduces the risk of infection. Although humidification of the air has this unwanted effects, routine removal of the humidifier is not recommended because it requires interrupting the circuit and waiting a few minutes for it to dry. This decrease of lung deposition is not significant so that justify withdrawing the humidification (Fink, et al., 2000; Walenga et al., 2017).

The position of the aerosol generator in the ventilatory circuit can influence its deposition in the lung. The administration of the aerosol between the ventilator and the humidification system seems to be better. According to a study by Fink and Dhand, the production of an aerosol is high in dry and cold atmosphere, before the humidification system, and so that can generate particles with smaller and more stable dimensions, improving the drug deposition in the lung (Fink & Dhand, 2000).

MDIs are frequently used because they are cost-effective, reproductive and safe. MDIs use must be synchronized with inspiration, improving its efficiency. Synchronizing the actuation of the MDI with the beginning of the inspiration increases lung drug deposition in 30%. Do not shake the doser reduces the respirable dose by

35%. There is also reduction when multiple quick shots are fired by the turbulence of the particles. These are some cautions to take with this type of devices. In NIV-dependent patients there is evidence that an MDI with a spacer is more efficient for bronchodilator administration than an MDI without a spacer.

Even in NIV-dependent patients, bronchodilators should preferentially be administered with the head of the bed elevated because sitting position seems to improve drug delivery to the lung.

High and turbulent flows can increase particle impaction that can increase particle deposition in the proximal airways. The density of the inhaled gas can also influence drug delivery to the lung.

Patient-ventilator synchrony also improves lung drug deposition. A delay between device actuation and the beginning of inhalation reduce significantly the efficiency of drug delivery in the lung. It is important that the extent of lung disease and the ability of patients to tolerate the mask and the ventilator also play a role in the success of treatment with NIV and inhalation therapy (Fink & Dhand, 2000).

Aerosol Therapy During NIV

Mechanical ventilation encompasses all procedures that use a mechanical device to assist or replace a patient's respiratory function. If the ventilatory support does not require inserting an endotracheal tube (by orotracheal or nasotracheal intubation or tracheostomy), it is called noninvasive ventilation (NIV). The early development of this therapeutic modality focused on patients with neuromuscular diseases, sequelae of tuberculosis, thoracic cage deformities, and hypoventilation-obesity syndrome. At the beginning of the 1980s, when the efficacy of continuous positive airway pressure (CPAP) applied through a nasal mask was described for patients with obstructive sleep apnea syndrome, the number of patients receiving NIV was not great. However, the demonstrated ability of NIV to give effective, comfortable, and well-tolerated mechanical ventilation through a nasal mask encouraged exponential growth in the number of patients using that modality for long periods. The 1990s can be considered the decade of NIV and home ventilation thanks to the important invention of the nasal mask (Hess, 2015).

The use of non-invasive ventilation (NIV) has markedly increased over the last decades, and NIV has now become an important alternative to invasive ventilation, and has gained popularity particularly as the treatment option for patients with obstructive sleep apnea, chronic obstructive pulmonary disease (COPD) and acute respiratory failure. However, its utilization is still controversial in determined pathologies like community acquired pneumonia, acute respiratory distress syndrome or pulmonary hypertension. The principal benefits of noninvasive ventilation application are to reduce work of breathing, diminish the rate of intubations and its possible consequences, prevent atelectasis and assist the failing heart. The selection of patients must be done very carefully because the risk of complications could be increased if noninvasive ventilation is used inappropriately, leading to an increase in mortality (DGS, 2011; França, et al., 2006).

The most prominent forms of NIV are noninvasive positive pressure ventilation (NPPV), such as CPAP or BPAP, and recently introduced high-flow nasal cannula (HFNC) therapy. CPAP uses a positive airway pressure and air flow is introduced into the airways to maintain a continuous pressure to constantly stent the airway open, in patients that are breathing spontaneously. It maintains the set pressure throughout the respiratory cycle, during both inspiration and expiration, preventing the airway collapse that can occur in many situations and maintaining airway patency (Maccari, et al., 2014).

NIV is a recognized intervention in the treatment of acute hypercapnic respiratory failure due to exacerbations of Chronic Obstructive Pulmonary Disease (COPD), in weaning in COPD, in immunocompromised patients, in post-operative respiratory failure and in cystic fibrosis. It is also used for the treatment of chronic hypercapnic respiratory failure in patients with neuromuscular diseases such as Duchenne's muscular dystrophy, myotonic dystrophy, motor neuron disease, chest wall diseases such as thoracoplasty and kyphoscoliosis, in the treatment of selected patients with COPD or bronchiectasis. This treatment may be used in conjunction with conventional or standard treatments which might include inhalers, oxygen therapy and antibiotics (Davies, et al., 2002; França, et al., 2006).

In patients with Chronic Respiratory Insufficiency (CRI), nocturnal ventilation should be prescribed when $PaCO_2$ is greater than 55mm Hg in the presence of hypoventilation symptoms. If $PaCO_2$ falls to between 50 and 55mmHg, the consensus is to recommend starting NIV if the patient had nocturnal desaturation defined as a pulse oximeter reading of less than 88% for longer than five consecutive minutes in spite of receiving oxygen at 2 L/min or if the patient had been hospitalized with hypercapnic respiratory insufficiency at least twice in one year (Davies et al., 2002).

The use of NIV is considered standard of care for some forms of acute respiratory failure such as acute cardiogenic pulmonary edema and COPD exacerbation, being the last the most common etiology of Acute Respiratory Insufficiency (ARI). NIV should be considered in these patients, when respiratory acidosis ($pH<7.35$, $pCO_2>45mmHg$) persists despite maximum medical treatment optimized and controlled oxygen therapy. With the application of NIV, there has been a considerable reduction on mortality and need for orotracheal intubation (OTI) both in intensive care units and on respiratory medicine wards. NIV is also indicated in acute or acute-on-chronic hypercapnia respiratory failures due to chest wall deformity or neuromuscular disease. A study of predictors of success for NIV in patients with ARI due to COPD found that unsuccessful episodes of treatment were associated with a severely deranged baseline pH and $PaCO_2$, a low body mass index, the presence of pneumonia, a severe level of neurological deterioration and an inability to comply with ventilation. In addition, copious respiratory secretions, poor nutritional status and the edentulous state have been associated with poor outcomes with NIV (Davies et al., 2002).

Most ventilators used for noninvasive ventilation deliver either volume or pressure-targeted ventilation. In the volume-targeted ventilation, the ventilator delivers a fixed volume during a given time and will generate whatever pressure is necessary to achieve this, regardless of the patient contribution to ventilation. In pressure-targeted ventilation, the ventilator is set to deliver airflow by generating a predefined positive pressure in the airways for a given time. Airflow is therefore adjusted in order to establish and maintain a constant pressure in the airways. Bi-level ventilators are the most commonly used for noninvasive ventilation. These devices cycle between a higher inspiratory positive airway pressure (IPAP) and a lower expiratory positive airway pressure (EPAP) that can be independently adjusted. IPAP is the maximum inspiratory pressure level to be reached after the onset of the cycle triggered by the individual or ventilator and it plays an important role in unloading respiratory muscles, reducing the work of breathing, controlling obstructive hypopnea or flow limitation, maintaining alveolar ventilation, and reducing the partial pressure of carbon dioxide. EPAP allows the maintenance of positive pressure in the airways after expiration, contributing to alveolar recruitment and oxygenation leading to a decrease in re-inhalation, work of breathing and corrects hypoxemia (Davies et al., 2002; Hess, 2015).

The success of NIV depends in great measure on the interface, the element of interaction between the patient and the respirator and a perfect balance of mask efficacy and patient comfort and tolerance must be achieved. There are many different interfaces available including nasal mask, nasal pillows, oronasal mask, hybrid devices, total face mask and helmet, being the selection of the interface to each patient based on the comfort that is variable and different from a patient to another. The mask-related complications that develop most often are rejection due to discomfort, claustrophobia, facial erythema, leaks, skin rashes, conjunctivitis and pressure sores (Davies et al., 2002).

The more commonly used are nasal masks and facial masks. Nasal mask is the main choice of patients who use NIV over long periods at home. Facial masks were developed in an effort to increase tolerance of NIV, particularly in patients with acute respiratory failure. A variety of factors converge to limit the utility of nasal masks in uncooperative patients, such as those with ARI, tachypnea, and anxiety. One is leakage, a problem of such major importance that it alone can compromise the efficacy of NIV. A stubborn mouth leak decreases alveolar ventilation, reduces the positive pressure that affects respiratory muscles, and renders NIV less effective in reducing work of breathing. The need to administer the high flows that are usual in patients with ARI can also increase nasal resistance and likewise diminish the efficacy of ventilation delivered through a nasal mask. The face mask, covering both the nose and mouth, allows the patient to receive gases through both natural routes, eliminating the problem of mouth leaks and the increase of nasal resistance. Face masks interfere with feeding, communication, and expectoration, and they can give rise to claustrophobia in a large number of patients. Modern face masks have an anti-asphyxia, anti-rebreathing valve that allows patients to continue breathing spontaneously in case the respirator malfunctions. Total face masks have been developed in order to make NIV more comfortable. It is sealed around the entire perimeter of the patient's face, thereby avoiding the placement of direct pressure on anatomical structures, resulting in less leaks and improving patients' well-being.

Aerosol and HFNC

HFNC appeared initially for use in neonates. With scientific advances interesting new modes of delivering NIV were studied, mainly because e of the awareness of the potential damage associated with the use of invasive ventilation like ventilator-associated pneumonia and excessive pulmonary stress. HFNC allows the maintaining of a high oxygen flows and the increased end-expiratory pressure (PEEP), without compromising blood flow to skin areas susceptible to pressure sores (Helviz & Sharon, 2018).

HFNC devices only have two variables that are percentage of oxygen (FiO_2 ranging between 21-100%) and rate of gas flow (until 60L/min). The gas is humidified and heated to approximately normal body temperature.

The main advantages of HFNC are its capacity in giving a constant FiO_2 from 21-100%, gas flow until 60L/min, generation of a positive PEEP, reduction of the anatomical dead space, improvement of mucociliary clearance, reduction in the work of breathing, better comfort of the patient given by humidified and heated gas.

This is a versatile, friendly and comfortable ventilator (Maccari, et al., 2014; Helviz & Sharon, 2018).

Some of this patient will need aerosol therapy too. The high flow nasal cannula is increasingly used for hypoxemic respiratory failure and can also be used for aerosol delivery in the intensive care unit. The results in vitro studies suggest that aerosols can be delivery by HFNC (Maccari et al., 2014).

So, aerosol therapy can also be administrated during NIV, using devices adapted for inline administration.

REFERENCES

Beeh, K. M., Burgel, P. R., Franssen, F. M., Lopez-Campos, J. L., Loukides, S., Hurst, J. R., ... Valipour, A. (2017). How do dual long-acting bronchodilators prevent exacerbations of chronic obstructive pulmonary disease? *American Journal of Respiratory and Critical Care Medicine*, *196*(2), 139–149. doi:10.1164/rccm.201609-1794CI PMID:27922741

Boer, A. H., Hagedoorn, P., Hoppentocht, M., Buttini, F., Grasmeijer, F., & Frijlink, H. W. (2017). Dry powder inhalation: Past, present and future. *Expert Opinion on Drug Delivery*, *14*(4), 499–512. doi:10.1080/17425247.2016.1224846 PMID:27534768

Borghardt, J. M., Kloft, C., & Sharma, A. (2018). Inhaled Therapy in Respiratory Disease: The Complex Interplay of Pulmonary Kinetic Processes. *Canadian Respiratory Journal*, *2732017*, 1–11. Advance online publication. doi:10.1155/2018/2732017 PMID:30018677

Bosnic-Anticevich, S., Chrystyn, H., Costello, R. W., Dolovich, M. B., Fletcher, M. J., Lavorini, F., Rodríguez-Roisin, R., Ryan, D., Wan Yau Ming, S., & Price, D. B. (2017). The use of multiple respiratory inhalers requiring different inhalation techniques has an adverse effect on COPD outcomes. *International Journal of Chronic Obstructive Pulmonary Disease*, *12*, 59–71. doi:10.2147/COPD.S117196 PMID:28053517

British Thoracic Society Standards of Care Committee. (2002). Non-invasive ventilation in acute respiratory failure. *Thorax*, *57*(3), 192–211. doi:10.1136/thorax.57.3.192 PMID:11867822

Calzetta, L., Rogliani, P., Matera, M. G., & Cazzola, M. (2016). A systematic review with meta-analysis of dual bronchodilation with LAMA/LABA for the treatment of stable COPD. *Chest*, *149*(5), 1181–1196. doi:10.1016/j.chest.2016.02.646 PMID:26923629

Deng, Q., Deng, L., Miao, Y., Guo, X., & Li, Y. (2019). Particle deposition in the human lung: Health implications of particulate matter from different sources. *Environmental Research*, *169*, 237–245. doi:10.1016/j.envres.2018.11.014 PMID:30476747

Direção Geral de Saúde. (2011). *Cuidados de Saúde Respiratórios Domiciliários em Portugal*. DGS.

Fink, J. B., & Dhand, R. (2000). Aerosol therapy in mechanically ventilated patients: Recent advances and new techniques. *Seminars in Respiratory and Critical Care Medicine*, *21*(03), 183–201. doi:10.1055-2000-9854 PMID:16088731

França, E. E., Dornelas de Andrade, A. F., Cabral, G., Almeida Filho, P., Silva, K. C., Galindo Filho, V. C., Marinho, P. E. M., Lemos, A., & Parreira, V. F. (2006). Nebulization associated with bi-level noninvasive ventilation: Analysis of pulmonary radioaerosol deposition. *Respiratory Medicine, 100*(4), 721–728. doi:10.1016/j.rmed.2005.07.012 PMID:16139491

Helviz Y.& Einav S. (2018). A systematic review of the high-flow nasal cannula for adult patients. *Crit Care, 22*(1), 71.

Hess, D. R. (2015). Aerosol therapy during noninvasive ventilation or high-flow nasal cannula. *Respiratory Care, 60*(6), 880–891. doi:10.4187/respcare.04042 PMID:26070581

Levy, M. L., Dekhuijzen, P. N. R., Barnes, P. J., Broeders, M., Corrigan, C. J., Chawes, B. L., ... Roche, N. (2016). Inhaler technique: Facts and fantasies. A view from the Aerosol Drug Management Improvement Team (ADMIT). *NPJ Primary Care Respiratory Medicine, 26*(1), 16017. doi:10.1038/npjpcrm.2016.17 PMID:27098045

Maccari, J. G., Teixeira, C., Savi, A., Oliveira, R. P., Machado, A. S., Tonietto, T. F., & .... (2014). Nebulization during spontaneous breathing, CPAP, and bi-level positive-pressure ventilation: A randomized analysis of pulmonary radioaerosol deposition. *Respiratory Care, 59*(4), 479–484. doi:10.4187/respcare.02518 PMID:24003242

Miguel, A. F. (2017). Penetration of inhaled aerosols in the bronchial tree. *Medical Engineering & Physics, 44*, 25–31. doi:10.1016/j.medengphy.2017.03.004 PMID:28373015

Price, D., Østrem, A., Thomas, M., & Welte, T. (2017). Dual bronchodilation in COPD: Lung function and patient-reported outcomes–a review. *International Journal of Chronic Obstructive Pulmonary Disease, 12*, 141–168. doi:10.2147/COPD.S116719 PMID:28115839

Walenga, R. L., Longest, P. W., Kaviratna, A., & Hindle, M. (2017). Aerosol Drug Delivery During Noninvasive Positive Pressure Ventilation:Efffects of Intersubject Variability and Excipient Enhanced Growth. *Journal of Aerosol Medicine and Pulmonary Drug Delivery, 30*(3), 190–205. doi:10.1089/jamp.2016.1343 PMID:28075194

Yang, I. A., Brown, J. L., George, J., Jenkins, S., McDonald, C. F., McDonald, V. M., Phillips, K., Smith, B. J., Zwar, N. A., & Dabscheck, E. (2017). COPD-X Australian and New Zealand guidelines for the diagnosis and management of chronic obstructive pulmonary disease: 2017 update. *The Medical Journal of Australia, 207*(10), 436–442. doi:10.5694/mja17.00686 PMID:29129177

Chapter 12
Person in Need of Airway Cleaning and Use of Mechanical Insufflator-Exsufflator

Ana Daniela Costa
Hospital Center of Setúbal, Portugal

Raquel Cruz Amorim
Hospital Center of Setúbal, Portugal

Rogério Ferrinho Ferreira
https://orcid.org/0000-0001-5180-2036
Polytechnic Institute of Beja, Portugal

João Vitor Vieira
https://orcid.org/0000-0002-3905-4802
Polytechnic Institute of Beja, Portugal

ABSTRACT

Clearing of the airways in patients undergoing invasive mechanical ventilation (IMV) or non-invasive mechanical ventilation (NIMV) is a fundamental intervention that should be performed regularly, not only to avoid accumulation of secretions, but also to prevent the accumulation of secretions. One of the most relevant interventions in this type of patients is the use of the mechanical insufflator-exsufflator (MI-E), commonly known as cough assist. On the other hand, respiratory functional reeducation (RFR) involves a set of non-invasive procedures that allow the secretion to be released. The efficacy of the RFR associated with the use of MI-E presents gains resulting from this conjugation, namely when the person does not cooperate, when he/she shows a decrease in muscle strength or fails to present an effective cough. The integrative review of the literature has made evident the gains that exist for the person in intensive care, using MI-E associated with airway clearance, ventilation performance, airway permeability, decreased complications, and rate mortality.

DOI: 10.4018/978-1-7998-3531-8.ch012

Copyright © 2020, IGI Global. Copying or distributing in print or electronic forms without written permission of IGI Global is prohibited.

INTRODUCTION

The evolution of care was the motto of the specialty of Rehabilitation Nursing. Thus, it began to be seen as a creative process, which starts its immediate preventive care after the onset of illness or accident, and is important to schedule a recovery phase for adaptation to a new life with acquired comorbidities, after such event in the person's health (Hoeman, 2011).

In an Intensive Care Unit (ICU), the average length of hospital stay is six to 13 days. In the study by Júnior, Martinez, & Neto (2014), it was found that 40.9% of the admission reasons were neurological pathologies, followed by gastro-hepatic (22.7%) and cardiological (13.6%) pathologies. In this same study, it is explained that about 68% of the people were subjected to some type of sedation with an average period of two to six days. Regarding IMV, the mean duration of this therapy was approximately six to 12 days.

One of the main reasons for the abrupt reduction of natural airway defenses is endotracheal intubation, despite the fact that the ventilatory mechanisms present a great evolution; the quality of the supplied air decreases the capacity of the lower airway defenses (Barros, 2008).

Airway permeability and pulmonary ventilation can be significantly conditioned by situations that cause functional alterations of the airways, muco-ciliary system function, inspiratory and expiratory muscle strength, or coughing efficacy impairment . Pathological conditions of the respiratory system, such as atelectasis and pneumonia result from this process (Cordeiro, Menoita & Mateus, 2012).

The techniques of cleaning the airways have the benefits of: reducing the progression of respiratory disease, optimizing the mechanisms of muco-ciliary clearance, preventing bronchial obstruction and bronchial secretion, improving pulmonary ventilation, reducing energy expenditure during ventilation, maintaining ventilation mobility of the rib cage and to promote a greater effectiveness of the coughing, and facilitate expectoration (Bradley, Moran, & Elborn, 2006).

To RFR techniques we can associate MI-E, a device that enables a non-invasive method of mobilization and elimination of secretions. The use of this device is important for patients undergoing IMV or non-invasive mechanical ventilation (NIMV), since both may present significant difficulties in adapting to these types of ventilation, often justified by excess secretions of the airways.

It should be noted that even in patients who do not present an artificial airway or require any type of mechanical ventilation, there are benefits of using mechanically assisted coughing, since this minimizes the need for endotracheal intubation or tracheostomy and therefore minimizes the successive occurrences of hospital infection (Barros, 2008).

MECHANICAL INSUFFLATOR-EXSUFLATOR ASSOCIATED WITH AIRWAY CLEANING TECHNIQUES

Muscle weakness is usually associated with shallow breathing with low tidal volumes associated with a small vital capacity and an ineffective coughing by reducing the capacity of the inspiratory and expiratory muscle. The MI-E emerges as a noninvasive device that promotes inflation and then rapid exsufflation. The rapid transition of these two pressures (insufflation - positive pressure and exsufflation - negative pressure) provides a high respiratory flow, which simulate the more natural mode of coughing, thus causing respiratory secretions to be moved to facilitate their elimination in patients with ineffective coughing (Mendes, Chorão, Martinho, & Gabriel, 2013).

MI-E has been an effective technique in patients with muscle weakness. This therapy is perhaps the most mechanical physiological re-creation of a natural coughing, and when applied after extubating can improve secretion elimination in patients with acute respiratory disease and produces positive results (Gonçalves, Honrado, Winck, & Paiva, 2012).

Secretions are one of the main causes of respiratory failure after extubating. MI-E provides an efficient method for increasing coughing in respiratory patients in ICU, either through an endotracheal tube or through a face mask. This device mobilizes secretions in abundance and helps prevent orotracheal re-enactment and improve the effectiveness of NIV in patients developing respiratory failure after extubating (Gonçalves et al., 2012).

The feasible adjustment parameters of the device and its recommendations are presented in Table 1, according to Mendes et al. (2013).

Excessive pulmonary secretions may lead to increased resistance in the airways, partial or total obstruction, which promotes alveolar hypoventilation and, by inheritance, contributes to the appearance of atelectasis, hypoxemia and increased respiratory effort. Bacterial colonization and lung infections occur through the presence of pulmonary secretion stasis and atelectasis with greater ease (Dias et al., 2011).

The use of MI-E should be associated with area-path cleaning techniques. For Cordeiro et al. (2012), the objective of the techniques of cleaning the airways are to reduce the evolution of respiratory disease, optimize muco-ciliary clearance mechanisms, prevent bronchial obstruction and accumulation of secretions, benefit pulmonary ventilation, reduce energy expenditure during ventilation, to preserve the movements of the rib cage and to improve the effectiveness of the coughing, promoting the expiration.

Table 1. Parameters of mechanical insufflator-exsufflator

Manual / Auto Mode	Manual - the performer manually controls the time of insufflation, exsufflation and pause (better patient / device synchronization). Automatic - Cycles are programmed with insufflation / exsufflation / pause time
Times of insufflation, exsufflation and pause	Manual - does not allow Automatic - Various times can be used, such as 2,3,1 seconds or 3,4,4 seconds or a 3-second blow-up and a 2-second blow-up. What is important is the maximum synchrony between the device and the patient for greater benefit to the patient.
Inspiratory and expiratory pressures	Pressures – 0 to 60 cmH_2O There should be a progressive increase of the pressures up to the recommended optimum value of +/- 40 cmH_2O. Example: six cycles at 15 cmH_2O, six cycles at 30 cmH_2O and six cycles at 40 cmH_2O. If there is high pressure in the airways or reduced pulmonary compliance, patients may favor a higher pressure of +/- 60 cmH_2O.
Flow	High – Adult Low - Children; patients with instability in the upper airways The low-flow mode should always be associated with respiratory functional rehabilitation techniques for efficacy.

The cleansing techniques of the airways allow the area to be cleared, ensuring the elimination of secretions and improving pulmonary function, preventing pathophysiological changes that may compromise the efficacy of coughing and, consequently, pulmonary ventilation (Gomes & Ferreira, 2017).

The use of MI-E is essential to be associated with RFR. The program to be instituted requires individualization, taking into account factors such as pathology, severity of the problem, age, learning ability, program objectives, available material, motivation of the patient, among others (Cordeiro & Menoita, 2014).

One of the main goals of RFR is to ensure airway permeability. The most common maneuvers for clearing the airways are: directed coughing and / or assisted coughing; classical postural drainage; modified postural drainage; accessory maneuvers such as, precursor, vibration, compression and vibro-compression; flutter / acapella; positive expiratory pressure; total slow expiration with the glottis open in lateral decubitus; active cycle of respiratory techniques (Cordeiro & Menoita, 2014). Table 2 shows the techniques that optimize airway clearance.

The contraindications or limitations for using this type of program are the presence of hemoptysis and digestive hemorrhages, fever, acute pulmonary edema, shock state, acute pulmonary embolism, active pulmonary tuberculosis and lung and pleural cancer (Cordeiro & Menoita, 2014).

Table 2. Techniques that optimize airway cleanliness

Techniques that improve airway cleanliness	• Coughing (directed and assisted) • Postural drainage (classical and modified) • Autogenic drainage • the use of shock waves (manual vibration, thoracic percussions, manual compression) • Forced expiratory technique or Huff • Acceleration of expiratory flow or expiratory pressure • The active cycle of breathing • Total slow expiration with the glottis open in the lateral decubitus position • Supporting products (*vest, smartvest, acapella, Flutter, Shaker*)

(Gomes & Ferreira, 2017)

Earnings from Rehabilitation Nursing Intervention

The integrative literature review has become an appropriate method to synthesize the information of studies that address it, allowing the analysis of the scientific evidence around the central question of this investigation. This study involved the definition of the objective, formulation of the research question, methodology, results and discussion and main conclusions.

Objective

Identify the gains of the Rehabilitation Nursing intervention for people in Intensive Care who need to clean the airways and undergo the use of MI-E.

Research Question

For the selection of articles and formulation of the research question, the PI [C] OD methodology was used, being the target population (P), the type of Intervention (I), the comparisons (C), the outcome - outcome (O) and the type of study - design (D). The following question was elaborated to answer the objective outlined and that served as the guiding thread for this integrative review of the literature: What are the gains that exist (Outcomes) for the patient in intensive care (Population) using MI-E (Intervention)?

METHODOLOGY

After the formulation of the departure question, a research was done on the topic under study. The EBSCOHOST database was used and the MEDLINE COMPLETE and CINHAL COMPLETE databases were selected, with the following descriptors:

- "Airway Clearance", "Physiotherapy", "Mechanical Ventilation" e "Mechanically Ventilated".

The descriptors were searched at EBSCO in the following order:

- [(Airway Clearance)] AND
- [(Physiotherapy)] AND
- [(Mechanical Ventilation)] OR
- [(Mechanically Ventilated)]

The descriptors were searched in full text and retrospectively searched until 2014.

As inclusion criteria, articles with quantitative and / or qualitative, full-text methodologies that focused on the subject of study, from academic journals (analyzed by specialists) were privileged, with available references and with date published between January 2014 and December 2018.

In the exclusion criteria, all articles with ambiguous methodology, repeated in both databases, without correlation with the object of study and with dates below 2014 were considered.

The selection of papers involved the evaluation of the title and analysis of the abstract to verify that they met the inclusion and exclusion criteria. When the title and the abstract were not illuminating, the article was read in its entirety to minimize the loss of important studies for the accomplishment of this integrative review of the literature.

Eighteen articles from databases, MEDLINE COMPLETE and CINHAL COMPLETE were identified. After the abstracts were read, the potential interest for ten articles was justified. From these, six articles were selected as a result of the methodological quality analysis, after reading the article.

Given the articles selected, the critical analysis of methodological quality focused on the appreciation of the levels of evidence of each article. We used the contributions of Melnyk and Fineout-Overholt (2005), in order to identify the types of production of knowledge implicit in it. These authors considered the following levels of evidence:

- Level I - Systematic reviews (meta-analyzes, guidelines for clinical practice based on systematic reviews);
- Level II - Experimental studies;
- Level III - Near-experimental studies;
- Level IV - Non-experimental studies;
- Level V - Program evaluation reports / literature reviews;
- Level VI - Opinions of authorities / consensus panels.

In the evaluation of methodological quality, two researchers were involved, using the tools recommended by Joana Briggs Institute (2014), which determined the incorporation of articles that obeyed more than 50% of the quality criteria. Where necessary, a third researcher was used to analyze the articles.

In this process, two synthesis tables were constructed: the first to describe the studies and the second one to synthesize the results. These synthesis tables were constructed jointly by the researchers, culminating in the incorporation of six articles in this integrative review of the literature.

Results

With the purpose of answering the question of departure, several articles were read, aiming the analysis of its content. The results obtained are summarized in Table 3.

Discussion

Following the analysis carried out, four categories emerged, supported by the indicators systematized in Table 4.

Ventilator Performance

In the study by Camillis et al. (2018) it was found that the mobilization and removal of secretions from the airways during the rehabilitation program played an important role in increasing bronchial hygiene and gas exchange, thus optimizing the respiratory mechanics of patients considered critical and submitted mechanical ventilation. In this sense, the absence of a correct cleaning of the airways is associated with an increased risk of adverse effects such as pneumonia associated with mechanical ventilation and ineffective ventilatory weaning.

Intrapulmonary ventilation therapy in patients with thicker and more abundant secretions is a reasonable and safe therapeutic option (Camillis et al., 2018).

Table 3. Results of literature review

Authors / Method / Level of Evidence	Objectives	Results
Camillis et al. (2018) **Method:** Experimental study, with participants randomly assigned to two groups (experimental group and control group). **Level of evidence:** II **Participants:** 180 participants (90 in each group), hospitalized in the ICU older than 18 years and submitted to mechanical ventilation for more than 24 hours, with ventilatory and hemodynamic stability and no history of primary neuromuscular disease, or in exclusive palliative treatment or with pneumothorax or subcutaneous emphysema.	To evaluate the effectiveness of the technique of insufflation-mechanical exsufflation in airway clearance in patients hospitalized in the ICU who underwent mechanical ventilation.	After five minutes of application of the technique under study, the amount of aspirated secretions of the airway (in weight measurement), as well as the variation obtained (five minutes before and after the application of the technique) in pulmonary compliance, airway, ventilatory work and occurrence of adverse ventilatory and hemodynamic events during the procedure. Comparatively, the amount of aspirated secretions was higher in the intervention group. Statistical values of pulmonary compliance were also higher in the intervention group. The values regarding ventilatory work and airway resistance did not differ between the two study groups. There were no adverse ventilatory or hemodynamic events during the study interventions.
Ntoumenopoulos et al. (2017) **Method:** Prospective observational study. **Level of evidence:** IV **Participants:** 47 ICUs collected data from 230 mechanically ventilated and intubated patients submitted to airway cleansing techniques on a pre-specified day in the period between September and October 2015.	To describe the airway clearance process in mechanically ventilated and adult adults hospitalized in Australian and New Zealand ICUs (establishing the frequency and type of airway cleansing technique for this type of patient, as well as the methods used in management removal of endotracheal tube secretions and in large).	In about 78% of patients, the use of a moist atmosphere in the fluidization of secretions was described as the most common method. Aspiration of secretions was the technique most commonly used in the removal of secretions (in about 96% of the patients under study). On average, patients received 8.8 aspirations in a 24-hour period (221 patients). In 84/230 (37%) of the patients, additional techniques were used to clean the airways - ancillary vibration maneuvers [34/84 (40%)], manual over inflation 24/84 (29%), accessory percussion maneuvers [20/84 (24%)], postural drainage and therapeutic placement [17/84 (20%)] and other techniques such as patient mobilization [15/84 (18%].
Wang et al. (2016) **Method:** Experimental prospective study with participants randomly assigned to two groups. **Level of evidence:** II **Participants:** 164 patients diagnosed with exacerbation of Chronic Obstructive Pulmonary Disease and hypercapnia encephalopathy admitted to the ICU of a University Hospital in China between October 2013 and August 2015 (divided into two groups: 74 patients received NIMV treatment and 90 patients underwent invasive mechanical ventilation).	To compare the treatment of patients with exacerbation of Chronic Obstructive Pulmonary Disease and hypercapnia encephalopathy undergoing invasive mechanical ventilation with NIMV treatment associated with noninvasive secretion cleaning strategies.	Compared with baseline data, arterial gasimetry values increased significantly in both groups after two hours of mechanical ventilation, but no significant differences were found in pH, PaO2 / FiO2 and PaCO2 values between the two groups in the first two hours of treatment. The sensory level of patients receiving NIMV had a significant increase in the first two hours, but did not evolve in the group undergoing invasive mechanical ventilation (due to the use of sedation). There was a higher rate of complications in patients receiving invasive mechanical ventilation (with correlation to the occurrence of nosocomial infections and use of more devices considered invasive). There was a lower hospital mortality rate in the group receiving NIMV, but the same mortality rate within one year after hospital discharge, as well as the need for invasive mechanical ventilation and administration of long-term oxygen therapy was similar in both groups. NIMV treatment failed in 12 of the 74 participants (16%) after a total of 5.9 days, due to worsening of arterial gasimetry (n = 5), retention of secretions (n = 3), facial mask intolerance (n = 2) or worsening of the state of consciousness (n = 2). Facial erythema occurred in 22 participants. It was verified that four patients refused endotracheal intubation after treatment with NIMV and died of septic shock (n = 2) and cardiac arrest (n = 2). The causes of death in the group receiving treatment with invasive mechanical ventilation were septic shock (n = 8), cardiovascular complications (n = 6) and renal failure (n = 2). It should be noted that three patients in the group receiving treatment with invasive mechanical ventilation underwent tracheostomy and mechanical ventilation at home. There were no differences in the duration of mechanical ventilation and length of hospital stay in both groups. However, data analysis shows that the percentage of failure of ventilatory weaning within 30 days was significantly lower in the group receiving NIMV than in the other study group.
Coutinho et al. (2018) **Method:** Experimental study, with randomly selected participants (only one group receiving two different techniques on two consecutive days). **Level of evidence:** II **Participants:** 43 adult patients of both sexes hospitalized in an ICU between February and April 2014 and submitted to invasive mechanical ventilation for more than 48 hours. The inclusion criteria applied were: absence of facial trauma and hemodynamic stability. Patients with a history of pulmonary emphysema, presence of barotrauma, thrombocytopenia, and infeasibility to apply the techniques under study were excluded.	To compare the psychological effects and the volume of secretions removed through the use of MI-E compared to conventional aspiration of secretions (without the association of other techniques) in patients undergoing invasive mechanical ventilation.	The analysis of respiratory mechanics during the study period revealed no statistical difference in the dynamics of pulmonary compliance (MI-E, P = 0.58, conventional aspiration, P = 0.78) or pulmonary vascular resistance (MI-E, P = 0.87, conventional aspiration, P = 0.85). Regarding the hemodynamic variables, there were also no significant differences. When comparing the volume of aspirated secretions (in grams): MI-E, 8.42; Conventional aspiration: 7.09.

continued on following page

Table 3. Continued

Authors / Method / Level of Evidence	Objectives	Results
Volpe, Naves, Ribeiro, Ruas & Amato (2018) **Method:** Laboratory study conducted in nine trials conducted in two experiments for each three of the different scenarios (pulmonary impedance simulation), totaling 81 different test conditions. **Level of evidence:** IV	To evaluate the effects on the mobilization of secretions between the use of two mechanical insufflation-mechanical exsufflation devices (conventional version vs optimized version), with variables in the inflation velocity and pressure parameters, in scenarios that simulate patients submitted to invasive mechanical ventilation.	The first result was the amount of secretions mobilized (in centimeters) obtained through the use of the two different devices (conventional version vs. optimized version). The second analyzed result was the evidence of the effects of other variables observed in the ventilation due to the mobilization of secretions. The pressure and flow curve of the two devices were also studied, where in the optimized version the inspiratory flow pressure was much lower and the expiratory flow pressure slightly decreased. Consequently, the ratio of both expiratory and inspiratory flow pressures was higher in the optimized device (2.8 and 2.5 times higher, respectively). The optimized device mobilized secretions at a difference of 2.6 cm when compared to the conventional version. Analysis of the results of the various tests reveals that the increase in inspiratory / expiratory pressures from +30 / -30 cmH2O to +40 / -40 or +50 / -50 cmH2O (i.e., increase only the inspiratory / expiratory pressure mode), did not clearly increase the mobilization of secretions in any of the scenarios under study with the two different devices. However, when the inspiratory / expiratory pressure gradient (for example, increase from +30 / -30 cmH2O to +30 / -40 cmH2O or to +30 / -50 cmH2O) increases, the mobilization of secretions. It was verified that the ratio of expiratory / inspiratory flow pressure was lower in the scenario attributed to the obstructive lung, which resulted in a low mobilization of secretions.
Rose, Adhikari, Poon, Leasa & McKim (2016) **Method:** Non-experimental study conducted after a national survey and questionnaires in all ICUs in Canada, as well as in other high-dependency units, ventilatory weaning centers and other units providing specific care for patients undergoing prolonged invasive mechanical ventilation. **Level of evidence:** IV **Participants:** 238 questionnaires were applied between August and December 2014 (in the region of Canada with English language), and between February and June 2015 (in French-speaking regions). Inclusion criteria included units that used manual techniques of assisted coughing or insufflation-mechanical exsufflation device.	To describe the use, indications, contraindications, interfaces, definitions, complications and barriers of implementation of techniques that increase the efficiency of the coughing reflex in the process of cleaning the airways.	The study reveals that the most common techniques used to release secretions and increase coughing reflex are: manually assisted coughing techniques, increase and expansion of lung volume and use of mechanical insufflator-exsufflator. The most frequent indications for the use of these techniques are: presence of secretions in cases of re-infection, re-infection prevention, ventilatory weaning (either invasive mechanical ventilation or non-invasive ventilation). The most frequent diagnoses in which these techniques are used are: neuromuscular diseases, acquired weakness in the ICU, presence of secretions in patients with reduced lung volumes and difficulty in secretions elimination, restrictive diseases, chronic obstructive pulmonary disease (COPD), and acute respiratory failure. Concerning contraindications, only two units (3%) reported that they would use the techniques described in all patients, regardless of their diagnosis. More than 50% of the surveyed units stated that they would not apply the techniques in patients with COPD or acute respiratory failure. Pneumothorax was the most frequently reported pathology as an absolute contraindication for the use of mechanical insufflator-exsufflator (n = 41.93%) and application of pulmonary volume recruitment techniques (n = 44.83%), while costal mesh fracture was identified as the most common diagnosis for absolute contraindication for the use of assisted manual coughing techniques (n = 31.69%). The interfaces most used in the application of techniques are: endotracheal tube, face mask, mouthpiece and tracheostomy. The mean of the parameters used in the mechanical insufflator-exsufflator was 31 cmH2O at inspiratory pressure, and -32 cmH2O at expiratory pressure. Concerning the complications, the great majority of the units surveyed reported that the occurrence of complications associated with coughing increase techniques was infrequent. Maintenance care to the tracheostomy cannula after the use of the mechanical insufflator-exsufflator was pointed out as a frequent complication (23%). 45.36% of the units reported that patients reported chest pain after the application of manually assisted coughing techniques. In the recruitment of lung volume, hypotension was described as the most common symptom (17%). The lack of experienced professionals (45 of 66.70%), knowledge (43 of 66.65%), resources (34 of 66.52% and lack of equipment (33 of 66.50%) were described as the most in the application and use of these techniques.

For better ventilatory performance, Volpe et al. (2018) state that MI-E in the optimized version, characterized by slow inflation, has been shown to be more effective in mobilizing secretions when compared to the conventional version of the same device (where a faster inflation typically applies). The results indicate that the mobilization of secretions is strongly related to the current expiratory flow and not only to the peak expiratory flow (PEF) and also that the MI-E therapy can be enhanced by the definition of higher parameters in the differentials pressure. The study by Volpe et al. (2018) also revealed that MI-E has the capacity to achieve PEF greater than 160 L / min, which is the reference value for an effective coughing reflex.

Table 4. Synthesis of gains for the patient in intensive care with the use of MI-E associated with airway clearance

Categories	Indicators
Ventilatory performance	• Improved lung compliance: Camillis et al. (2018); • Improvement of sensory level in patients with NIMV in the first two hours: Wang et al. (2016); • Decreased inspiratory and expiratory flow pressure: Volpe et al. (2018); • Improvement in the relationship between expiratory and inspiratory flow pressures: Volpe et al. (2018).
Permeability of the airways	• Contributes to the release of secretions and increased coughing reflex: Rose et al. (2016); • Improvement in the volume of aspirated secretions: Camillis et al. (2018); Coutinho et al. (2018); • Improvement in the amount of mobilized secretions: Volpe et al. (2018).
Complications	• Reduced complication rate in patients with NIMV (compared to patients with IMV): Wang et al. (2016); • Reduction in the percentage of failure in ventilatory weaning within 30 days in patients with NIMV: Wang et al. (2016); • Decreased occurrence of complications of coughing-raising techniques: Rose et al. (2016).
Mortality rate	• Decrease in mortality rate in patients with NIMV (compared to patients with IMV): Wang et al. (2016).

These authors state that there are studies indicating that MI-E is more effective than manually assisted coughing, in terms of achieving this PEF target.

In the study by Rose et al. (2016), it was found that in a patient under controlled mechanical ventilation (i.e. without spontaneous ventilation) it is necessary to control the expiratory current flow, since in the use of MI-E in the removal of secretions, PEF control by itself just is not enough. Extubation of patients undergoing NIMV, in combination with manually assisted coughing and MI-E use, has been shown to decrease the need for re-enactment and tracheostomy in patients with neuromuscular disease. These authors further affirm that a rehabilitation program is strongly recommended in mechanically ventilated patients who exhibit decreased coughing reflex with muscle weakness but with hemodynamic stability since it prevents atelectasis, pneumonia and respiratory failure.

One of the main results obtained in the study presented by Wang et al. (2016), which states that noninvasive techniques for cleaning the airways in the first two hours in patients undergoing NIMV were considered safe and effective when applied to patients with acute exacerbation of COPD and hypercapnic encephalopathy. In fact, after two hours of use of the technique of cleaning of airways in the patients with NIMV, an improvement of the gasometric values was verified, and no complications were observed. In both groups, Wang et al. (2016), improvements in pH, PaO2 / FiO2 and PaCO2, as well as decreased duration of hospitalization were recorded.

However, in the group submitted to NIMV, a significantly shorter time was observed in the effective ventilatory weaning process.

Permeability of the Airways

During voluntary coughing, the importance of current expiratory flow in the removal of secretions may be concealed by the fact that peak inspiratory flow (PIF) is often much lower than PEF. However, the influence of PIF is minimized and PEF emerges as the key determinant for eliminating secretions present in the pathways (Volpe et al., 2018). The difference between PEF-PIF is referred to as the variable that best demonstrates the mobilization of secretions and above the reference value (17L / min) the larger the difference between PEF-PIF, the greater amount of secretions are mobilized.

Regarding the cleansing of the airways, it is demonstrated that the inspiratory flow cannot be neglected especially in mechanically ventilated patients who are sedated. The use of MI-E minimizes the risk of hypersecretion after extubating when applied immediately before the extubating process (Volpe et al., 2018).

Coughing is the largest and most important component of the cleansing of the areas. The efficacy of coughing is related to the peak flow of coughing (Coutinho et al., 2018). In order to increase the efficacy of this reflex in patients undergoing mechanical ventilation, we have as main therapeutic target, the optimization of peak expiratory coughing flow, which can be provided through the devices, and this is often the reason for its use. In this process, we must take into account the various clinical conditions (decreased coughing reflex, neuromuscular disease and polyneuropathies). The presence of artificially-via pathway may influence the decrease in peak coughing flow, reducing the ability to remove secretions.

The results obtained through the study of Ntoumenopouls et al. (2017), show that 37% of ventilated patients used additional secretion removal techniques. The most common techniques for cleaning the pathways include chest wall vibration followed by manual hyperinflation, percussion maneuvering, postural drainage / positioning, and mobilization of the patient.

In the study Coutinho et al. (2018), we compared the effects of MI-E vs. endotracheal aspiration, the relationship between hemodynamic stability and respiratory mechanics, as well as the ability of each technique to remove secretions. After evaluating the efficacy of the use of the device, and after adjustment of the parameters, the results obtained were significantly positive, with the re-exposure rate being only 17% in the study group compared to 49% in the control group. However, the main result obtained through this study reveals that there is no significant difference in the amount of aspirated secretions when compared to the use of MI-E with conventional tracheal aspiration, 8.42 g vs. 7.09gr, respectively.

The use of the MI-E device during the rehabilitation program applied to critically ill patients submitted to mechanical ventilation has the potential to increase the occurrence of relevant outcomes, such as reduction of ventilation-associated pneumonia, decreased duration of mechanical ventilation and length of stay in the ICU (Camillis et al., 2018).

Coughing enhancement techniques, which lead to increased lung volume capacity or assisted manual or mechanical coughing techniques, may be used to prevent and manage respiratory complications associated with chronic complications, in particular in neuromuscular diseases in patients with tracheal devices, allowing a short and long term increase in the positive results of patients with acute respiratory failure (Camillis et al., 2018).

In the study developed by Ntoumenopouls et al. (2017), a rehabilitation program including RFR techniques was applied in 89% of 100 patients admitted to the ICU. The techniques most used to clean the airways were postural repositioning / drainage (55%) and hyperinflation using the ventilator (27%).

Complications

Although the potential advantages of using NIMV on VMI are well documented, NIMV is usually not recommended in patients with altered consciousness, with stasis of secretions secondary to coughing reflex depression, and risk of aspiration as the protection of the area. The ineffectiveness of NIMV is usually attributed to a reflection of ineffective coughing, excess secretions, hypercapnic encephalopathy, tolerance, and asynchrony (Wang et al., 2016).

In the study by Wang et al. (2016), it was found that the use of NIMV combined with non-invasive area-path cleansing strategies was more effective in the first two hours of treatment of patients with acute exacerbation of COPD complicated by hypercapnic encephalopathy. Also in this study, it is reported that 78% of patients treated with NIMV showed improvement in their state of consciousness and a stabilization of the pH value within 48% for reference values and that 69% survived. NIMV was successfully used in 72% of patients with acute exacerbation of COPD and hypercapnic encephalopathy with a survival rate of 86%. It was pointed out as the main reason for failure the excessive presence of secretions (Wang et al., 2016).

NIMV was associated with a reduced incidence of complications (nosocomial infections or sepsis) and a shorter time of need for ventilation (Wang et al., 2016).

Decreased coughing reflex leads to inefficient pathway clearance and is the most common cause of NIMV use failure. This is considered a relative contraindication, especially in patients with altered consciousness and suppressed coughing reflex (Wang et al., 2016).

Contrary to the person submitted to IMV with artificial airway, the person undergoing NIMV does not have direct access to the areas, which is a disadvantage in the removal of secretions. The implementation of a rehabilitation program increases the muco-ciliary clearance during the use of this technique.

The adoption of techniques for increasing coughing reflex associated with alveolar recruitment are the most frequently used techniques. The efficacy and the reduced number of complications with respect to these techniques when applied to critically ill patients is recognized from the perspective of Rose et al. (2016). Patients with neuromuscular disease had a significantly low re-intubation.

In this study by Rose et al. (2016), it is demonstrated that the use of MI-E associated with manual coughing techniques, before and after, of the extubating process in NIV reveals a 100% success rate in extubating in patients with peak coughing greater than 160 l / min and 80% success in extubating patients with peak coughing flow of 160 l / min or less.

Mortality Rate

The study by Wang et al. (2016) demonstrated that the use of NIMV significantly reduced mortality rates, intubation, complications related to invasive ventilation and duration of ventilation. The group in which this technique was used presented a lower rate of complications due to nosocomial infections, as well as a lower percentage of hospital mortality.

CONCLUSION

The integrative review of the literature has made explicit the gains that exist for the patient in intensive care, using MI-E associated with airway clearance, ventilation performance, airway permeability, complications and mortality rate.

Evidence demonstrates that in terms of ventilatory performance, there is an improvement in pulmonary compliance, a sensory improvement in patients with NIMV in the first two hours, a decrease in inspiratory and expiratory flow pressure, and an improvement in the relationship between expiratory flow pressures and inspiratory.

The use of the MI-E device during a respiratory functional rehabilitation program is considered safe and more effective in the cleaning of the area routes than a rehabilitation program without the use of it. The MI-E, when applied with slower inflation, is more effective in the mobilization of secretions compared to its use with higher values. This fact results in an increase in the expiratory tidal volume, being this determinant in the removal of secretions, independently of the expiratory flow pressure. The efficacy of coughing enhancement techniques in the management of hypersecretion, as well as gains in the volume of mobilized and aspirated secretions.

The rate of complications and the mortality rate decreased particularly in patients with NIMV, compared to patients with IMV.

The nurse specialist in rehabilitation nursing is a professional with a set of specific skills to provide care to people in intensive care, needing airway clearance and involving the use of MI-E. Its integration into the dynamics of a multidisciplinary team is a key factor in the implementation of rehabilitation programs that allow to promote the association between the use of airway cleansing techniques and the use of this device.

Considering the reality of ICUs, where only 1/3 of the mechanically ventilated and intubated patients receive additional techniques for clearing the airways, there is a need to modify potential barriers to RFR interventions. The development of research projects in the reality of intensive care with people requiring airway clearance and involving the use of MI-E are crucial to substantiate the efficacy and relevance of these techniques and the need to value the use of less invasive procedures.

It is fundamental to carry out research that makes it possible to highlight the importance of nursing specialists in rehabilitation in the quality of life of these patients with airway clearance problems, undoubtedly contributing to the development of knowledge related to nursing care in this domain of knowledge in Nursing.

Given the importance of the intervention of the specialist rehabilitation nurse in the development of specialized care for these people, it is essential that health institutions value their skills in the prevention of complications and in the rehabilitation of people, in a multidisciplinary team dynamics.

The professional development of rehabilitation nurses should involve a continuous process of learning in programs and strategies of professional intervention that ensure gains in the care to the people in intensive care and in need of cleaning of the airways. It is a process that must reconcile the needs and interests of the people, in the organizational perspective, with the motivations of these professionals specialized in rehabilitation nursing.

We believe that this path will be decisive for the development of nursing discipline and profession, in favor of improving care for the person with airway cleaning needs.

REFERENCES

Barros, L. (2008). *Dipositivo Mecânico que Promove Insuflação e Exsuflação Pulmonar* (Dissertação de Mestrado não publicada). Universidade Federal de Minas Gerais, Belo Horizonte. Retrieved from: http://www.bibliotecadigital.ufmg.br/dspace/bitstream/handle/1843/MDAD-7VRJD2/tese_completa.pdf?sequence=1

Bradley, J., Moran, F., & Elborn, J. (2006). Evidence for physical therapies (airway clearance and physical training) in cystic fibrosis: An overview of five Cochrane systematic reviews. *Respiratory Medicine*, *100*(2), 191–201. doi:10.1016/j.rmed.2005.11.028 PMID:16412951

Camillis, M., Savi, A., Rosa, R., Figueiredo, M., & Wickert, R. (2018). Effects of Mechanical Insufflation-Exsufflation on Airway Mucus Clearance Among Mechanically Ventilated ICU Subjects. *Respiratory Care*, *63*(12), 1471–1477. doi:10.4187/respcare.06253 PMID:30018175

Cordeiro, M., & Menoita, E. (2012). *Manual de boas práticas na reabilitação respiratória: conceitos, princípios e técnicas*. Loures: Lusociência.

Cordeiro, M., Menoita, E., & Mateus, D. (2012). Limpeza das Vias Aéreas: Conceitos, Técnicas e Princípios. *Journal of Aging & Innovation*, *1*(5), 30–44. http://www.journalofagingandinnovation.org/wp-content/uploads/4-Limpeza-das-vias-aereas.pdf

Coutinho, W., Vieira, P., Kutchak, F., Dias, A., Rieder, M., & Forgarini, L. (2018). Comparison of Mechanical Insufflation-Exsufflation and Endotracheal Suctioning in Mechanically Ventilated Patients: Effects on Respiratory Mechanics, Hemodynamics, and Volume of Secretions. *Indian Journal of Critical Care Medicine: Peer-Reviewed, Official Publication of Indian Society of Critical Care Medicine*, *22*(7), 485–490. doi:10.4103/ijccm.IJCCM_164_18 PMID:30111922

Dias, C., Siqueira, T., Faccio, T., Gontijo, L., Salge, J., & Volpe, M. (2011). Efetividade e segurança da técnica de higiene brônquica: Hiperinsuflação manual com compressão torácica. *Revista Brasileira de Terapia Intensiva*, *23*(2), 190–198. doi:10.1590/S0103-507X2011000200012 PMID:25299720

Gomes, B., & Ferreira, D. (2017). Enfermagem de Reabilitação à Pessoa submetida a Ventilação Mecânica. In C. Marques-Vieira & L. Sousa (Eds.), Cuidados de Enfermagem de Reabilitação à Pessoa ao Longo da Vida (pp. 365-380). Loures: Lusodidacta.

Gonçalves, M. R., Honrado, T., Winck, J. C., & Paiva, J. A. (2012). Effects of mechanical insufflation-exsufflation in preventing respiratory failure after extubation: A randomized controlled trial. *Critical Care (London, England)*, *16*(2), R48. doi:10.1186/cc11249 PMID:22420538

Hoeman, S. P. (2011). História, Controvérsias e Tendências. In S. P. Hoeman (Coord., Enfermagem de Reabilitação. Prevenção, Intervenção e Resultados Esperados (4th ed., pp. 1-13). Loures: Lusodidacta.

Joana Briggs Institute. (2014). *Joana Briggs Institute Reviewers' Manual* (2014 edition). Joana Briggs Institute.

Júnior, B., Martinez, B., & Neto, M. (2014). Impacto do Internamento em Unidade de Cuidados Intensivos na Amplitude de Movimento de Pacientes Graes: Estudo Piloto. *Revista Brasileira de Terapia Intensiva*, *26*(1), 65–70. doi:10.5935/0103-507X.20140010 PMID:24770691

Mendes, R., Chorão, R., Martinho, F., & Gabriel, J. (2013). In-exsuflação mecânica em cuidados intensivos a propósito de um caso clínico de atelectasia pulmonar. *Revista de Saúde Amato Lusitano, 32*, 47-51. Retrieved from: http://portaisuls.azurewebsites.net/ulscb/wp-content/uploads/sites/9/2017/02/Revista-32-1.trimestre-2013.pdf

Ntoumenopoulos, G., Hammond, N., Watts, N., Thompson, K., Hanlon, G., Paratz, J., & Thomas, P. (2018). Secretion clearance Strategies in Australian and New Zealand Intensive Care Units. *Australian Critical Care*, *31*(4), 191–196. doi:10.1016/j.aucc.2017.06.002 PMID:28662942

Rose, L., Adhikari, N., Poon, J., Leasa, D., & McKim, D. (2016). Cough Augmentation Techniques in the Critically Ill: A Canadian National Survey. *Respiratory Care*, *61*(10), 1360–1368. doi:10.4187/respcare.04775 PMID:27624630

Volpe, M., Naves, J., Riberio, G., Ruas, G., & Amato, M. (2018). Airway Clearance with na Optimized Mechanical Insufflation-Exsufflation Maneuver. *Respiratory Care*, *63*(10), 1214–1222. doi:10.4187/respcare.05965 PMID:30018177

Wang, J., Cui, Z., Liu, S., Gao, X., Gao, P., Shi, Y., Guo, S., & Li, P. (2016). Early use of noninvasive techniques for clearing respiratory secretions during noninvasive positive-pressure ventilation in patients with acute exacerbation of chronic obstructive pulmonary disease and hypercapnic encephalopathy: A prospective cohort study. *Medicine*, *96*(12), e6371. doi:10.1097/MD.0000000000006371 PMID:28328824

Compilation of References

Aboussouan, L. S. (2009). Mechanisms of exercise limitation and pulmonary rehabilitation for patients with neuromuscular disease. *Chronic Respiratory Disease, 6*(4), 231–249. doi:10.1177/1479972309345927 PMID:19858353

Acker, G. M. (2011). Burnout among mental health care providers. *Journal of Social Work, 24*(2), 112–119.

Agudelo, D., Buela-Casal, G., & Mental, C. (2007). Ansiedad y depresión: el problema de la diferenciación a través de los síntomas. *Medigraphic.Com.* Retrieved from https://www.medigraphic.com/cgi-bin/new/resumen.cgi?IDARTICULO=16113

Akyil, F. T., Gunen, H., Agca, M., Gungor, S., Yalcinsoy, M., Sucu, P., Akyil, M., & Sevim, T. (2016). Patient outcome after COPD exacerbations requiring non-invasive ventilation during hospitalization. *Archivos de Bronconeumologia, 52*(9), 470–476. doi:10.1016/j.arbr.2016.03.012 PMID:27156204

Albuquerque, I., Machado, A., Carvalho, M., & Soares, J. (2015). Impact of early mobilization in Intensive care patient. *Salud(i)Ciencia, 21*, 403-406. Retrieved from: https://www.siicsalud.com/dato/sic/214/146066.pdf

Alcántara Santaigo, Z. R., Torres Amengual, M., Martinez Fernandez, C. A., & García Jiménez, E. (2014). ¿Somos conscientes de nuestras creencias? Estudio piloto. *Paraninfo Digital.* Recuperado de: http://www.index-f.com/para/n20/pdf/381.pdf

Alencar, T. A. M. D., & Matias, K. F. D. S. (2010). Princípios fisiológicos do aquecimento e alongamento muscular na atividade esportiva. *Revista Brasileira de Medicina do Esporte, 16*(3), 230–234. doi:10.1590/S1517-86922010000300015

Allué, M. (2002). *Temporarily valid: an ethnography on the environment of disability* (PhD thesis). Universitat Rovira i Virgili.

Alonso, J., & Sobradillo, V. (2004). Continuous home oxygen therapy: A good treatment if it is done well. *Anales de Medicina Interna (Madrid, Spain), 21*, 5–7.

Álvarez-Sala, J., Cimas, E., Masa, J., Miravitlles, M., Molina, J., Naberan, K. . . . of Pneumology, E. (2001). Recommendations for the care of patients with chronic obstructive pulmonary disease. *Bronchopneumology Archives, 37*(7), 269-278.

Ambrosino, N., & Cigni, P. (2015). Non invasive ventilation as an additional tool for exercise training. *Multidisciplinary Respiratory Medicine, 10*(1), 14. doi:10.118640248-015-0008-1 PMID:25874110

Ambrosino, N., Venturelli, E., Vagheggini, G., & Clini, E. (2012). Rehabilitation, weaning and physical therapy strategies in chronic critically ill patients. *The European Respiratory Journal, 39*(2), 487–492. doi:10.1183/09031936.00094411 PMID:22135278

American Association of Cardiovascular & Pulmonary Rehabilitation. (2011). Guidelines for Pulmonary Rehabilitation Programs. In Human Kinetics (4th ed.). Author.

American College of Sports Medicine (2014). *Diretrizes do ACSM para os testes de esforço e sua prescrição* (9th ed.). Guanabara Koognan Ltda.

American College of Sports Medicine. (2009). American College of Sports Medicine position stand. Progression models in resistance training for healthy adults. *Medicine and Science in Sports and Exercise, 41*(3), 687–708. doi:10.1249/MSS.0b013e3181915670 PMID:19204579

American Psychological Association. (2010). *Publication Manual of the American Psychological Association* (6th ed.). Author.

Ancochea, J., Badiola, C., Duran-Tauleria, E., Rio, F. G., Miravitlles, M., Muñoz, L., ... Soriano, J. (2009). EPI-SCAN study: Summary of the protocol of a study to estimate the prevalence of COPD in people aged 40 to 80 in Spain. *Bronchopneumology Archives, 45*(1), 41–47. doi:10.1016/j.arbres.2008.06.001

Andretta, G., & Genske, J. H. (2018). Índice de sucesso da ventilação não invasiva em um hospital universitário e o perfil desses pacientes. *Revista Varia Scientia: Ciências da Saúde, 1*(4), 1–9.

Ankjaergaard, K., Tonnesen, P., Laursen, L., Hansen, E., Andreassen, H., & Wilcke, J. (2016). *Home Non Invasive Ventilation (NIV) treatment for COPD patients with a history of NIV- treated exacerbation; a randomized, controlled, multi-center study*. BioMed Central. doi:10.118612890-016-0184-6

Anne, B., Didier, T., Jean-paul, J., Jean-bernard, M., Samir, J., & Philippe, J. (2005). laboratory and animal investigations Performance Characteristics of 10 Home Mechanical Ventilators in. *Chest, 127*(5), 1784–1792. doi:10.1378/chest.127.5.1784 PMID:15888859

Antonio, J., Fernández-Fidalgo, M., & Cieza, A. (2010). Los conceptos de calidad de vida, salud y bienestar analizados desde la perspectiva de la Clasificación Internacional del Funcionamiento (CIF). In *Revista española de salud pública. Revista Española de Salud Pública* (Vol. 84). Ministerio de Sanidad y Consumo. Retrieved from http://scielo.isciii.es/scielo.php?script=sci_arttext&pid=S1135-57272010000200005

Araújo, R. B., Camisasca, M. T., Britto, R. R., & Parreira, V. F. (2017). O uso da ventilação não-invasiva na reabilitação pulmonar em pacientes portadores da doença pulmonar obstrutiva crônica: Uma revisão de literatura. *Fisioterapia em Movimento*, *18*(1), 49–57.

Arbillaga-Etxarri, A., Gimeno-Santos, E., Barberan-Garcia, A., Benet, M., Borrell, E., Dadvand, P., Foraster, M., Marín, A., Monteagudo, M., Rodriguez-Roisin, R., Vall-Casas, P., Vilaró, J., & Garcia-Aymerich, J. (2017). Socio-environmental correlates of physical activity in patients with chronic obstructive pulmonary disease (COPD). *Thorax*, *72*(9), 796–802. doi:10.1136/thoraxjnl-2016-209209 PMID:28250201

Ardila, R. (2003). Quality of life: An inclusive definition. *Revista Latinoamericana de Psicología*, *35*(2), 161–164.

Area, G. L., Janssens, J., Derivaz, S., & Breitenstein, E. (2003). *Changing Patterns in Long-term Noninvasive Ventilation: A 7-Year Prospective Study in the*. doi:10.1378/chest.123.1.67

Asaba, E., Nakamura, M., Asaba, A., & Kottorp, A. (2017). Integrating Occupational Therapy Specific Assessments in Practice: Exploring Practitioner Experiences. *Occupational Therapy International*, *7602805*, 1–8. Advance online publication. doi:10.1155/2017/7602805 PMID:29333112

Bach, J. R., & Martinez, D. (2011). Duchenne muscular dystrophy: Continuous noninvasive ventilatory support prolongs survival. *Respiratory Care*, *56*(6), 744–750. doi:10.4187/respcare.00831 PMID:21333078

Balachandran, S., D'Souza, M., Radhakrishnan, J., & Venkatesaperumal, R. (2013). Role of a nurse in non-invasive positive Pressure ventilation: A conceptual model for clinical practice. *International Journal of Nursing Education*, *1*(5), 119–123.

Balady, G. J., Arena, R., Sietsema, K., Myers, J., Coke, L., Fletcher, G. F., Forman, D., Franklin, B., Guazzi, M., Gulati, M., Keteyian, S. J., Lavie, C. J., Macko, R., Mancini, D., & Milani, R. V. (2010). Clinician's guide to cardiopulmonary exercise testing in adults. A scientific statement from the American Heart Association. *Circulation*, *122*(2), 191–225. doi:10.1161/CIR.0b013e3181e52e69 PMID:20585013

Balbo, N. A., Acosta, M. A., & Kevorkof, G. V. (2012). *Calidad de vida en pacientes EPOC con oxigenoterapia crónica domicialiaria* (Vol. 69). Retrieved from http://www.revista2.fcm.unc.edu.ar/2012.69.2/Epoc/EPOC.pdf

Balboa, M., Pérez, M., & Sarasola, J. L. (2012). Propuestas saludables para el envejecimiento activo. *Revista de Educación Hekademos.*, *11*(5), 29–36.

Banfi, P., Cappuccio, A., Latella, M. E., Reale, L., Muscianisi, E., & Marini, M. G. (2018). Narrative medicine to improve the management and quality of life of patients with COPD: The first experience applying parallel chart in Italy. *International Journal of Chronic Obstructive Pulmonary Disease*, *13*, 287–297. doi:10.2147/COPD.S148685 PMID:29391786

Barros, L. (2008). *Dipositivo Mecânico que Promove Insuflação e Exsuflação Pulmonar* (Dissertação de Mestrado não publicada). Universidade Federal de Minas Gerais, Belo Horizonte. Retrieved from: http://www.bibliotecadigital.ufmg.br/dspace/bitstream/handle/1843/MDAD-7VRJD2/tese_completa.pdf?sequence=1

Basheer, R., & Shiromani, P. J. (2001). Effets of prolonged wakefulness on c-fos and AP1 activity in Young and old rats. *Brain Research. Molecular Brain Research*, *89*(1-2), 153–157. doi:10.1016/S0169-328X(01)00045-6 PMID:11311986

Beeh, K. M., Burgel, P. R., Franssen, F. M., Lopez-Campos, J. L., Loukides, S., Hurst, J. R., ... Valipour, A. (2017). How do dual long-acting bronchodilators prevent exacerbations of chronic obstructive pulmonary disease? *American Journal of Respiratory and Critical Care Medicine*, *196*(2), 139–149. doi:10.1164/rccm.201609-1794CI PMID:27922741

Bellido Vallejo, J. C., & Lendínez Cobo, J. F. (2010). *Proceso Enfermero desde el modelo de cuidados de Virginia Henderson y los Lenguajes NNN*. Ilustre Colegio Oficial de Enfermería de Jaén. España. Primera Edición. Disponible en: www.index-f. com/lascasas/documentos/lc0714.pdf

Bello, S., Naranjo, C., Hinrichsen, J., & Morales, M. (2002). Oxigenoterapia domiciliaria a largo plazo, necesidad apremiante en enfermos con insuficiencia respiratoria crónica. *Revista Chilena de Enfermedades Respiratorias*, *18*(3), 175–181. doi:10.4067/S0717-73482002000300007

Benner, P. (2001). *De iniciado a perito: excelência e poder na prática clínica de enfermagem*. Quarteto Editora.

Betancourt-Peña, J., & Tonguino-Rosero, S. (2016). Impacto de la oxigenoterapia domiciliaria en la capacidad funcional de pacientes con enfermedad pulmonar obstructiva crónica. *Rehabilitacion*, *50*(1), 13–18. doi:10.1016/j.rh.2015.10.001

Bhushan, B., Ayub, B., Thompson, D. M., Abdullah, F., & Billings, K. R. (2016). *Impact of Short Sleep on Metabolic Variables in Obese Children With Obstructive Sleep Apnea*. doi:10.1002/lary.26420

Bielicki, P., Byskniewicz, K., Kumor, M., Korczynski, P., & Chazan, R. (2006). Obstructive sleep apnoa syndrome in yourger and older age groups –differences and similarities. *Pneumonologia i Alergologia Polska*, *74*(1), 56–58.

Blanco, J. B., Ribeiro, R., & Alves, I. (2011). Protocolo de Início da VMNI. In A. M. Esquinas (Eds.), Princípios da Ventilação Mecânica Não Invasiva – Do Hospital ao Domicílio. Vila do Conde: Gasin Médica.

Blanco, J. B., Ribeiro, R., & Alves, I. (2011). Protocolo de início da VMNI. In A. M. Esquinas (Ed.), *Princípios da Ventilação Mecânica Não Invasiva - Do Hospital ao Domicílio* (pp. 173–185). Gasin Médica.

Bloom, H. G., Ahmed, I., Alessi, C. A., Ancoli-Israel, S., Buysse, D. J., Kryger, M. H., Phillips, B. A., Thorpy, M. J., Vitiello, M. V., & Zee, P. C. (2009). Evidence-based recommendations for the assessment and management of sleep disorders in older persons. *Journal of the American Geriatrics Society*, *57*(5), 761–789. doi:10.1111/j.1532-5415.2009.02220.x PMID:19484833

Bobak, M., Bobrova, N., West, R., Malyutina, D., & Malyutina, S. (2010). Gender differences in drinking practices in middle aged and older Russians. *Alcohol and Alcoholism (Oxford, Oxfordshire)*, *45*(6), 573–580. doi:10.1093/alcalc/agq069 PMID:21075855

Boer, A. H., Hagedoorn, P., Hoppentocht, M., Buttini, F., Grasmeijer, F., & Frijlink, H. W. (2017). Dry powder inhalation: Past, present and future. *Expert Opinion on Drug Delivery*, *14*(4), 499–512. doi:10.1080/17425247.2016.1224846 PMID:27534768

Bohannon, R. W. (1995). Sit-to-stand test for measuring performance of lower extremity muscles. *Perceptual and Motor Skills*, *80*(1), 163–166. doi:10.2466/pms.1995.80.1.163 PMID:7624188

Bonsaksen, T., Fagermoen, M. S., & Lerdal, A. (2016). Trajectories of physical and mental health among persons with morbid obesity and persons with COPD: A longitudinal comparative study. *Journal of Multidisciplinary Healthcare*, *9*, 191. doi:10.2147/JMDH.S102630 PMID:27175082

Borel, J., Tamisier, R., Gonzalez-bermejo, J., Baguet, J., Pharmd, D. M., Arnol, N., ... Pépin, J. (2012). Noninvasive Ventilation in Mild Obesity. *Chest*, *141*(3), 692–702. doi:10.1378/chest.10-2531 PMID:21885724

Borg, G. A. (1982). Psychophysical bases of perceived exertion. *Medicine and Science in Sports and Exercise*, *14*(5), 377–381. doi:10.1249/00005768-198205000-00012 PMID:7154893

Borghardt, J. M., Kloft, C., & Sharma, A. (2018). Inhaled Therapy in Respiratory Disease: The Complex Interplay of Pulmonary Kinetic Processes. *Canadian Respiratory Journal*, *2732017*, 1–11. Advance online publication. doi:10.1155/2018/2732017 PMID:30018677

Bosnic-Anticevich, S., Chrystyn, H., Costello, R. W., Dolovich, M. B., Fletcher, M. J., Lavorini, F., Rodríguez-Roisin, R., Ryan, D., Wan Yau Ming, S., & Price, D. B. (2017). The use of multiple respiratory inhalers requiring different inhalation techniques has an adverse effect on COPD outcomes. *International Journal of Chronic Obstructive Pulmonary Disease*, *12*, 59–71. doi:10.2147/COPD.S117196 PMID:28053517

Boticario, C., & Angosto, M. C. (2010). Hypoxia and cancer. *Annals of the Royal National Academy of Pharmacy*, *76*(3).

Bott, J., Blumenthal, S., Buxton, M., Ellum, S., Falconer, C., Garrod, R., ... Potter, C. (2009). Guidelines for the physiotherapy management of the adult, medical, spontaneously breathing patient. *Thorax*, *64*(Suppl 1), i1–i52. doi:10.1136/thx.2008.110726 PMID:19406863

Bourdieu, P., Passeron, J. C., & Chamboredon, J.-C. (1968). *Le Métier de sociologue*. Mouton, Bordas.

Bradley, J. & O'Neill, B. (2007). Short-term ambulatory oxygen for chronic obstructive pulmonary disease. *Cochrane Library Plus, 4*.

Bradley, J., Moran, F., & Elborn, J. (2006). Evidence for physical therapies (airway clearance and physical training) in cystic fibrosis: An overview of five Cochrane systematic reviews. *Respiratory Medicine*, *100*(2), 191–201. doi:10.1016/j.rmed.2005.11.028 PMID:16412951

Branco, P., Barata, S., Barbosa, J., Cantista, M., Lima, A., & Maia, J. (2012). *Temas de Reabilitação–Reabilitação Respiratória*. Servier.

British Thoracic Society Standards of Care Committee. (2002). Non-invasive ventilation in acute respiratory failure. *Thorax*, *57*(3), 192–211. doi:10.1136/thorax.57.3.192 PMID:11867822

Bronc, A. (2005). Documento consenso español sobre el síndrome de apneas-hipopneas del sueño. *Grupo Español de Sueño*, *41*, 4.

Cafarella, P. A., Effing, T. W., Usmani, Z.-A., & Frith, P. A. (2012). Treatments for anxiety and depression in patients with chronic obstructive pulmonary disease: A literature review. *Respirology (Carlton, Vic.)*, *17*(4), 627–638. doi:10.1111/j.1440-1843.2012.02148.x PMID:22309179

Calzada, N., Soro, E., Gomez, L., Bulta, E., Izquierdo, A., Panades, M., Sargatal, J., & Muñoz, E. (2016). *Factors predicting survival in amyotrophic lateral sclerosis patients on non-invasive ventilation*. Taylor & Francis Group.

Calzetta, L., Rogliani, P., Matera, M. G., & Cazzola, M. (2016). A systematic review with meta-analysis of dual bronchodilation with LAMA/LABA for the treatment of stable COPD. *Chest*, *149*(5), 1181–1196. doi:10.1016/j.chest.2016.02.646 PMID:26923629

Camargo, F. C., Iwamoto, H. H., Galvão, C. M., Monteiro, D. A. T., Goulart, M. B., & Garcia, L. A. A. (2017). Modelos para a implementação da prática baseada em evidências na enfermagem hospitalar: Revisão narrativa. *Texto & Contexto Enfermagem*, *26*(4), 1–12.

Cameron, S., Ball, I., Cepinskas, G., Choong, K., Doherty, T. J., Ellis, G. C., Martin, C. M., Mele, T. S., Sharpe, M., Shoemaker, J. K., & Fraser, D. D. (2015). Early mobilization in the critical care unit: A review of adult and pediatric literature. *Journal of Critical Care*, *30*(4), 664–672. doi:10.1016/j.jcrc.2015.03.032 PMID:25987293

Camillis, M., Savi, A., Rosa, R., Figueiredo, M., & Wickert, R. (2018). Effects of Mechanical Insufflation-Exsufflation on Airway Mucus Clearance Among Mechanically Ventilated ICU Subjects. *Respiratory Care*, *63*(12), 1471–1477. doi:10.4187/respcare.06253 PMID:30018175

Cano, W. (2013). Evidence and narratives in health care: An anthropological perspective. *The Journal of Pain and the Survival of Illness in Patients with Pain, 11*, 357.

Cano-Pumarega, I., Durán-Cantolla, J., Aizpuru, F., Miranda-Serrano, E., Rubio, R., Martínez-Null, C., de Miguel, J., Egea, C., Cancelo, L., Álvarez, A., Fernández-Bolaños, M., & Barbé, F. (2011). Obstructive Sleep Apnea and Systemic Hypertension: Longitudinal Study in the General Population: The Vitoria Sleep Cohort. *American Journal of Respiratory and Critical Care Medicine*, *184*(11), 1299–1304. doi:10.1164/rccm.201101-0130OC PMID:21868499

Canteiro, M., & Heitor, M. (2003). Reabilitação respiratória. *Tratado de Pneumologia. lisboa: Sociedade Portuguesa de Pneumologia*, 1785-1896.

Cantero, A. R. (2011). Control del riesgo cardiovascular en el anciano. *Revista Clínica Española, 211*, 2–7. doi:10.1016/S0014-2565(11)70002-9

Carreño, S. P., & Chaparro, L. (2016). Calidad de vida de los cuidadores de personas con enfermedad crónica. *Aquichan, 16*(4), 447–461. doi:10.5294/aqui.2016.16.4.4

Cavalleri, M. A., Barbagelata, E., Scudeletti, M., & Nicolini, A. (2018). Effectiveness of non-invasive ventilation in acute respiratory failure of obese patients: A brief narrative review. *Italian Journal of Medicine, 12*(1), 5–9. doi:10.4081/itjm.2018.916

Cedano, S. (2013). Qualidade de vida e sobrecarga dos cuidadores de portadores de Doença Pulmonar Obstrutiva Crônica em oxigenoterapia. *Revistas.Usp.Br.* Retrieved from https://www.revistas.usp.br/rlae/article/view/75996

Cederwall, C., Plos, K., Rose, L., Dübeck, A., & Ringdal, M. (2014). Critical care nurses management of prolonged weaning: An interview study. *Nursing in Critical Care, 19*(5), 236–242. doi:10.1111/nicc.12092 PMID:24809683

Ceriana, P., & Nava, S. (2006). Hypoxic and hypercapnic respiratory failure. *European Respiratory Society Monograph, 36*, 1–15. doi:10.1183/1025448x.00036001

Chan, M. (2015). Prefácio. In Organização Mundial de Saúde (Ed.), Relatório Mundial de Envelhecimento e Saúde, (p. vii). Genebra: Autor.

Charon, R. (2001). Narrative medicine: A model for empathy, reflection, profession, and trust. *Journal of the American Medical Association, 286*(15), 1897–1902. doi:10.1001/jama.286.15.1897 PMID:11597295

Charon, R. (2005). Narrative medicine: Attention, representation, affiliation. *Narrative, 13*(3), 261–270. doi:10.1353/nar.2005.0017

Charon, R. (2008). *Narrative medicine: Honoring the stories of illness*. Oxford University Press.

Çiftci, F., Çiledağ, A., Erol, S., & Kaya, A. (2017). Non-invasive ventilation for acute hypercapnic respiratory failure in older patients. *Wiener Klinische Wochenschrift, 129*(19-20), 680–686. doi:10.100700508-017-1182-2 PMID:28283771

Çiftci, F., Çiledağ, A., Erol, S., & Kaya, A. (2017). Non-invasive ventilation for acute hypercapnic respiratory failure in older patients. *Wiener klinische Wochenschrift. Central European Journal of Medicine, 129*, 680–686. PMID:28283771

Clèries, X., Solà, M., Chiner, E., & Escarrabill, J. (2016). Approach to the experience of the patient and their caregivers in home oxygen therapy. *Bronchopneumology Archives, 52*(3), 131–137. doi:10.1016/j.arbr.2016.01.005

Codinardo, C., Cáneva, J., Gil, B., & Echevarría, M. (2018). Recomendaciones sobre el uso de oxigenoterapia ambulatoria. *Vitalaire.Com.Ar.* Retrieved from https://www.vitalaire.com.ar/sites/vitalaire_ar/files/2018/09/19/recomendaciones_sobre_el_uso_de_oxigenoterapia_ambulatoria.pdf

Codinardo, C., Cáneva, J. O., Montiel, G., Uribe Echevarría, M. E., Lisanti, R., Larrateguy, L., ... Torres, R. (2016). Recommendations on the use of oxygen therapy in special situations. *American Journal of Respiratory Medicine*, *16*(2), 150–162.

Collado-Mateo, D., Adsuar, J. C., Olivares, P. R. & García-Gordillo, M. Á. (2017). Health-related quality of life in Chilean patients with chronic obstructive pulmonary disease. *Medical Journal of Chile, 145*(2), 147-155.

Collop, N. A. (1997). The significance of sleep-disordered breathing and obstructive sleep apnea in the elderly. *Chest*, *112*(4), 867–868. doi:10.1378/chest.112.4.867 PMID:9377944

Consejería de Sanidad de Madrid. (2013). *Plan Estratégico en EPOC de la Comunidad de Madrid 2013/2017*. Retrieved from http://www.madrid.org/es/transparencia/sites/default/files/plan/document/307_158_planepocmadrid_1abr13_lowres_0.pdf

Conti, G., Costa, R., Craba, A., Festa, V., & Catarci, S. (2004). Non-invasive ventilation in COPD patients. *Minerva Anestesiologica*, *70*(4), 145–150. PMID:15173688

Cordeiro, M. & Menoita, E. (2014). *Manual de boas praticas na reabilitação respiratória. Conceitos, princípios e técnicas*. Loures: Lusociência.

Cordeiro, M., & Menoita, E. (2012). *Manual de boas práticas na reabilitação respiratória: conceitos, princípios e técnicas*. Loures: Lusociência.

Cordeiro, M. D. C. O., & Menoita, E. C. P. C. (2012). *Manual de boas práticas na reabilitação respiratória: Conceitos, princípios e técnicas*. Lusociência.

Cordeiro, M., & Menoita, E. (2012). *Manual de Boas Práticas na Reabilitação Respiratória – Conceitos, princípios e técnicas*. Lusociência.

Cordeiro, M., Menoita, E., & Mateus, D. (2012). Limpeza das Vias Aéreas: Conceitos, Técnicas e Princípios. *Journal ofAging & Innovation*, *1*(5), 30–44. http://www.journalofagingandinnovation.org/wp-content/uploads/4-Limpeza-das-vias-aereas.pdf

Cordero del Castillo, P. (2013). *2012, Año Europeo del Envejecimiento Activo y la Solidaridad Intergeneracional.* Academic Press.

Corhay, J.-L., Dang, D. N., Van Cauwenberge, H., & Louis, R. (2014). Pulmonary rehabilitation and COPD: Providing patients a good environment for optimizing therapy. *International Journal of Chronic Obstructive Pulmonary Disease*, *9*, 27–39. doi:10.2147/COPD.S52012 PMID:24368884

Corner, E., & Garrod, R. (2009). Does the addition of noninvasive ventilation during pulmonary rehabilitation in patients with chronic obstructive pulmonary disease augment patient outcome in exercise tolerance? A literature review. *Fisiotherapy Research International*, *15*(1), 5–15. doi:10.1002/pri.451 PMID:20033880

Corner, E., & Garrod, R. (2010). Does the addition of non-invasive ventilation during pulmonary rehabilitation in patients with chronic obstructive pulmonary disease augment patient outcome in exercise tolerance? A literature review. *Physiotherapy Research International*, *15*(1), 5–15. PMID:20033880

Cortés Duque, C., Uribe, C. A., & Vásquez, R. (2005). Clinical ethnography and disease narratives of patients with obsessive-compulsive disorder. *Colombian Journal of Psychiatry*, *34*(2).

Costa-Dias, M.J.M.D., Ferreira, P.L., & Oliveira, A.S. (2014). Adaptação cultural e linguística e validação da Escala de Quedas de Morse. *Revista de Enfermagem Referência*, (2), 7-17.

Costa, J. C., Machado, J. N., Costa, J., Fortuna, J., Gama, J., & Rodrigues, C. (2018). Ventilação Não Invasiva: Experiência de um Serviço de Medicina Interna. *Medicina Interna*, *25*(1), 18–22. doi:10.24950/rspmi/original/78/1/2018

Costa, M. F. D. L., Barros, M. P. D., & Lima, J. H. M. (2010). O Impacto do CPAP na Reabilitação Cardíaca de Pacientes com ICC: Relato de caso. *Arquivos Brasileiros de Cardiologia*, *95*(1), e7–e9. doi:10.1590/S0066-782X2010001100023 PMID:20694398

Costa, X., Gómez-Batiste, X., Pla, M., Martínez Muñoz, M., Blay, C., & Vila, L. (2016). Living with advanced chronic obstructive pulmonary disease: The impact of dyspnoea on patients and caregivers. *Primary Care*, *48*(10), 665–673. PMID:27288085

Costa, X., Gómez-Batiste, X., Pla, M., Martínez-Muñoz, M., Blay, C., & Vila, L. (2016). Vivir con la enfermedad pulmonar obstructiva crónica avanzada: El impacto de la disnea en los pacientes y cuidadores. *Atencion Primaria*, *48*(10), 665–673. doi:10.1016/j.aprim.2016.02.008 PMID:27288085

Coutinho, W., Vieira, P., Kutchak, F., Dias, A., Rieder, M., & Forgarini, L. (2018). Comparison of Mechanical Insufflation-Exsufflation and Endotracheal Suctioning in Mechanically Ventilated Patients: Effects on Respiratory Mechanics, Hemodynamics, and Volume of Secretions. *Indian Journal of Critical Care Medicine: Peer-Reviewed, Official Publication of Indian Society of Critical Care Medicine*, *22*(7), 485–490. doi:10.4103/ijccm.IJCCM_164_18 PMID:30111922

Coventry, P., Panagioti, M., Scott, C., & Blakemore, A. (2014). Overview of the prevalence, impact, and management of depression and anxiety in chronic obstructive pulmonary disease. *International Journal of Chronic Obstructive Pulmonary Disease*, *9*, 1289. doi:10.2147/COPD.S72073 PMID:25419126

Crawford, E. (2013). Le sommeil physiologique et pathologique du sujet âge: impact sur la qualité du vieillissement et le vieillissement cognitif. Médecine humaine et pathologie. *Archives-Ouvertes: Université Jean Monnet – Saint-Etienne.*

Crepo, M., & López, M. (2007). *El apoyo a los cuidadores familiares mayores dependientes en el hogar: desarrollo del programa "cómo mantener su bienestar."* Recuperado en: https://www.imserso.es/InterPresent1/groups/imserso/documents/binario/apoyocuidadores.pdf

Cueva Chenche, M. E. (2018). *Enfermedad pulmonar obstructiva crónica (EPOC): método diagnóstico de elección y tratamiento indicado usado con mayor frecuencia para evitar agudizaciones*. Retrieved from http://repositorio.utmachala.edu.ec/handle/48000/12585

Da Silva, L., Fierro Jordán, N., Guitérrez Monclus, P., & Rodriguez, O. (2011). Ciencia de la ocupación y Terapia Ocupacional: Sus relaciones y aplicaciones a la práctica clínica. *Revista Chilena de Terapia Ocupacional*, *11*(1), 79. doi:10.5354/0719-5346.2011.17084

Dalal, A. A., Shah, M., Lunacsek, O., & Hanania, N. A. (2011). Clinical and Economic Burden of Depression/Anxiety in Chronic Obstructive Pulmonary Disease Patients within a Managed Care Population. *COPD*, *8*(4), 293–299. doi:10.3109/15412555.2011.586659 PMID:21827298

Darío, I., & Andrés, E. (2017). *Tratamiento médico-quirúrgico de la obesidad en el síndrome de apnea-hipopnea obstructiva del sueño (SAHOS)*. Academic Press.

Davidson, A. C., Banham, S., Elliot, M., Kennedy, D., Gelder, C., Glossop, A., Church, A. C., Creagh-Brown, B., Dodd, J. W., Felton, T., Foëx, B., Mansfield, L., McDonnell, L., Parker, R., Patterson, C. M., Sovani, M., & Thomas, L.BTS Standards of Care Committee Member, British Thoracic Society/Intensive Care Society Acute Hypercapnic Respiratory Failure Guideline Development Group. (2015). BTS/ICS guideline for the ventilatory management of acute hypercapnic respiratory failure in adults. *Thorax Journal*, *71*, 1–35. PMID:26976648

De la Campa. (2014). Actualización en oxigenoterapia. *Revista de Patología Respiratoria*, *17*(1).

De la Cuesta, C. (2005). La artesanía del cuidado. Cuidar en la casa de un familiar con demencia avanzada. *Enfermeria Clinica*, *15*(6), 335–342. doi:10.1016/S1130-8621(05)71140-2

De Llano, L. A. P., Golpe, R., Piquer, M. O., Racamonde, A. V., Caruncho, M. V., Muinelos, O. C., & Carra, C. A. (2005). Short-term and long-term effects of nasal intermittent positive pressure ventilation in patients with obesity-hypoventilation syndrome. *Chest*, *128*(2), 587–594. doi:10.1378/chest.128.2.587 PMID:16100142

De Pablos, C. M., & Lozano, S. G. (2012). *Funciones del Terapeuta Ocupacional en el ámbito de la Salud Mental*. Retrieved from www.revistatog.com

Demoule, A., Chevret, S., Carlucci, A., Kouatchet, A., Jaber, S., Meziani, F., ... Rabbat, A. (2016). Changing use of noninvasive ventilation in critically ill patients: Trends over 15 years in francophone countries. *Intensive Care Medicine*, *42*(1), 82–92. doi:10.100700134-015-4087-4 PMID:26464393

Deng, Q., Deng, L., Miao, Y., Guo, X., & Li, Y. (2019). Particle deposition in the human lung: Health implications of particulate matter from different sources. *Environmental Research*, *169*, 237–245. doi:10.1016/j.envres.2018.11.014 PMID:30476747

DesJardins, T., Burton, G., & Timothy, P. (2015). Clinical manifestations and assessment of respiratory disease. Mosby Elsevier.

DGS. (2009). *Orientações Técnicas sobre Reabilitação Respiratória na Doença Pulmonar Obstrutiva Crónica (DPOC)*. Circular Normativa nº: 40A/DSPCD de 27/10/09. Acedido a 19 de Novembro de 2018. Disponível em: https://www.dgs.pt/directrizes-da- dgs/normas-e-circulares-normativas.aspx

DGS. (2012) *Programa Nacional para as Doenças Respiratórias*. Acedido a 17 de Novembro de 2018. Disponível em: https://www.dgs.pt/pns-e-programas/programas-de- saude-prioritarios/doencas-respiratorias.aspx

DGS. (2015) Norma 022/2011, actualizada a 11/09/2015: *Cuidados Respiratórios Domiciliários: Prescrição de Ventiloterapia e outros Equipamentos*. Acedido a 09 de Dezembro de 2018. Disponível em: https://www.dgs.pt/directrizes-da-dgs/Fnormas-e- circulares-normativas/norma-n-0222011-de-28092011-jpg.aspx

Diário da República. (2011). Regulamento das Competências Comuns do Enfermeiro Especialista. *Regulamento, 122*.

Dias, C., Siqueira, T., Faccio, T., Gontijo, L., Salge, J., & Volpe, M. (2011). Efetividade e segurança da técnica de higiene brônquica: Hiperinsuflação manual com compressão torácica. *Revista Brasileira de Terapia Intensiva*, *23*(2), 190–198. doi:10.1590/S0103-507X2011000200012 PMID:25299720

Díaz Lobato, S., García González, J. L., & Mayoralas Allses, S. (2015). Controversias en oxigenoterapia continua domiciliaria. *Archivos de Bronconeumologia*, *51*(1), 31–37. doi:10.1016/j.arbres.2014.05.002 PMID:24976235

Digby, G. C., Keenan, S. P., Parker, C. M., Sinuff, T., Burns, K. E., Mehta, S., ... Berthiaume, L. R. (2015). Noninvasive ventilation practice patterns for acute respiratory failure in Canadian tertiary care centres: A descriptive analysis. *Canadian Respiratory Journal*, *22*(6), 331–340. doi:10.1155/2015/971218 PMID:26469155

Direção Geral da Saúde. (2015). *A Saúde dos Portugueses: perspetiva 2015*. Autor.

Direção Geral da Saúde. (2016). *Aprenda a viver com a DPOC: Doença Pulmonar Obstrutiva Crónica*. Autor.

Direção Geral da Saúde. (2017). *Programa Nacional para as Doenças respiratórias*. Autor.

Direção Geral de Saúde. (2011). *Cuidados de Saúde Respiratórios Domiciliários em Portugal*. DGS.

Direção-Geral da Saúde. (2009). Orientações técnicas sobre reabilitação respiratória na doença pulmonar obstrutiva crónica (DPOC). *Circular Informativa, 40*.

Domínguez, R. S., Rodríguez, Z. N., & Mendoza, Y. L. (2015). Caracterización de la ventilación no invasiva en pacientes con enfermedad pulmonar obstructiva crónica agudizada. *Medisan (Santiago de Cuba)*, *18*(9), 1085–1092.

Donaldson, G. C., Ambrosino, N., Escarabill, J., Farre, R., Fauroux, B., Robert, D., ... Wedzicha, J. A. (2005). *Patterns of home mechanical ventilation use in Europe: results from the Eurovent survey*. doi:10.1183/09031936.05.00066704

Dong, Z., Yu, B., Sun, Y., Fang, W., & Li, L. (2014). Effects of early rehabilitation therapy on patients with mechanical ventilation. *World Journal of Emergency Medicine*, *5*(1), 48–52. doi:10.5847/wjem.j.issn.1920-8642.2014.01.008 PMID:25215147

dos Enfermeiros, O. (2011). *Regulamento dos Padrões de Qualidade dos Cuidados Especializados em Enfermagem de Reabilitação*. Retrieved from: https://www.ordemenfermeiros.pt/colegios/documents/pqceereabilitacao.pdf

dos Enfermeiros, O. (2018). Guia Orientador de Boa Prática - Reabilitação Respiratória. Ordem dos Enfermeiros.

Dourado, V. Z. (2011). Equações de referência para o teste de caminhada de seis minutos em indivíduos saudáveis. *Arquivos Brasileiros de Cardiologia*, *96*(6), e128–e138. doi:10.1590/S0066-782X2011005000024 PMID:22262150

Dourado, V. Z., & Godoy, I. (2004). Recondicionamento muscular na DPOC: Principais intervenções e novas tendências. *Revista Brasileira de Medicina do Esporte*, *10*(4), 331–334. doi:10.1590/S1517-86922004000400010

Dueñas-Espín, I., Demeyer, H., Gimeno-Santos, E., Polkey, M., Hopkinson, N., Rabinovich, R., Dobbels, F., Karlsson, N., Troosters, T., & Garcia-Aymerich, J. (2016). Depression symptoms reduce physical activity in COPD patients: A prospective multicenter study. *International Journal of Chronic Obstructive Pulmonary Disease*, *11*, 1287. doi:10.2147/COPD.S101459 PMID:27354787

Duffy, J. F., Zeitzer, J. M., Rimmer, D. W., Klerman, E. B., Dijk, D. J., & Czeisler, C. A. (2002). Peak of circadian melatonin rhythm occurs later within the sleep of older subjects. *American Journal of Physiology. Endocrinology and Metabolism*, *282*(2), E297–E303. doi:10.1152/ajpendo.00268.2001 PMID:11788360

Duiverman, M. L., Wempe, J. B., Bladder, G., Vonk, J. M., Zijlstra, J. G., Kerstjens, H. A., & Wijkstra, P. J. (2011). Two-year home-based nocturnal noninvasive ventilation added to rehabilitation in chronic obstructive pulmonary disease patients: A randomized controlled trial. *Respiratory Research*, *12*(1), 112. doi:10.1186/1465-9921-12-112 PMID:21861914

Dunn, H., Quinn, L., Corbridge, J. S., Eldeirawi, K., Kapella, M., & Collins, G. E. (2017). Mobilization of prolonged mechanical ventilation patients: An integrative review. *Heart & Lung*, *46*(4), 221–233. doi:10.1016/j.hrtlng.2017.04.033 PMID:28624337

Dyer, F., Flude, L., & Bazari, F. (2018). Noninvasive ventilation (NIV) as an aid to rehabilitation in acute respiratory disease. *BioMedCentral Pulmonary Medicine*, *11*(58). Advance online publication. doi:10.1186/1471-2466-11-58 PMID:22177338

Eguía, V. M., & Cascante, J. A. (2007). Síndrome de apnea-hipopnea del sueño. Concepto, diagnóstico tratamiento médico. *Anales del Sistema Sanitario de Navarra*, *30*(1), 53–74. doi:10.4321/S1137-66272007000200005 PMID:17491608

Epstein, S. K., & Durbin, C. G. (2010). Should a patient be extubated and placed on noninvasive ventilation after failing a spontaneous breathing trial? *Respiratory Care*, *55*(2), 198–206. PMID:20105345

Escarrabill, J. (2003). *Enfermedad pulmonar obstructiva crónica (EPOC): visión global y continuidad de cuidados*. Retrieved from www.coldcopd.org

Escobar, J. C., Ruiz, C. C., & Muela, P. G. (2013). *Protocolo de intervención desde Terapia Ocupacional*. Retrieved from www.madridsalud.es

Esquinas, A. M. (2011). *Princípios de Ventilação Mecânica Não Invasiva: do Hospital ao Domicílio*. GASINMédica.

European Respiratory Society. (2013). *Respiratory disease in the world*. Autor.

Evans, M., & Sweeney, K. (1998). The human side of medicine. *Occasional Paper (Royal College of General Practitioners)*, 76. PMID:9707989

Falque-Madrid, L. (2014). La evidencia científica y el arte de envejecer. *Anales Venezolanos de Nutrición*, *27*(1), 110 118.

Fanelli, A., Cabral, A. L., Neder, J. A., Martins, M. A., & Carvalho, C. R. (2007). Exercise training on disease control and quality of life in asthmatic children. *Medicine and Science in Sports and Exercise*, *39*(9), 1474–1480. doi:10.1249/mss.0b013e3180d099ad PMID:17805077

Farmakis, D., Parissis, J., Lekakis, J., & Filippatos, G. (2015). Insuficiencia cardiaca aguda: Epidemiología, factores de riesgo y prevención. *Revista Espanola de Cardiologia*, *68*(3), 245–248. doi:10.1016/j.recesp.2014.11.009 PMID:25659507

Faverio, P., Giacomi, F., & Sardella, L. (2018). Management of acute respiratory failure in interstitial lung diseases: Overview and clinical insights. *BioMedCentral Pulmonary Medicine*, *18*(70), 70. Advance online publication. doi:10.118612890-018-0643-3 PMID:29764401

Fazekas, A., Aboulghaith, M., Kriz, R., Urban, M., Breyer, M., Kohansal, R., Burghuber, O., Harti, S., & Funk, G. (2017). *Long-term outcomes after acute hypercapnic COPD exacerbation –first-ever episode of non-invasive ventilation*. The Central European Jounal of Medicine. Taylor & Francis Group.

Felgueiras, J., Lohmann, C., Delerue, F., & Barata, J. (2006). Ventilação não invasiva numa unidade de cuidados intermédios. *Revue de Médecine Interne*, *13*(21), 73–78.

Ferenhof, H. A., & Fernandes, R. F. (2016). Desmistificando a revisão de literatura como base para redação científica: Método SSF. *Revista ACB*, *21*(3), 550–563.

Fernández Mayoralas, G., & Rojo Pérez, F. (2005). *Calidad de vida y salud: planteamientos conceptuales y métodos de investigación*. Retrieved from https://www.raco.cat/index.php/Territoris/article/viewFile/117017/147939

Fernández, V., & Sánchez, M. (2017). *Roles a través de la ocupación, justificación bajo el modelo de atención centrada en la persona*. Retrieved from https://dialnet.unirioja.es/servlet/articulo?codigo=5915166

Ferreira, C. A. C. (2017). Um percurso de especialização em urgência e cuidados intensivos: relevância da ventilação mecânica no tratamento da insuficiência respiratória (Relatório de estágio não publicado). Escola Superior de Enfermagem de São José de Cluny, Funchal.

Ferreira, H., & Santos, F. (2008). *Aspectos Gerais da Ventilação Não-Invasiva*. Disponível em http://www.hce.eb.mil.br/rev/rev2008/aspectosgerais.pdf

Ferreira, S., Nogueira, C., Conde, S., & Taveira, N. (2009). Ventilação não invasiva. *Revista Portuguesa de Pneumologia*, *15*(4), 655–667. doi:10.1016/S0873-2159(15)30162-8 PMID:19547897

Fink, J. B., & Dhand, R. (2000). Aerosol therapy in mechanically ventilated patients: Recent advances and new techniques. *Seminars in Respiratory and Critical Care Medicine*, *21*(03), 183–201. doi:10.1055-2000-9854 PMID:16088731

Fioretti, C., Mazzocco, K., Riva, S., Oliveri, S., Masiero, M., & Pravettoni, G. (2016). Research studies on patients' illness experience using the Narrative Medicine approach: A systematic review. *BMJ Open*, *6*(7), e011220. doi:10.1136/bmjopen-2016-011220 PMID:27417197

Florence, J. M., & Hagberg, J. M. (1984). Effect of training on the exercise responses of neuromuscular disease patients. *Medicine and Science in Sports and Exercise*, *16*(5), 460–465. doi:10.1249/00005768-198410000-00007 PMID:6513764

Fontanella, L., Rigon, L. A., Serena, P. & Munarin, F. (2010). Rischio clinico per le persone che utilizzano a domicilio ossigenoterapia e ventilazione meccanica: indagine di prevalenza. *SCENARIO: Official Italian Journal of ANIARTI, 27*(4).

Fortin. (2009). Fundamentos e etapas do processo de investigação. Lisboa: Lusodidacta.

França, E. E., Dornelas de Andrade, A. F., Cabral, G., Almeida Filho, P., Silva, K. C., Galindo Filho, V. C., Marinho, P. E. M., Lemos, A., & Parreira, V. F. (2006). Nebulization associated with bi-level noninvasive ventilation: Analysis of pulmonary radioaerosol deposition. *Respiratory Medicine*, *100*(4), 721–728. doi:10.1016/j.rmed.2005.07.012 PMID:16139491

Fritzsche, A., Clamor, A., & von Leupoldt, A. (2011). Effects of medical and psychological treatment of depression in patients with COPD – A review. *Respiratory Medicine*, *105*(10), 1422–1433. doi:10.1016/j.rmed.2011.05.014 PMID:21680167

Gabbay, I. E., & Lavie, P. (2012). Age- and gender-related characteristics of obstructive sleep apnea. *Sleep and Breathing*, *16*(2), 453–460. doi:10.100711325-011-0523-z PMID:21499842

Gabriel, R., Figueiredo, D., Jácome, C., Cruz, J., & Marques, A. (2014). Day-to-day living with severe chronic obstructive pulmonary disease: Towards a family-based approach to the illness impacts. *Psychology & Health, 29*(8), 967–983. doi:10.1080/08870446.2014.902458 PMID:24617821

Gaio, Antunes, Barreto, Gil, Kislaya, Namorado, Rodrigues, Santos, & Nunes. (2018). Prevalência de excesso de peso e de obesidade em Portugal: resultados do primeiro Inquérito Nacional de Saúde com Exame Físico (INSEF 2015). *Boletim Epidemiológico Observações, 22*(7), 29–33.

Ganga, H., Thangaraj, V., y Puppala, N. (2009). Obstructive Sleep Apnea in the ederly Population: Atypical Presentation and Diagnostic Challenges. *The Internet Journal of Internal Medicine, 8*(2).

Garber, C. E., Blissmer, B., Deschenes, M. R., Franklin, B. A., Lamonte, M. J., Lee, I.-M., Nieman, D. C., & Swain, D. P. (2011). American College of Sports Medicine Position Stand. The quantity and quality of exercise for developing and maintaining cardiorespiratory, musculoskeletal, and neuromotor fitness in apparently healthy adults: Guidance for prescribing exercise. *Medicine and Science in Sports and Exercise, 43*(7), 1334–1359. doi:10.1249/MSS.0b013e318213fefb PMID:21694556

Garcia Oliva, M., Sala, E., & Coscolla Aisa, R. (2009). *La calidad de vida de las cuidadoras informales: bases para un sistema de valoración.* Recuperado en: http://www.segsocial.es/prdi00/groups/public/documents/binario/119780.pdf

García, D. A. R., & Martínez, E. G. (2015). El síndrome de apnea obstructiva del sueño en el anciano: características específicas. Investigación en Salud y Envejecimiento, 3, 77-84.

Garcia, S., Rocha, M., Pinto, P., Lopes, A. M., & Bárbara, C. (2008). Treino de músculos inspiratórios em doentes com DPOC. *Revista Portuguesa de Pneumologia, 14*(2), 177–194. doi:10.1016/S0873-2159(15)30229-4 PMID:18363017

Garrod, R., Bestall, J. C., Paul, E. A., Wedzicha, J. A., & Jones, P. W. (2000). Development and validation of a standardized measure of activity of daily living in patients with severe COPD: The London Chest Activity of Daily Living scale (LCADL). *Respiratory Medicine, 94*(6), 589–596. doi:10.1053/rmed.2000.0786 PMID:10921765

Gastrointestinal surgery for severe obesity. (2018). *National Institutes of Health Consensus Development Conference.*

Gatti, V., Banfi, P., Centanni, S., D'Antonio, S., Giustini, S., Piraino, A., Zibellini, M., & Marini, M. G. (2018). Enlightening chronic obstructive pulmonary disease through patients' and caregivers' narratives. *International Journal of Chronic Obstructive Pulmonary Disease, 13*, 3095–3105. doi:10.2147/COPD.S172214 PMID:30323580

Gefael, C. V. (2009). Patients bleed stories: A narrative approach to decrease clinical misunderstandings. *North Mental Health, 8*(34), 9.

Gellish, R. L., Goslin, B. R., Olson, R. E., McDonald, A., Russi, G. D., & Moudgil, V. K. (2007). Longitudinal modeling of the relationship between age and maximal heart rate. *Medicine and Science in Sports and Exercise, 39*(5), 822–829. doi:10.1097/mss.0b013e31803349c6 PMID:17468581

Georges, M., Goldmard, J., Llontop, C., Shoukri, A., Salachas, F., Similowski, T., … Bermejo, J. (2017). *Initiation of non-invasive ventilation in amyotrophic lateral sclerosis and clinical practice guedelines: Single-centre, retrospective, descriptive study in a national referece centre.* Academic Press.

Global Iniciative for Chronic Obstructive Lung Disease. (2019). *Global Strategy for the diagnosis, management and prevention of COPD-Pocket Guide to COPD Diagnosis, Management, and Prevention, 2019 Report.* Author.

Gluzmann, P. (2013). Bienestar Subjetivo y Crecimiento Económico: Analizando La Paradoja Del Crecimiento Infeliz En La Encuesta Mundial Gallup. *Económica, 59*, 231–258.

Godoy. (2007). El efecto del ejercicio sobre los niveles de ansiedad, depresión y autoconcepto de pacientes con dolencia pulmonar obstructiva crónica. *Rpd-Online.Com.* Retrieved from https://www.rpd-online.com/article/view/158

Göktas, S., Kiraner, E., Dogan, P., & Tunali, B. (2017). *Effects of Provided Trainings Regarding Non-Invasive Mechanical Ventilation on the Knowledge Level of Nurses.* Eurasian Pulmonol. doi:10.5152/ejp.2016.05706

Gomes, B., & Ferreira, D. (2017). Enfermagem de Reabilitação à Pessoa submetida a Ventilação Mecânica. In C. Marques-Vieira & L. Sousa (Eds.), Cuidados de Enfermagem de Reabilitação à Pessoa ao Longo da Vida (pp. 365-380). Loures: Lusodidacta.

Gómez Sánchez, A. (n.d.). Intervenciones de enfermería en el cuidador informal del adulto dependiente. *Nuberos Científica, 2*(11), 21-26. Recuperado de: http://nc.enfermeriacantabria.com/index.php/nc/article/view/35/33

Gómez, S., Duque, T. C., & Sukkarieh, N. S. (2015). Otras unidades multiprofesionales en la formación sanitaria especializada desde el punto de vista de la enfermería. Principios de Educación Médica. Desde el grado hasta el desarrollo profesional. *Editorial médica Panamericana. S.A., 20*(6), 439-440.

Gómez, L., Verdugo, M., Arias, B., & Navas, P. (2008). Evaluation of the quality of life in elderly and disabled people: The Fumat Scale. *Intervención Psicosocial, 17*(2), 189–199.

Gonçalves, M. R., Honrado, T., Winck, J. C., & Paiva, J. A. (2012). Effects of mechanical insufflation-exsufflation in preventing respiratory failure after extubation: A randomized controlled trial. *Critical Care (London, England), 16*(2), R48. doi:10.1186/cc11249 PMID:22420538

González Castro, U., & Reyes, A. (2012). Algunos aspectos del proceso que viven los cuidadores primarios de un enfermo crónico-degenerativo. *Revista Electrónica de Psicología Iztacala, 15*(2), 636–661.

Gosselink, R. (2003). Controlled breathing and dyspnea in patients with chronic obstructive pulmonary disease (COPD). *Journal of Rehabilitation Research and Development, 40*(5), 25-34.

Gosselink, R., De Vos, J., Van den Heuvel, S. P., Segers, J., Decramer, M., & Kwakkel, G. (2011). Impact of inspiratory muscle training in patients with COPD: What is the evidence? *The European Respiratory Journal, 37*(2), 416–425. doi:10.1183/09031936.00031810 PMID:21282809

Gouda, P., Chua, J., Langan, D., Hannon, T., Scott, A., & O'Regan, A. (2016). *A decade of domiciliary non-invasive ventilation in the west of Ireland.* Royal Academy of Medicine in Ireland.

Granger, C. V., Hamilton, B. B., Keith, R. A., Zielezny, M., & Sherwin, F. S. (1986). Advances in functional assessment for medical rehabilitation. *Topics in Geriatric Rehabilitation, 1*(3), 59–74. doi:10.1097/00013614-198604000-00007

Greenhalgh, T., & Hurwitz, B. (1998). *Narrative Based Medicine Dialogue and discourse in clinical practice*. PhilPapers.

Grupo Anima Educação. (2014). *Manual de Revisão Bibliográfica Sistemática Integrativa: A Pesquisa Baseada em Evidências*. Grupo Anima Educação.

Grupo Español de sueño. (2005). Consenso Nacional sobre el síndrome de apneas-hipopneas del sueño. *Archivos de bronconeumología, 41*(4).

Güell Rous, M. R., Díaz Lobato, S., Rodríguez Trigo, G., Morante Vélez, F., San Miguel, M., Cejudo, P., Ortega Ruiz, F., Muñoz, A., Galdiz Iturri, J. B., García, A., & Servera, E. (2014). Rehabilitación respiratoria. *Archivos de Bronconeumologia, 50*(8), 332–344. doi:10.1016/j.arbres.2014.02.014 PMID:24845559

Gulati, M., Shaw, L. J., Thisted, R. A., Black, H. R., Merz, C. N., & Arnsdorf, M. F. (2010). Heart rate response to exercise stress testing in asymptomatic women. The St. James Women Take Heart Project. *Circulation, 122*(2), 130–137. doi:10.1161/CIRCULATIONAHA.110.939249 PMID:20585008

Gunnarsson, A., Wagman, P., Hedin, K., & Håkansson, C. (2018). Treatment of depression and/or anxiety - outcomes of a randomised controlled trial of the tree theme method® versus regular occupational therapy. *BMC Psychology, 6*(1), 25. doi:10.118640359-018-0237-0 PMID:29792226

Haarmann, H., Folle, J., Nguyen, X., Herrmann, P., Heusser, K., Hasefub, G., … Raupach, T. (2016). *Impact of Non-Invasive Ventilation on Sympathetic Nerve Activity in Chronic Obtrutive Pulmunary Disease.* Springer Science + Business Media.

Hare, D.L., Ryan, T.M., Selig, S.E., Pellizzer, A.M., Wrigley, T.V., & Krum, H. (1999) Resistance exercise training increases muscle strength, endurance, and blood flow in patients with chronic heart failure. *Am J Cardiol. 83*(12), 1674–7.

Hashem, M. D., Nelliot, A., & Needham, D. (2016). Early Mobilization and Rehabilitation in the ICU: Moving Back to the Future. *Respiratory Care, 61*(7), 971–979. doi:10.4187/respcare.04741 PMID:27094396

Haskell, W. L., Lee, I. M., Pate, R. R., Powell, K., Blair, S. N., Franklin, B. A., Macera, C. A., Heath, G. W., Thompson, P. D., & Bauman, A. (2007). Physical activity and public health: Updated recommendation for adults from the American College of Sports Medicine and the American Heart Association. *Medicine and Science in Sports and Exercise*, *39*(8), 1423–1434. doi:10.1249/mss.0b013e3180616b27 PMID:17762377

Helviz Y.& Einav S. (2018). A systematic review of the high-flow nasal cannula for adult patients. *Crit Care, 22*(1), 71.

Hernan Silva, I. (2014). DSM-5 Nueva clasificación de los trastornos mentales. *Revista Chilena de Neuro-psiquiatría, 52*. www.sonepsyn.cl

Hernández Hernández, J. (2016). *Enfermedad Pulmonar Obstructiva Crónica (EPOC) en pacientes ambulatorios*. Retrieved from https://www.semg.es/doc/documentos_SEMG/consenso_epoc_cyl.pdf

Hess, D. R. (2013). Noninvasive ventilation for acute respiratory failure. *Respiratory Care*, *58*(6), 950–969. doi:10.4187/respcare.02319 PMID:23709194

Hess, D. R. (2015). Aerosol therapy during noninvasive ventilation or high-flow nasal cannula. *Respiratory Care*, *60*(6), 880–891. doi:10.4187/respcare.04042 PMID:26070581

Heuer, A., & Scanlan, C. L. (2013). *Wilkins' Clinical Assessment in Respiratory Care-E-Book*. Elsevier Health Sciences.

Hill, K., & Holland, A. E. (2014). Strategies to enhance the benefits of exercise training in the respiratory patient. *Clinics in Chest Medicine*, *35*(2), 323–336. doi:10.1016/j.ccm.2014.02.003 PMID:24874128

Hoeman, S. P. (2011). História, Controvérsias e Tendências. In S. P. Hoeman (Coord., Enfermagem de Reabilitação. Prevenção, Intervenção e Resultados Esperados (4th ed., pp. 1-13). Loures: Lusodidacta.

Holland, A. E., Wadell, K., & Spruit, M. A. (2013). How to adapt the pulmonary rehabilitation programme to patients with chronic respiratory disease other than COPD. Pulmonary Rehabilitation, 577-586. doi:10.1183/09059180.00005613

Hollandl, A. E., & Buttonl, B. M. (2006). Is there a role for airway clearance techniques in chronic obstructive pulmonary disease? *Chronic Respiratory Disease*, *3*(2), 83–91. doi:10.1191/1479972306cd097rs PMID:16729766

Hoo, G. W. S. (2003). Nonpharmacologic adjuncts to training during pulmonary rehabilitation: the role of supplemental oxygen and noninvasive ventilation. *Journal of rehabilitation research and development, 40*(5), 81-98.

Hoo, G. W. S. (2016). Determinants of Utilization of Noninvasive Mechanical Ventilation in Hospitals: Key Technical and Nontechnical Issues. In *Noninvasive Mechanical Ventilation* (pp. 839–850). Springer. doi:10.1007/978-3-319-21653-9_97

Hough, A. (2001). *Physiotherapy in respiratory care: an evidence-based approach to respiratory and cardiac management*. Nelson Thornes.

Huerta, J. A. L., Romo, R. A. G., & Tayabas, J. M. T. (2017). Propiedades Psicométricas de la Versión en Español de la Escala de Calidad de Vida WHO QoL BREF en una Muestra de Adultos Mexicanos. *Revista Iberoamericana de Diagnóstico y Evaluación-e Avaliação Psicológica, 2*(44), 105–115. doi:10.21865/RIDEP44.2.09

Ides, K., Vissers, D., De Backer, L., Leemans, G., & De Backer, W. (2011). Airway clearance in COPD: Need for a breath of fresh air? A systematic review. *COPD, 8*(3), 196–205. doi:10.3109/15412555.2011.560582 PMID:21513439

Inouye, K., Silva, E., Iost, S., & Yoshie, C. (2009). Perceived quality of life of elderly patients with dementia and family caregives: Evaluation and correlation. *Revista Latino-Americana, 17*(3), 35–41.

Instituto Nacional de Estadística. (2013). *Proyecciones de población a largo plazo*. Recuperado en: https://www.ine.es/jaxi/menu.do?type=pcaxis&path=%Ft20%Fp251&file=inebase&L=0

Instituto Nacional de Estatística. (2015). *Envelhecimento da população residente em Portugal e na União Europeia*. Autor.

Instituto Nacional de Estatística. (2018). *Estimativas de População Residente - A redução da população residente atenuou-se - 2017*. Acedido a 7 de Dezembro de 2018. Disponível em: https://www.ine.pt/xportal/xmain?xpid=INE&xpgid=ine_destaques&DESTAQUESdest_boui=315156710&DESTAQUESmodo=2&xlang=pt

Inzunza, M., Moreno, C., & Vallejos, M. J. (2016). Nuevas estrategias de intervención desde Terapia Ocupacional para personas con Enfermedad Pulomar Obstructiva Crónica (EPOC). *Revista Chilena de Terapia Ocupacional, 16*(2), 77–91. Retrieved from https://revistas.uchile.cl/index.php/RTO/article/view/44753

Ivziku, D., Clari, M., Piredda, M., De Marinis, M. G., & Matarese, M. (2018). Anxiety, depression and quality of life in chronic obstructive pulmonary disease patients and caregivers: An actor–partner interdependence model analysis. *Quality of Life Research: An International Journal of Quality of Life Aspects of Treatment, Care and Rehabilitation*. Advance online publication. doi:10.100711136-018-2024-z PMID:30341578

Jackson, C., & Wenger, N. (2011). Enfermedad cardiovascular en el anciano. *Revista Espanola de Cardiologia, 64*(8), 697–712.

Jacqueline, S., Espinoza, N., Alexandra, K., Lozano, A., Geovanny, C., & Rivera, A. (n.d.). *S índrome de hipoventilación del obeso : revisión de la literatura*. Academic Press.

Janssens, J., Metzger, M., & Sforza, E. (2009). Impact of volume targeting on efficacy of bi-level non-invasive ventilation and. *Respiratory Medicine, 103*(2), 165–172. doi:10.1016/j.rmed.2008.03.013 PMID:18579368

Jarillo Quijada, A. (2004). *Oxigenoterapia*. Retrieved from http://himfg.com.mx/descargas/documentos/planeacion/guiasclinicasHIM/oxigenotrepia.pdf

Jennum, P., & Kjellberg, J. (2011). *Health, social and economical consequences of sleep-disordered breathing : a controlled national study*. doi:10.1136/thx.2010.143958

Joana Briggs Institute. (2014). *Joana Briggs Institute Reviewers' Manual* (2014 edition). Joana Briggs Institute.

Joanna Briggs Institute. (2014). *Joanna Briggs Institute Reviewers' Manual* (2014 edition). Autor.

Johnson, C., Connolly, M., & Clover, S. (2013). Audit of acute exacerbations of chronic obstructive pulmonary disease at Waitemata District Health Board, New Zealand. *The New Zealand Medical Journal, 126*(1378), 15–25. PMID:24045312

Jones, P. W., Quirk, F. H., & Baveystock, C. M. (1991). The St George's Respiratory Questionnaire. *Respiratory Medicine, 85*(B), 25–27.

Jørgensen, M., Mainz, J., Lange, P., & Paaske Johnsen, S. (2018). Quality of care and clinical outcomes of chronic obstructive pulmonary disease in patients with schizophrenia. A Danish nationwide study. *International Journal for Quality in Health Care, 30*(5), 351–357. doi:10.1093/intqhc/mzy014 PMID:29432585

Júnior, B., Martinez, B., & Neto, M. (2014). Impacto do Internamento em Unidade de Cuidados Intensivos na Amplitude de Movimento de Pacientes Graes: Estudo Piloto. *Revista Brasileira de Terapia Intensiva, 26*(1), 65–70. doi:10.5935/0103-507X.20140010 PMID:24770691

Kalitzkus, V., & Matthiessen, P. (2009). Narrative-based medicine: Potential, pitfalls, and practice. *The Permanente Journal, 13*(1), 80. doi:10.7812/TPP/08-043 PMID:21373252

Kaw, R., Hernandez, A. V., Walker, E., Aboussouan, L., & Mokhlesi, B. (2009). Determinants of Hypercapnia in Obese Patients With Obstructive Sleep Apnea A Systematic Review and Metaanalysis of Cohort. *Chest, 136*(3), 787–796. doi:10.1378/chest.09-0615 PMID:19567489

Keenan, S. P., Sinuff, T., Burns, K. E., Muscedere, J., Kutsogiannis, J., Mehta, S., ... Scales, D. C. (2011). Clinical practice guidelines for the use of noninvasive positive-pressure ventilation and noninvasive continuous positive airway pressure in the acute care setting. *Canadian Medical Association Journal, 183*(3), E195–E214. doi:10.1503/cmaj.100071 PMID:21324867

Kendall, A. R., Lewy, A. J., & Sack, R. L. (2001). Effects of aging on the intrinsic circadian period of totally blind humans. *Journal of Biological Rhythms, 16*(1), 87–95. doi:10.1177/074873040101600110 PMID:11220783

Khan, M. U. (2011). Noninvasive positive pressure ventilation in hospital setting. *JPMA. The Journal of the Pakistan Medical Association, 61*(6), 592–597. PMID:22204218

Kielhofner, G. (2004). *Terapia ocupacional : modelo de ocupación humana : teoría y aplicación*. Médica Panamericana.

Kleinman, A. (1988). *Suffering, healing and the human condition.* New York: Basic Book Publication.

Kleisiaris, C. F., Kritsotakis, E. I., Danil, Z., Tzanakis, N., Papaioannou, A., & Gourgoulianis, K. I. (2014). The prevalence of obstructive sleep apnea-hypopnea syndrome-related symptoms and their relation to airflow limitation in and elderly population receiving home care. *International Journal of Chronic Obstructive Pulmonary Disease, 10*(9), 1111–1117. doi:10.2147/COPD.S67779 PMID:25336942

Kovelis, D., Segretti, N. O., Probst, V. S., Lareau, S. C., Brunetto, A. F., & Pitta, F. (2008). Validação do Modified Pulmonary Functional Status and Dyspnea Questionnaire e da escala do Medical Research Council para o uso em pessoas com doença pulmonar obstrutiva crónica no Brasil [Validation of the Modified Pulmonary Functional Status and Dyspnea Questionnaire and the Medical Research Council scale for use in Brazil patients with chronic obstructive pulmonary disease]. *Jornal Brasileiro de Pneumologia, 34*(12), 1008–1018. doi:10.1590/S1806-37132008001200005 PMID:19180335

Lai, C., Chou, W., Chan, K., Cheng, K., Yuan, K., Chao, C., & Chen, C. (2016). Early Mobilization Reduces Duration of Mechanical Ventilation and Intensive Care Unit Stay in Patients with Acute Respiratory Failure. *Archives of Physical Medicine and Rehabilitation, 98*(5), 931–939. doi:10.1016/j.apmr.2016.11.007 PMID:27979608

Langer, D., Probst, V. S., Pitta, F., Burtin, C., Hendriks, E., Schans, C. P. V. D., ... Troosters, T. (2009). Guia para prática clínica: Fisioterapia em pacientes com Doença Pulmonar Obstrutiva Crônica (DPOC). *Brazilian Journal of Physical Therapy, 13*(3), 184–204. doi:10.1590/S1413-35552009005000034

Lara, G., González-Pedraza, A., & Blanco, L. (2008). Perfil del cuidador: Sobrecarga y apoyo familiar e institucional del cuidador primario en el primer nivel de atención. *Revista de Especialidades Médico-Quirúrgicas, 3*(1), 159–166.

Launois, S. H., Pepin, J. L., & Levy, P. (2007). Sleep apnea in the elderly: A especific entity? *Sleep Medicine Reviews, 11*(2), 87–97. doi:10.1016/j.smrv.2006.08.005 PMID:17276106

Lee, C., Simmonds, M., Novy, D., & Jones, S. (2002). Functional self-efficacy, perceived gait ability and perceived exertion in walking performance of individuals with low back pain. *Physiotherapy Theory and Practice, 18*(4), 193–203. doi:10.1080/09593980290058553

Leibold, M., Holm, M. B., Raina, K. D., Reynolds, C. F. III, & Rogers, J. C. (2014). Activities and adaptation in late-life depression: A qualitative study. *The American Journal of Occupational Therapy : Official Publication of the American Occupational Therapy Association, 68*(5), 570–577. doi:10.5014/ajot.2014.011130 PMID:25184470

Leiton-Espinoza, Z. E. (2016). El envejecimiento saludable y el bienestar: Un desafío y una oportunidad para enfermería. *Enfermería Universitaria, 13*(3), 139–141. doi:10.1016/j.reu.2016.06.002

Leland, N. E., Crum, K., Phipps, S., Roberts, P., & Gage, B. (2015). Advancing the value and quality of occupational therapy in health service delivery. *The American Journal of Occupational Therapy, 69*(1), 1-7. . doi:10.5014/ajot.2015.691001

Leland, N. E., Fogelberg, D. J., Halle, A. D., & Mroz, T. M. (2017). Occupational Therapy and Management of Multiple Chronic Conditions in the Context of Health Care Reform. *The American Journal of Occupational Therapy, 71*(1), 6. . doi:10.5014/ajot.2017.711001

Levy, M. L., Dekhuijzen, P. N. R., Barnes, P. J., Broeders, M., Corrigan, C. J., Chawes, B. L., ... Roche, N. (2016). Inhaler technique: Facts and fantasies. A view from the Aerosol Drug Management Improvement Team (ADMIT). *NPJ Primary Care Respiratory Medicine, 26*(1), 16017. doi:10.1038/npjpcrm.2016.17 PMID:27098045

Livi-Bacci, M. (2002). *Historia mínima de la población mundial.* Ariel.

López Riolobos, C., García del Castillo, E., Gómez Punter, R. M., & Fernandes de Vasconcelos, G. M. (2014). Indicaciones de la oxigenoterapia domiciliaria. Regulación y seguimiento clínico. *Medicine - Programa de Formación Médica Continuada Acreditado, 11*(63), 3777–3781. doi:10.1016/S0304-5412(14)70843-1

López, S. H., & Cob, L. H. (2018). *Proyecto de educación para la salud para personas con EPOC.* Retrieved from https://repositorio.uam.es/handle/10486/684884

López-Dávalos, G., Domínguez-Guedea, M., & Ochoa, M. (2010). Validación de la Escala de Bienestar Subjetivo en cuidadores familiares de adultos mayores. *Revista Psicologia e Saúde, 1*(1), 13–22.

López-Gil, M., Orueta, R., Gómez-Caro, S., Sánchez-Oropesa, A., Carmona, J., & Alonso-Moreno, F. (2009). El rol del cuidador de personas dependientes y sus repercusiones sobre su calidad de vida y su salud. *Revista Clínica Médica Familiar, 2*(1), 332–339.

López-Jiménez, M. J., Masa, J. F., Corral, J., Terán, J., Ordaz, E., Troncoso, M. F., ... Cancelo, L. (2016). Mid- and Long-Term Efficacy of Non-Invasive Ventilation in Obesity Hypoventilation Syndrome: The Pickwick's Study. *Archivos de Bronconeumologia, 52*(3), 158–165. doi:10.1016/j.arbr.2016.01.012 PMID:26656679

Lorenzi, C. M., Cilione, C., Rizzardi, R., Furino, V., Bellantone, T., Lugli, D., & Clini, E. (2004). Occupational Therapy and Pulmonary Rehabilitation of Disabled COPD Patients. *Respiration, 71*(3), 246–251. doi:10.1159/000077422 PMID:15133344

Lun, C. T., Chan, V. L., Leung, W. S., Cheung, A. P. S., Cheng, S. L., Tsui, M. S. N., & Chu, C. M. (2013). A pilot randomized study comparing two methods of non-invasive ventilation withdrawal after acute respiratory failure in chronic obstructive pulmonary disease. *Respirology (Carlton, Vic.), 18*(5), 814–819. doi:10.1111/resp.12080 PMID:23490403

Maccari, J. G., Teixeira, C., Savi, A., Oliveira, R. P., Machado, A. S., Tonietto, T. F., & … . (2014). Nebulization during spontaneous breathing, CPAP, and bi-level positive-pressure ventilation: A randomized analysis of pulmonary radioaerosol deposition. *Respiratory Care*, *59*(4), 479–484. doi:10.4187/respcare.02518 PMID:24003242

Maceiras, M., Juan, F., Navarro, M., Ramón, C., & García, R. (2016). *Proyecto Editorial Terapia Ocupacional*. Retrieved from http://www.sintesis.com

MacIntyre, N. R., Epstein, S. K., Carson, S., Scheinhorn, D., Christopher, K., & Muldoon, S. (2005). Management of patients requiring prolonged mechanical ventilation: Report of a NAMDRC consensus conference. *Chest*, *128*(6), 3937–3954. doi:10.1378/chest.128.6.3937 PMID:16354866

Maekura, R., Hiraga, T., Miki, K., Kitada, S., Miki, M., Yoshimura, K., Yamamoto, H., Kawabe, T., & Mori, M. (2015). Personalized pulmonary rehabilitation and occupational therapy based on cardiopulmonary exercise testing for patients with advanced chronic obstructive pulmonary disease. *International Journal of Chronic Obstructive Pulmonary Disease*, *10*, 1787–1800. doi:10.2147/COPD.S86455 PMID:26366071

Magano, C., Reis, M., Guedes, P. & Brito, R. M. (2007). Ventilação Não Invasiva. *Sinais Vitais, 72*, 13-19.

Mahoney, F. I., & Barthel, D. (1965). Functional evaluation: The Barthel Index. *Maryland State Medical Journal*, *14*, 56–61. PMID:14258950

Maraffi, T., Brambilla, A. M., & Cosentini, R. (2018). Non-invasive ventilation in acute cardiogenic pulmonary edema: How to do it. *Internal and Emergency Medicine*, *13*(1), 107–111. doi:10.100711739-017-1751-4 PMID:28952011

Mariano Juárez, L. (2012). *Definitions of evidence between signs and words. From Medical Anthropology to Narrative-Based Medicine. In Medicine and narratives. From theory to practice*. Editorial Círculo Rojo.

Mariano Juárez, L., Rodríguez Martín, B., & Conde, D. (2013). Narrative-based care: Redefining the hierarchy of evidence. *Nursing Index*, *22*(1-2), 55–59.

Márquez Romero, M. (2010). From the narratives of madness: I'm not mad! Why am I here? Approach to the narratives of illness in a mental health unit. *Periphery: Journal of Research and Training in Anthropology,* (12).

Martínez Muñiz, F. B., Esperanza Barrios, A., Pérez Labour, R. A., & Rodríguez González-Moro, J. M. (2017). Tratamiento de la insuficiencia respiratoria crónica. Oxigenoterapia. *Medicine - Programa de Formación Médica Continuada Acreditado, 12*(46), 2755–2765. . doi:10.1016/j.med.2017.12.003

Martinez Rivera, C., Costan Galicia, J., Alcázar Navarrete, B., Garcia-Polo, C., Ruiz Iturriaga, L. A., Herrejón, A., Ros Lucas, J. A., García-Sidro, P., Tirado-Conde, G., López-Campos, J. L., Mayoralas Alises, S., de Miguel-Díez, J., Esquinas, C., & Miravitlles, M. (2016). Factors Associated with Depression in COPD: A Multicenter Study. *Lung, 194*(3), 335–343. doi:10.100700408-016-9862-7 PMID:26932809

Martínez, L., Martín-Bejarano, L., Diéguez, Mª. D., Garrido, Mª. V., Romero, L., & Carrasco, Mª. A. (2018). Pincipales causas de la no adherencia al tratamiento con CPAP (Presión continua positiva de aire). *Hygia de enfermería: revista científica del colegio,* (98), 19–21.

Martínez, M., & De la Cuesta, C. (2016). La experiencia del cuidado de las mujeres cuidadoras con procesos crónicos de salud de familiares dependientes. *Atención primaria: Publicación oficial de la Sociedad Española de Familia y Comunitaria, 48*(2), 77-84.

Martínez-García, M. A., Durán-Cantolla, J., & Montserrat, J. M. (2010). El síndrome de apneas-hipopneas durante el sueño en edades avanzadas. *Archivos de Bronconeumologia, 46*(9), 479–488. doi:10.1016/j.arbres.2010.05.003 PMID:20580480

Mas, A., & Masip, J. (2014). Noninvasive ventilation in acute respiratory failure. *International Journal of COPD, 9*, 837–852. PMID:25143721

Masa, J. F., Utrabo, I., de Terreros, J. G., Aburto, M., Esteban, C., Prats, E., ... Farrero, E. (2016). Noninvasive ventilation for severely acidotic patients in respiratory intermediate care units. *BMC Pulmonary Medicine, 16*(1), 97. doi:10.118612890-016-0262-9 PMID:27387544

Masana, L. (2013). Between doctors and anthropologists. Attentive and committed listening to the narrated experience of chronic disease. In Evidence and narratives in health care: an anthropological perspective. Tarragona: Publicacions URV.

Masclans, J., Pérez-Terán, P., & Roca, O. (2015). Role of high flow oxygen therapy in acute respiratory failure. *Intensive Medicine, 39*(8), 505–515. doi:10.1016/j.medin.2015.05.009 PMID:26429697

McCarthy, B., Casey, D., Devane, D., Murphy, K., Murphy, E., & Lacasse, Y. (2015). Pulmonary rehabilitation for chronic obstructive pulmonary disease. *Cochrane Database of Systematic Reviews*, (2), 1–22. doi:10.1002/14651858.CD003793.pub3 PMID:25705944

McHugh, M. P., & Cosgrave, C. H. (2010). To stretch or not to stretch: The role of stretching in injury prevention and performance. *Scandinavian Journal of Medicine & Science in Sports, 20*(2), 169–181. PMID:20030776

McMillan, A., Bratton, D. J., Faria, R., Laskawiec-Szkonter, M., Griffin, S., Davies, R. J., Nunn, A. J., Stradling, J. R., Riha, R. L., & Morrell, M. J. (2014). Continuous Positive Airway Pressure in Older People with Obstructive Sleep Apnoea Syndrome (PREDICT): A 12-Month, Multicentre, Randomised Trial. *The Lancet. Respiratory Medicine, 2*(10), 804–812. doi:10.1016/S2213-2600(14)70172-9 PMID:25172769

Mctigue, K., Larson, J. C., Burke, G., Kotchen, J., Lewis, C. E., & Stefanick, M. L. (2006). Article. *Mortality and Cardiac and Vascular Outcomes in Extremely Obese Women, 296*(1), 79–86.

Megido, J. A., & Franco, Á. G. (2014). Ventilación Mecánica No Invasiva En El Tratamiento de La Insuficiencia Cardíaca Aguda. *Medicina Clínica, 142*, 55–58. doi:10.1016/S0025-7753(14)70084-3

Menadue, C., Piper, A., Van 't Hul, A., & Wong, K. (2014). Non-invasive ventilation during exercise training for people with chronic obstructive pulmonary disease. *Cochrane Database of Systematic Reviews, 5*. Advance online publication. doi:10.1002/14651858.CD007714.pub2 PMID:24823712

Mendes, R., Chorão, R., Martinho, F., & Gabriel, J. (2013). In-exsuflação mecânica em cuidados intensivos a propósito de um caso clínico de atelectasia pulmonar. *Revista de Saúde Amato Lusitano, 32*, 47-51. Retrieved from: http://portaisuls.azurewebsites.net/ulscb/wp-content/uploads/sites/9/2017/02/Revista-32-1.trimestre-2013.pdf

Mendes, F. A., Almeida, F. M., Cukier, A., Stelmach, R., Jacob-Filho, W., Martins, M. A., & Carvalho, C. R. F. (2011). Effects of aerobic training on airway inflammation in asthmatic patients. *Medicine and Science in Sports and Exercise, 43*(2), 197–203. doi:10.1249/MSS.0b013e3181ed0ea3 PMID:20581719

Mendes, J. (2015). Ventilação Mecânica Não Invasiva. In P. Ponce (Ed.), *J. Mendes. Manual de Medicina Intensiva* (pp. 113–122). Lidel.

Mercado, R. (2010). *Los entornos y contextos dentro del proceso de valoración. Evaluación e intervención en Terapia Ocupacional* (Vol. 7). Retrieved from www.revistatog.com

Miguel, A. F. (2017). Penetration of inhaled aerosols in the bronchial tree. *Medical Engineering & Physics, 44*, 25–31. doi:10.1016/j.medengphy.2017.03.004 PMID:28373015

Miravitlles, M., Izquierdo, J. L., Esquinas, C., Pérez, M., Calle, M., López-Campos, J. L., Rodríguez González-Moro, J. M., Casanova, C., Esteban, C., & de Lucas, P. (2017). The variability of respiratory symptoms and associated factors in COPD. *Respiratory Medicine, 129*, 165–172. doi:10.1016/j.rmed.2017.06.017 PMID:28732827

Miravitlles, M., & Ribera, A. (2017). Understanding the impact of symptoms on the burden of COPD. *Respiratory Research, 18*(1), 67. doi:10.118612931-017-0548-3 PMID:28431503

Miravitlles, M., Soler-Cataluña, J. J., Cataluña, C., Calle, M., Molina, J., Almagro, P., ... Ancocheã, J. (2017). Guía española de la enfermedad pulmonar obstructiva crónica (GesEPOC) 2017. Tratamiento farmacológico en fase estable. *Archivos de Bronconeumologia, 53*(6), 324–335. doi:10.1016/j.arbres.2017.03.018 PMID:28477954

Molina-Linde, J., Iáñez, M., & Iáñez, B. (2005). El apoyo social como modulador de la carga del cuidador de enfermos de Alzheimer. *Revista Psicologia e Saúde, 9*(1), 33–42.

Montserrat-Capdevila, J., Godoy, P., Marsal, J. R., Ortega, M., Pifarré, J., Alsedà, M., Castañ, M. T., & Barbé, F. (2018). Mental disorders in chronic obstructive pulmonary diseases. *Perspectives in Psychiatric Care, 54*(3), 398–404. doi:10.1111/ppc.12274 PMID:29577318

Moran, F., Bradley, J. M., & Piper, A. J. (2017). Non-invasive ventilation for cystic fibrosis. *Cochrane Database of Systematic Reviews*, (2), 1–21. PMID:28218802

Moreno, R. (2015). Terapias ventilatorias en el manejo del edema agudo de pulmón cardiogénico. *Revista Patología Respiratoria, 18*(1).

Moreno, S., Recio, C., Borrás, V., & Torns, T. (2016). Significados e imaginarios de los cuidados de larga duración en España. *Una aproximación cualitativa desde el discurso de las cuidadoras, 1*, 1-28.

Mortimore, I. L., Whittle, A. T., & Douglas, N. J. (1998). Comparison of Nose and Face Mask CPAP Therapy for Sleep Apnoea. *Thorax, 53*(4), 290–292. doi:10.1136/thx.53.4.290 PMID:9741373

Moruno Miralles, P., & Talavera Valverde, M. A. (2012). *Terapia ocupacional en salud mental.* Elsevier Masson.

Moxon, A., & Lee, G. (2015). Non-invasive ventilation in the emergency department for patients in type II respiratory failure due to COPD exacerbations. *Elsevier: International Emergency Nursing, 23*(3), 232–236. doi:10.1016/j.ienj.2015.01.002 PMID:25665756

Muñoz-Cobos, F., Acero-Guasch, N., Cuenca-del-Moral, R., Barnestein-Fonseca, P., Leiva-Fernández, F., & García-Ruiz, A. (2015). Cómo vivir con EPOC: Percepción de los pacientes. *Anales de Psicología, 32*(1), 18. doi:10.6018/analesps.32.1.186211

Murphy, P. B., Davidson, C., Hind, M. D., Simonds, A., Williams, A. J., Hopkinson, N. S., ... Hart, N. (2012). *Volume targeted versus pressure support non-invasive ventilation in patients with super obesity and chronic respiratory failure : a randomised controlled trial.* doi:10.1136/thoraxjnl-2011-201081

Nápolis, L. M., Dal Corso, S., Neder, J. A., Malaguti, C., Gimenes, A. C. O., & Nery, L. E. (2011). Neuromuscular electrical stimulation improves exercise tolerance in chronic obstructive pulmonary disease patients with better preserved fat-free mass. *Clinics (São Paulo), 66*(3), 401–406. doi:10.1590/S1807-59322011000300006 PMID:21552662

Naresh, M., & Punjabi, S. (2008). The Epidemiology of Adult Obstructive Sleep Apnea. *Proceedings of the American Thoracic Society, 5*(2), 136–143. doi:10.1513/pats.200709-155MG PMID:18250205

Nelson, M. E., Rejeski, W. J., Blair, S. N., Duncan, P. W., Judge, J. O., King, A. C., Macera, C. A., & Castaneda-Sceppa, C. (2007). Physical activity and public health in older adults: Recommendation from the American College of Sports Medicine and the American Heart Association. *Medicine and Science in Sports and Exercise, 39*(8), 1435–1445. doi:10.1249/mss.0b013e3180616aa2 PMID:17762378

Neves, J. T., & Lobão, M. J. (2012). Estudo multicêntrico de oxigenoterapia – uma auditoria nacional aos procedimentos de oxigenoterapia em enfermarias de medicina interna. *Revista Portuguesa de Pneumologia, 18*(2), 80–85. doi:10.1016/j.rppneu.2012.01.001 PMID:22280829

Nici, L., Donner, C., Wouters, E., Zuwallack, R., Ambrosino, N., Bourbeau, J., & Garvey, C. (2006). American thoracic society/European respiratory society statement on pulmonary rehabilitation. *American Journal of Respiratory and Critical Care Medicine*, *173*(12), 1390–1413. doi:10.1164/rccm.200508-1211ST PMID:16760357

Nicollini, A., Santo, M., Ferrera, L., Ferrari-Bravo, M., Barlascini, C., & Perazzo, A. (2014). The use of non-invasive ventilation in very old patients with hypercapnic acute respiratory failure because of COPD exacerbation. *International Journal of Clinical Practice*, *68*(12), 1523–1529. doi:10.1111/ijcp.12484 PMID:25283150

Nogueira, F., Nigro, C., Cambursano, H., Borsini, E., Silio, J., & Ávila, J. (2013). Practical guidelines for the diagnosis and treament of obstructive sleep apnea síndrome. *Medicine*, *73*(4), 349–362. PMID:23924537

Norma 028/2011. (2013). *Norma do Diagnóstico e Tratamento da Doença Pulmonar Obstrutiva Crónica*. Lisboa: Direção Geral de Saúde.

NOTT. (1980). Continuous or nocturnal oxygen therapy in hypoxemic chronic obstructive lung disease. *Annals of Internal Medicine*, *93*(3), 391–398. doi:10.7326/0003-4819-93-3-391 PMID:6776858

Nowbar, S., Burkart, K. M., Gonzales, R., Fedorowicz, A., Gozansky, W. S., Gaudio, J. C., Taylor, M. R. G., & Zwillich, C. W. (2004). Obesity-Associated hypoventilation in hospitalized patients: Prevalence, effects, and outcome. *The American Journal of Medicine*, *116*(1), 1–7. doi:10.1016/j.amjmed.2003.08.022 PMID:14706658

Ntoumenopoulos, G. (2015). Rehabilitation during mechanical ventilation: Review of the recent literature. *Intensive & Critical Care Nursing*, *31*(3), 125–132. doi:10.1016/j.iccn.2015.02.001 PMID:26026495

Ntoumenopoulos, G., Hammond, N., Watts, N., Thompson, K., Hanlon, G., Paratz, J., & Thomas, P. (2018). Secretion clearance Strategies in Australian and New Zealand Intensive Care Units. *Australian Critical Care*, *31*(4), 191–196. doi:10.1016/j.aucc.2017.06.002 PMID:28662942

Observatório Nacional das Doenças Respiratórias. (2017). *Relatório do Programa Nacional para as Doenças Respiratórias*. Autor.

OCD. (2015). *Indicación y empleo de la oxigenoterapia continua domiciliaria.* Retrieved from https://www.fisiorespiracion.es/indicacion_y_empleo_de_la_oxigenoterapia_continua_domiciliaria.pdf

Ojeda Castillejo, E., de Lucas Ramos, P., López Martin, S., Resano Barrios, P., Rodríguez Rodríguez, P., Morán Caicedo, L., Bellón Cano, J. M., & Rodriguez Gonzalez-Moro, J. M. (2015). Noninvasive Mechanical Ventilation in Patients with Obesity Hypoventilation Syndrome. Long-term Outcome and Prognostic Factors. *Archivos de Bronconeumologia*, *51*(2), 61–68. doi:10.1016/j.arbr.2014.06.016 PMID:24703500

Olmedo, P., & Sierra, A. (2004). Oxigenoterapia domiciliaria. *Neumosur.Net*. Retrieved from http://www.neumosur.net/files/EB02-20 ocd.pdf

Onen, F., & Onen, H. (2010). Syndrome d'apnées obstructives du sommeil et troubles cognitifs chez les sujets âgés. *Psychologie & Neuropsychiatrie du Vieillissement*, *8*(3), 9–163. PMID:20739254

Ordem Dos Enfermeiros. (2001). *Padrões de Qualidade dos Cuidados de Enfermagem - enquadramento conceptual enunciados descritivos*. Acedido a 9 de Dezembro de 2018. Disponível em: https://www.ordemenfermeiros.pt/media/8903/divulgar- padroes-de-qualidade-dos-cuidados.pdf

Ordem dos Enfermeiros. (2016). *Instrumentos de recolha de dados para a documentação dos cuidados especializados em Enfermagem de Reabilitação*. Ordem dos Enfermeiros.

Ordem dos Enfermeiros. (2018). *Guia Orientador de Boas Práticas – Reabilitação Respiratória*. Lisboa: Ordem dos Enfermeiros.

Orfanos, S., Jaffuel, D., Perrin, C., Molinari, N., Chanez, P., & Palot, A. (2017). Switch of noninvasive ventilation (NIV) to continuous positive airway pressure (CPAP) in patients with obesity hypoventilation syndrome: A pilot study. *BMC Pulmonary Medicine*, *17*(1), 1–11. doi:10.118612890-017-0391-9 PMID:28288605

Organização Mundial de Saúde. (2009). *World Health Organization Guidelines on Hand Hygiene in Health Care*. Autor.

Ortega Ruiz, F., Díaz Lobato, S., Galdiz Iturri, J. B., García Rio, F., Güell Rous, R., Morante Velez, F., ... Tàrrega Camarasa, J. (2014). Oxigenoterapia continua domiciliaria. *Archivos de Bronconeumologia*, *50*(5), 185–200. doi:10.1016/J.ARBRES.2013.11.025 PMID:24461631

Ortega, F., Lobato, S. D., Iturri, J. B. G., Rio, F. G., Rous, R. G., Velez, F. M., ... Camarasa, J. T. (2014). Continuous home oxygen therapy. *Archives of Bronchopneumology, 50*(5), 185-200.

Ortiz, M. M., Aguilera, A., & Hernández, C. (2016). Analizando las patologías más prevalentes en la edad avanzada. In *Investigación en salud y envejecimiento* (pp. 129–133). ASUNIVEP.

Ou, Y., Lin, Z., Wu, W., Luo, Q., & Chen, R. C. (2016). Efficacy of non-invasive ventilation as a rescue therapy for relieving dyspnea in patients with stable severe COPD. *Elsevier: Respiratory Medicine*, *121*, 74–80. PMID:27888995

Overbeek, J. (1984). *Historia de las teorías demográficas*. México: Fondo de Cultura Económica.

Ozyilmaz, E., Ugurlu, A. O., & Nava, S. (2014). Timing of noninvasive ventilation failure: Causes, risk factors and potential remedies. *BMC Pulmonary Medicine*, *14*(19), 1–10. doi:10.1186/1471-2466-14-19 PMID:24520952

Pamplona, P., & Morais, L. (2007). Treino de exercício na doença pulmonar crónica. [English Edition]. *Revista Portuguesa de Pneumologia*, *13*(1), 101–128. doi:10.1016/S0873-2159(15)30340-8 PMID:17315093

Papp, M. E., Wändell, P. E., Lindfors, P., & Nygren-Bonnier, M. (2017). Effects of yogic exercises on functional capacity, lung function and quality of life in participants with obstructive pulmonary disease: A randomized controlled study. *European Journal of Physical and Rehabilitation Medicine*, *53*(3), 447–461. doi:10.23736/S1973-9087.16.04374-4 PMID:27830924

Paranhos, W. Y., & Santos, V. L. C. G. (1999). Avaliação de risco para úlceras de pressão por meio da escala de Braden, na língua portuguesa. *Revista da Escola de Enfermagem da U S P.*, *33*(1), 191–206.

Paredes, M. C., & Aznar, I. (2009). *Fundamentos de la oxigenoterapia en situaciones agudas y crónicas: indicaciones, métodos, controles y seguimiento.* Elsevier. Retrieved from https://www.sciencedirect.com/science/article/pii/S1695403309003294

Paredes, M. L., De la Cruz, O. A., Aznar, I. C., Carrasco, M. M., de Agüero, M. B. G., Ruiz, E. (2009). Fundamentals of oxygen therapy in acute and chronic situations: indications, methods, controls and follow-up. *Annals of Pediatrics Peneumology.*

Parra, O., Sánchez-Armengol, A., Capote, F., Bonnin, M., Arboix, A., Campos-Rodríguez, F., & Macarrón, J. (2015). Efficacy of Continuous Positive Airway Pressure Treatment on 5-Year Survival in Patients with Ischaemic Stroke and Obstructive Sleep Apnea: A Randomized Controlled Trial. *Journal of Sleep Research*, *24*(1), 47–53. doi:10.1111/jsr.12181 PMID:25040553

Party, M. W. (1981). Long term domiciliary oxygen therapy in chronic hypoxic cor pulmonale complicating chronic bronchitis. *Lancet*, *1*, 681–685. PMID:6110912

Pelgrim, C. E., Peterson, J. D., Gosker, H. R., Schols, A. M. W. J., van Helvoort, A., Garssen, J., Folkerts, G., & Kraneveld, A. D. (2019). Psychological co-morbidities in COPD: Targeting systemic inflammation, a benefit for both? *European Journal of Pharmacology*, *842*, 99–110. doi:10.1016/j.ejphar.2018.10.001 PMID:30336140

Pépin, J. L., Leger, P., Veale, D., Langevin, B., Robert, D., & Lévy, P. (1995). Side Effects of Nasal Continuous Positive Airway Pressure in Sleep Apnea Syndrome: Study of 193 Patients in Two French Sleep Centers. *Chest*, *107*(2), 375–381. doi:10.1378/chest.107.2.375 PMID:7842764

Pereira, J., Sequeira, R., Marques, M. D. C., Oliveira, N., & Realista, S. (2016). Ventilação não-invasiva: opção terapêutica nos cuidados ao doente com dispneia em contexto pré-hospitalar. *Nursing Magazine Digital*. Available in: http://hdl.handle.net/10174/20492

Perrin, C., Rolland, F., Berthier, F., Duval, Y., & Jullien, V. (2015). Ventilation non invasive dans l'insuffisance respiratoire aiguë en service de pneumologie. *Elsevier Masson: Revue des Maladies Respiratoires*, *32*(9), 895–902. doi:10.1016/j.rmr.2015.03.002

Petersen, A., & Larsen, S. (2011). Occupational therapy intervention for patients with COPD rehabilitation at home. *International Journal of Integrated Care, 11*(Suppl). Retrieved from https://www.ncbi.nlm.nih.gov/pmc/articles/PMC3184825

Peterson, M. D., Rhea, M. R., & Alvar, B. A. (2005). Applications of the dose-response for muscular strength development: Areview of meta-analytic efficacy and reliability for designing training prescription. *Journal of Strength and Conditioning Research*, *19*(4), 950–958. doi:10.1519/00124278-200511000-00038 PMID:16287373

Pıhtılı, A., Bingöl, Z., & Kıyan, E. (2017). *The Predictors of Obesity Hypoventilation Syndrome in Obstructive Sleep Apnea*. doi:10.4274/balkanmedj.2015.1797

Pinto, C. J. C., & Sousa, P. M. L. (2016). *Ventilação Não Invasiva: desenvolvimento de linhas orientadoras recorrendo à metodologia Delphi* (Artigo baseado em Dissertação de Mestrado). Leiria: Instituto Politécnico de Leiria.

Pinto, C. J. C., & Sousa, P. M. L. (2016). *Ventilação não invasiva: uma revisão integrativa da literatura* (Artigo baseado em Dissertação de Mestrado). Leiria: Instituto Politécnico de Leiria.

Pinto. (2013). Ventilação Não Invasiva – Uma prática fundamentada em evidência científica. *Revista Nursing Edição, 25*(288).

Pinto, S. (2013). Ventilação Não Invasiva: Uma prática fundamentada em evidência científica. *Nursing Magazine Digital*, *288*, 1–14.

Podsiadlo, D., & Richardson, S. (1991). The timed "Up & Go": A test of basic functional mobility for frail elderly persons. *Journal of the American Geriatrics Society*, *39*(2), 142–148. doi:10.1111/j.1532-5415.1991.tb01616.x PMID:1991946

Porcel, A. (2011). *Construcción y validación de un sistema de evaluación del nivel de dependencia para el cuidado de los pacientes hospitalizados*. Universidad de Granada.

Price, D., Østrem, A., Thomas, M., & Welte, T. (2017). Dual bronchodilation in COPD: Lung function and patient-reported outcomes–a review. *International Journal of Chronic Obstructive Pulmonary Disease*, *12*, 141–168. doi:10.2147/COPD.S116719 PMID:28115839

Rabinovich, R. A., & Vilaró, J. (2010). Structural and functional changes of peripheral muscles in COPD patients. *Current Opinion in Pulmonary Medicine*, *16*(2), 123. doi:10.1097/MCP.0b013e328336438d PMID:20071991

Ram, F. S., Robinson, S. M., Black, P. N., & Picot, J. (2005). Physical training for asthma. *Cochrane Database of Systematic Reviews*, (4), CD001116. PMID:16235280

Ramírez-Molina, V. R., Gómez-de-Terreros, F. J., Barca-Durán, J., & Masa, J. F. (2017). Non-invasive Positive Airway Pressure in Obesity Hypoventilation Syndrome and Chronic Obstructive Pulmonary Disease: Present and Future Perspectives. *COPD*, *14*(4), 418–428. doi:10.1080/15412555.2017.1317730 PMID:28485989

Rapsey, C. M., Lim, C. C. W., Al-Hamzawi, A., Alonso, J., Bruffaerts, R., Caldas-de-Almeida, J. M., Florescu, S., de Girolamo, G., Hu, C., Kessler, R. C., Kovess-Masfety, V., Levinson, D., Medina-Mora, M. E., Murphy, S., Ono, Y., Piazza, M., Posada-Villa, J., ten Have, M., Wojtyniak, B., & Scott, K. M. (2015). Associations between DSM-IV mental disorders and subsequent COPD diagnosis. *Journal of Psychosomatic Research, 79*(5), 333–339. doi:10.1016/j.jpsychores.2015.08.005 PMID:26526305

Real, B. A., Jiménez, M. M., & Castro, E. M. (2016). Factores que predisponen al incumplimiento terapéutico en el anciano. In *Investigación en salud y envejecimiento* (pp. 111–115). ASUNIVEP.

Reeves, S., Kuper, A., & Hodges, B. D. (2008). Qualitative research methodologies: Ethnography. *BMJ (Clinical Research Ed.), 337*(3), a1020. doi:10.1136/bmj.a1020 PMID:18687725

Respiratorias Observatório Nacional Das Doenças. (2017). *Relatório de 2017.* Acedido a 19 de Novembro de 2018. Disponível em: http://respirarmelhor.pt/wp- content/uploads/2017/11/Relat%C3%B3rio-Completo-ONDR-2017.pdf

Ribeiro, M. B. S., & de Oliveira, L. R. (2005). *Interface: Comunicacao, saude, educacao. Interface - Comunicação, Saúde, Educação* (Vol. 9). Fundacao UNI. Retrieved from https://www.scielosp.org/scielo.php?pid=S1414-32832005000200023&script=sci_arttext&tlng=en

Ries, A. L., Make, B. J., & Reilly, J. J. (2011). Pulmonary Rehabilitation. *Respiratory Journal, 38*, 971-975.

Ries. (2008). Pulmonary Rehabilitation in Emphysema. *American Thoracic Society Journal. 5*(4), 524–529.

Ries, A. L., Bauldoff, G. S., Carlin, B. W., Casaburi, R., Emery, C. F., Mahler, D. A., Make, B., Rochester, C. L., ZuWallack, R., & Herrerias, C. (2007). Pulmonary rehabilitation: Joint ACCP/AACVPR evidence-based clinical practice guidelines. *Chest, 131*(5), 4S–42S. doi:10.1378/chest.06-2418 PMID:17494825

Río, F. G., Clau, L. B., Macario, C. C., Celli, B. R., Sanglás, J. E., Mangado, N. G., ... Romero, F. U. (2007). Respiratory pathology and airplane flights. *Bronchopneumology Archives, 43*(2), 101–125.

Rocha, S. M. P. (2017). *Impacto de um programa de reabilitação respiratória na qualidade de vida e nas atividades de vida diária de pessoas com doença pulmonar obstrutiva crónica* (Doctoral dissertation). Porto: Escola Superior de Enfermagem do Porto.

Rodríguez Ibagué, L.-F., Díaz Castillo, L. Á., Martinez-Santa, J., Rodríguez Ibagué, L. F., Díaz Castillo, L. Á., & Martínez Santa, J. (2008). Oxigenoterapia. *Instname:Universidad Del Rosario.* Retrieved from http://repository.urosario.edu.co/handle/10336/3696

Rodríguez, J. B., Carrión, M. R., Espina, M. A., Jiménez, J. P., Oliver, M. C., Péculo, J. A., & ... . (2005). *Marco conceptual, proceso enfermero en EPES.* Empresa Pública de Emergencias Sanitarias.

Roll, S. C. (2015). Role of sonographic imaging in occupational therapy practice. *The American Journal of Occupational Therapy, 69*(3), 1-8. . doi:10.5014/ajot.2015.015941

Roque. (2014). Ventilação Não-Invasiva. Vital Aire: Centro Hospitalar Lisboa Norte.

Rosalía. (2016). *La ansiedad de la EPOC*. Retrieved February 1, 2019, from https://www.tucuentasmucho.com/cuidarse/ansiedad-en-epoc/

Rosas Jiménez, C. A. (2017). Narrative medicine: The patient as "text", object and subject of compassion. *Bioethical Act, 23*(2), 351–359.

Rose, L., Adhikari, N., Poon, J., Leasa, D., & McKim, D. (2016). Cough Augmentation Techniques in the Critically Ill: A Canadian National Survey. *Respiratory Care, 61*(10), 1360–1368. doi:10.4187/respcare.04775 PMID:27624630

Rubio, M. C., Hermosa, J. L. R., & Nebreda, M. J. G. (2009). Ansiedad y EPOC. *Archivos de Bronconeumologia, 45*(SUPPL.5), 51–53. doi:10.1016/S0300-2896(09)72865-0 PMID:20116751

Ruiz López, M. (2013). *Ni familiares ni profesionales: cuidadoras inmigrantes contratadas* (Tesis doctoral). Serie: Salud.

Ruiz, F. O., Lobato, S. D., Iturri, J. B. G., Rio, F. G., Rous, R. G., Velez, F. M., . . . Camarasa, J. T. (2014). Continuous home oxygen therapy. *Archives of Bronchopneumology, 50*(5), 185-200.

Sainburg, R. L., Liew, S.-L., Frey, S. H., & Clark, F. (2017). Promoting Translational Research Among Movement Science, Occupational Science, and Occupational Therapy. *Journal of Motor Behavior, 49*(1), 1–7. doi:10.1080/00222895.2016.1271299 PMID:28166469

Salcedo Posadas, A., Neira Rodnguez, M., Beltrán Bengoechea, B., Albi Rodnguez, S., & Sequeiros González, A. O. (2001). *Diagnostic and therapeutic protocols at pediatrna*. Spanish Association of Pediatrna.

Salech, M. F., Jara, L. R., & Michea, A. L. (2012). Cambios fisiológicos asociados al envjecimiento. *Revista Médica Clínica Las Condes, 23*(1), 19–29. doi:10.1016/S0716-8640(12)70269-9

Santos Del Riego, S. (2005). *El ser humano como ser ocupacional* (Vol. 39). Retrieved from https://ruc.udc.es/dspace/bitstream/handle/2183/16961/SantosRiego_SerHumano.pdf?sequence=3

Santos, L. A., de Oliveira Sanchez, M., Pinto, R. G. S., da Luz Filho, A. C., Luz, K. R. G., & Soares, J. L. (2017). Efeitos da ventilação não invasiva em pacientes com insuficiência respiratória aguda: Uma revisão integrativa. *Revista Ciência & Saberes-Facema, 3*(3), 642–648.

Saraiva, P., Moreira, M. H., Santos, R., & Martins, R. (2014). Qualidade de Vida do Doente Submetido a Ventilação Não Invasiva. *Millenium, 46*, 179–195.

Scheerens, C., Deliens, L., Van Belle, S., Joos, G., Pype, P., & Chambaere, K. (2018). A palliative end-stage COPD patient does not exist: A qualitative study of barriers to and facilitators for early integration of palliative home care for end-stage COPD. *NPJ Primary Care Respiratory Medicine, 28*(1), 23. doi:10.103841533-018-0091-9 PMID:29925846

Schlosshan, D., & Elliott, M. W. (2004). Sleep·3: Clinical presentation and diagnosis of the obstructive sleep apnoea hypopnoea syndrome. *Thorax*, *59*(4), 347–352. doi:10.1136/thx.2003.007179 PMID:15047962

Schubert, C., Cruickshanks, K., & Dalton, D., Klein, Klein, B., & Nondahl D. (2002). Prevalence of Sleep Problems and Quality of Life in an Older Population. *Sleep*, *25*(8), 48–52. PMID:12489896

Schuler, M., Strohmayer, M., Mühlig, S., Schwaighofer, B., Wittmann, M., Faller, H., & Schultz, K. (2018). Assessment of depression before and after inpatient rehabilitation in COPD patients: Psychometric properties of the German version of the Patient Health Questionnaire (PHQ-9/PHQ-2). *Journal of Affective Disorders*, *232*, 268–275. doi:10.1016/j.jad.2018.02.037 PMID:29499510

Severino, S. (2017). Enfermagem de Reabilitação à Pessoa submetida a Ventilação Mecânica. In. C. Marques Vieira & L. Sousa (Eds.), Cuidados de Enfermagem de Reabilitação à Pessoa ao Longo da Vida (pp. 365-380). Loures: Lusodidacta.

Shiromani, J., Lu, J., Wagner, D., Thakkar, J., Greco, M. A., Basheer, R., & Thakkar, M. (2000). Compensatory sleep response to 12h wakefulness in Young and ol rats. *American Journal of Physiology. Regulatory, Integrative and Comparative Physiology*, *278*(1), 125–133. doi:10.1152/ajpregu.2000.278.1.R125 PMID:10644630

Sillen, M. J., Janssen, P. P., Akkermans, M. A., Wouters, E. F., & Spruit, M. A. (2008). The metabolic response during resistance training and neuromuscular electrical stimulation (NMES) in patients with COPD, a pilot study. *Respiratory Medicine*, *102*(5), 786–789. doi:10.1016/j.rmed.2008.01.013 PMID:18294832

Silva, L. C. (2012). *Validação do questionário clínico para a doença pulmonar obstrutiva crónica (CCQ) para a língua portuguesa*. Academic Press.

Silva, E. G. D., & Dourado, V. Z. (2008). Treinamento de força para pacientes com doença pulmonar obstrutiva crônica. *Revista Brasileira de Medicina do Esporte*, *14*(3), 231–238. doi:10.1590/S1517-86922008000300014

Silva, G. A. (2006). *Obesidade-Hipoventilação Alveolar.* Ribeirão Preto: Medicina.

Simmonds, A. K. (2003). Home Ventilation. *The European Respiratory Journal*, *22*(47, Supplement 47), 38–46. doi:10.1183/09031936.03.00029803

Skidmore, P. M. L., & Yarnell, J. W. G. (2004). *Commentary The obesity epidemic : prospects for prevention.* doi:10.1093/qjmed/hch136

Sociedad Española de Neumología y Cirugía torácica. (2018). Retrieved from https://www.separ.es/sites/default/files/SEPAR_NP_muertes_anuales_EPOC.pdf

Society of Critical Care Medicine. (2008). Fundamental Critical Care Suporte (2nd ed.). São Paulo: AWWE.

Soleimanpour, H., Taghizadieh, A., Salimi, S., Golzari, S. E., Mahmoodpoor, A., Safari, S., Esfanjani, R. M., & Heshmat, Y. (2014). Rapid shallow Breathing Index Survey, a predictor of non-Invasive Ventilation Necessity in Patients with Chronic Obstructive Pulmonary Disease Exacerbation: An Analytical Descriptive Prospective Study. *Red Crescent Medical Journal, 16*(2), 1–6. doi:10.5812/ircmj.13326 PMID:24719729

Sousa, L. M. M., Severino, S., & Pestana, H. C. F. C. (2018). Revisões da literatura científica: tipos, métodos e aplicações em enfermagem. *Rev Port Enferm Reabil*, 46-55. Disponível na Internet: https://www.aper.pt/ficheiros/revista/rpern0.pdf

Sousa, L., & Duque, H. (2012). Reabilitação respiratória na pessoa com Ventilação Não Invasiva. In *Manual de boas práticas na reabilitação respiratória – Conceitos* (pp. 211–225). Princípios e Técnicas. Lusociência.

Sousa, L., Duque, H., & Ferreira, A. (2012). Reabilitação respiratória na pessoa submetida a ventilação invasiva. In *Manual de boas práticas na reabilitação respiratória – Conceitos* (pp. 194–211). Princípios e Técnicas. Lusociência.

Sousa, M. M. D., Oliveira, J. D. S., Soares, M. J. G. O., Bezerra, S. M. M. D. S., Araújo, A. A. D., & Oliveira, S. H. D. S. (2017). Associação das condições sociais e clínicas à qualidade de vida de pacientes com insuficiência cardíaca. *Revista Gaúcha de Enfermagem, 38*(2). Advance online publication. doi:10.1590/1983-1447.2017.02.65885 PMID:28700025

Souza deMelo, F. E., Nogueira, I. D. B., Felismino, A. S., dosSantos Vicente, R. N. I., & Soares daSilva, I. (2015). Use of noninvasive ventilation for acute respiratory failure in intensive care unit. *Manual Therapy, Posturology & Rehabilitation Journal= Revista Manual Therapy*, 13.

Spruit, M. A., Singh, S. J., Garvey, C., ZuWallack, R., Nici, L., Rochester, C., & Pitta, F. (2013). An official American Thoracic Society/European Respiratory Society statement: Key concepts and advances in pulmonary rehabilitation. *American Journal of Respiratory and Critical Care Medicine, 188*(8), e13–e64. doi:10.1164/rccm.201309-1634ST PMID:24127811

Stone, R., Harrison, B., Lowe, D., Buckingham, R. J., Pursey, N. A., Hosker, H. S. R., Potter, J. M., & Roberts, C. M. (2009). Introducing the national COPD resources and outcomes project. *BioMedCentral Health Services Research., 9*(173), 173. Advance online publication. doi:10.1186/1472-6963-9-173 PMID:19778416

Strang, S., Osmanovic, M., Hallberg, C., & Strang, P. (2018). Family Caregivers' Heavy and Overloaded Burden in Advanced Chronic Obstructive Pulmonary Disease. *Journal of Palliative Medicine, 21*(12), 1768–1772. doi:10.1089/jpm.2018.0010 PMID:30118371

Strumpf, D. A., Millman, R. P., Carlisle, C. C., Grattan, L. M., Ryan, S. M., Erickson, A. D., & Hill, N. S. (1991). *Nocturnal Positive-Pressure Ventilation via Nasal Mask in Patients with Severe Chronic Obstructive Pulmonary Disease*. Academic Press.

Sturm, R. Ã. (2007). *Increases in morbid obesity in the USA*. doi:10.1016/j.puhe.2007.01.006

Sugerman, H. J., Baron, P. L., Fairman, R. P., & Evans, C. R. (1987). *Hemodynamic Dysfunction in Obesity Hypoventilation Syndrome and the Effiects of Treatment with Surgically Induced Weight Loss*. Academic Press.

Suh, E., Mandal, S., & Hart, N. (2013). Admission prevention in COPD: Nonpharmacological management. *BioMedCentral Medicine*, *11*(247). Advance online publication. doi:10.1186/1741-7015-11-247 PMID:24252219

Sullivan, C. E., & Ph, D. (n.d.). *Effects of Short-term NIPPY in the Treatment of Patients With Severe Obstructive Sleep Apnea and Hypercapnia*. doi:10.1378/chest.105.2.434

Sullivan, C. E., Berthon-Jones, M., Issa, F. G., & Eves, L. (1981). Reversal of obstructive sleep apnoea by continuous positive airway pressure applied through the nares. *Lancet*, *317*(8225), 862–865. doi:10.1016/S0140-6736(81)92140-1 PMID:6112294

Suzuki, T., Kurazumi, T., Toyonaga, S., Masuda, Y., Morita, Y., Masuda, J., Kosugi, S., Katori, N., & Morisaki, H. (2014). Evaluation of nonivasive positive pressure ventilation after extubation from moderate positive end-expiratory pressure level in patients undergoing cardovasicular surgery: A prospective observational study. *Journal of Intensive Care*, *2*(1), 5. Advance online publication. doi:10.1186/2052-0492-2-5 PMID:25520822

Tanaka, H., Monahan, K. D., & Seals, D. R. (2001). Age-predicted maximal heart rate revisited. *Journal of the American College of Cardiology*, *37*(1), 153–156. doi:10.1016/S0735-1097(00)01054-8 PMID:11153730

The Joanna Briggs Institute. (n.d.a). *Critical Appraisal Tools*. The University Adelaide. 2014. Acedido a 8 de Novembro de 2018. Disponível em: https://joannabriggs.org/research/critical-appraisal-tools.html

The Joanna Briggs Institute. (n.d.b). *Levels of Evidence*. The University Adelaide. 2014. Acedido a 8 de Novembro de 2018. Disponível em: http://joannabriggs.org/jbi- approach.html#tabbed-nav=Levels-of-Evidence

The Joanna Briggs Institute. (n.d.c). *Grades of Recommendations*. The University Adelaide. 2014. Acedido a 8 de Novembro de 2018. Disponível em: http://joannabriggs.org/jbi-approach.html#tabbed-nav=Grades-of-Recommendation

Troosters, T., Casaburi, R., Gosselink, R., & Decramer, M. (2005). Pulmonary rehabilitation in chronic obstructive pulmonary disease. *American Journal of Respiratory and Critical Care Medicine*, *172*(1), 19–38. doi:10.1164/rccm.200408-1109SO PMID:15778487

Tselebis, A., Pachi, A., Ilias, I., Kosmas, E., Bratis, D., Moussas, G., & Tzanakis, N. (2016). Strategies to improve anxiety and depression in patients with COPD: A mental health perspective. *Neuropsychiatric Disease and Treatment*, *12*, 297–328. doi:10.2147/NDT.S79354 PMID:26929625

Turner, S., Eastwood, P., Cook, A., & Jenkins, S. (2011). Improvements in symptoms and quality of life following exercise training in older adults with moderate/severe persistent asthma. *Respiration*, *81*(4), 302–310. doi:10.1159/000315142 PMID:20501982

Tzeng, A. C., & Bach, J. R. (2000). Prevention of pulmonary morbidity for patients with neuromuscular disease. *Chest*, *118*(5), 1390–1396. doi:10.1378/chest.118.5.1390 PMID:11083691

Ugarte, I. (2012). Narrative evidence and quality of care in the National Health System. In *Medicine and Narratives. From theory to practice*. Editorial Círculo Rojo.

Ugurlu, A. O., Sidhom, S. S., Khodabandeh, A., Ieong, M., Mohr, C., Lin, D. Y., ... Hill, N. S. (2015). Where is noninvasive ventilation actually delivered for acute respiratory failure? *Lung*, *193*(5), 779–788. doi:10.100700408-015-9766-y PMID:26210474

Ugurlu, A. O., Sidhom, S. S., Khodabandeh, A., Ieong, M., Mohr, C., Lin, D. Y., ... Hill, N. S. (2016). Use and outcomes of noninvasive ventilation for acute respiratory failure in different age groups. *Respiratory Care*, *61*(1), 36–43. doi:10.4187/respcare.03966 PMID:26374908

Usmani, Z. A., Carson, K. V., Cheng, J. N., Esterman, A. J., & Smith, B. J. (2011). Pharmacological interventions for the treatment of anxiety disorders in chronic obstructive pulmonary disease. *Cochrane Database of Systematic Reviews*, (11), CD008483. doi:10.1002/14651858.CD008483.pub2 PMID:22071851

Vaca, B., & Elizabeth, G. (2019). *Prevalencia y factores asociados a la Malnutrición en pacientes con Enfermedad Pulmonar Obstructiva Crónica*. Hospital José Carrasco Arteaga.

Van der Molen, T., Willemse, B. W. M., Schokker, S., ten Hacken, N. H. T., Postma, D. S., & Juniper, E. F. (2003). Development, validity and responsiveness of the Clinical COPD Questionnaire. *Health and Quality of Life Outcomes*, *1*(1), 13. doi:10.1186/1477-7525-1-13 PMID:12773199

Vargas Escobar, L. M. (2012). Aporte de enfermería a la calidad de vida del cuidador familiar del paciente con alzheimer. *Aquichan*, *12*(1), 62–76. http://www.scielo.org.co/pdf/aqui/v12n1/v12n1a07.pdf

Velasco, H., & Díaz de Rada, A. (1997). *The logic of Ethnographic Research*. Trotta.

Velloso, M., & Jardim, J. R. (2006). Study of energy expenditure during activities of daily living using and not using body position recommended by energy conservation techniques in patients with COPD. *Chest*, *130*(1), 126–132. doi:10.1378/chest.130.1.126 PMID:16840392

Verdugo, M. A., Canal, R., Jenaro, M. C., Badía, M., & Aguado-Díaz, A. L. (2012). *Application of the paradigm quality of life to the intervention with people with disabilities from a holistic perspective*. INICO.

Verdugo, M. A., Gómez, L., & Arias, B. (2007). The integral scale of quality of life: Development and preliminary study of its psychometric properties. *Zero Century*, *38*(4), 37–56.

Vieira, P. J., Chiappa, A. M. G., Cipriano, G. Jr, Umpierre, D., Arena, R., & Chiappa, G. R. (2014). Neuromuscular electrical stimulation improves clinical and physiological function in COPD patients. *Respiratory Medicine*, *108*(4), 609–620. doi:10.1016/j.rmed.2013.12.013 PMID:24418570

Vilardell, M. (2014). *Envejecer Bien*. Plataforma.

Vilaró, J., Resqueti, V. R., & Fregonezi, G. A. F. (2008). Avaliação clínica da capacidade do exercício em pacientes com doença pulmonar obstrutiva crônica. *Brazilian Journal of Physical Therapy, 12*(4). Advance online publication. doi:10.1590/S1413-35552008000400002

Villaescusa, C., Pinares, M., & Pieras, E. (2014). *Oxygen management systems. SEPAR procedures manual*. Oxygen Therapy Systems.

Vinaccia, S. & Quiceno, J. M. (2011). Health-related quality of life and psychological factors: a study from chronic obstructive pulmonary disease-EPOC. *Psychological Therapy, 29*(1), 65-75.

Vital, F. M. R., Ladeira, M. T., & Atallah, A. N. (2013). Non-Invasive Positive Pressure Ventilation (CPAP or Bilevel NPPV) for Cardiogenic Pulmonary Oedema. *Cochrane Database of Systematic Reviews*, (5), CD005351. doi:10.1002/14651858.CD005351.pub3 PMID:23728654

Volpato, E., Banfi, P., & Pagnini, F. (n.d.). *A psychological intervention to promote acceptance and adherence to non-invasive ventilation in people with chronic obstrutive pulmonary disease: study protocol of a randomised controlled trial*. BioMed Central.

Volpe, M., Naves, J., Riberio, G., Ruas, G., & Amato, M. (2018). Airway Clearance with na Optimized Mechanical Insufflation-Exsufflation Maneuver. *Respiratory Care, 63*(10), 1214–1222. doi:10.4187/respcare.05965 PMID:30018177

Walenga, R. L., Longest, P. W., Kaviratna, A., & Hindle, M. (2017). Aerosol Drug Delivery During Noninvasive Positive Pressure Ventilation: Efffects of Intersubject Variability and Excipient Enhanced Growth. *Journal of Aerosol Medicine and Pulmonary Drug Delivery, 30*(3), 190–205. doi:10.1089/jamp.2016.1343 PMID:28075194

Wang, J., Cui, Z., Liu, S., Gao, X., Gao, P., Shi, Y., Guo, S., & Li, P. (2016). Early use of noninvasive techniques for clearing respiratory secretions during noninvasive positive-pressure ventilation in patients with acute exacerbation of chronic obstructive pulmonary disease and hypercapnic encephalopathy: A prospective cohort study. *Medicine, 96*(12), e6371. doi:10.1097/MD.0000000000006371 PMID:28328824

Weatherspoon, D., Weatherspoon, C. A., & Abbott, B. (2015). Pharmacology Update on Chronic Obstructive Pulmonary Disease, Rheumatoid Arthritis, and Major Depression. *The Nursing Clinics of North America, 50*(4), 761–770. doi:10.1016/j.cnur.2015.07.006 PMID:26596663

Weaver, T. E., Kribbs, N. B., Pack, A. I., Kline, L. R., Chugh, D. K., Maislin, G., Smith, P. L., Schwartz, A. R., Schubert, N. M., Gillen, K. A., & Dinges, D. F. (1997). Night-To-Night Variability in CPAP Use Over the First Three Months of Treatment. *Sleep, 20*(4), 278–283. doi:10.1093leep/20.4.278 PMID:9231953

Wilkinson, T. M. A., Aris, E., Bourne, S., Clarke, S. C., Peeters, M., Pascal, T. G., Schoonbroodt, S., Tuck, A. C., Kim, V., Ostridge, K., Staples, K. J., Williams, N., Williams, A., Wootton, S., & Devaster, J.-M. (2017). A Prospective, Observational Cohort Study of the Seasonal Dynamics of Airway Pathogens in the Aetiology of Exacerbations in COPD. *Thorax, 72*(10), 919–927. doi:10.1136/thoraxjnl-2016-209023 PMID:28432209

Willard, H. S., Spackman, C. S., Crepeau, E. B., Cohn, E. S., & Schell, B. A. B. (2005). *Terapia ocupacional*. Médica Panamericana.

Windisch, W., Walterspacher, S., Siemon, K., Geiseler, J., & Sitter, H. (2010). Guidelines for non-invasive and invasive mechanical ventilation for treatment of chronic respiratory failure. *Pneumologie (Stuttgart, Germany)*, *64*(10), 640–652. doi:10.1055-0030-1255558 PMID:20799159

World Health Organization. (2002). *Active Ageing: a police framework*. Contribuição na 2.ª Assembleia das Nações Unidas sobre o Envelhecimento, Madrid.

Yang, I. A., Brown, J. L., George, J., Jenkins, S., McDonald, C. F., McDonald, V. M., Phillips, K., Smith, B. J., Zwar, N. A., & Dabscheck, E. (2017). COPD-X Australian and New Zealand guidelines for the diagnosis and management of chronic obstructive pulmonary disease: 2017 update. *The Medical Journal of Australia*, *207*(10), 436–442. doi:10.5694/mja17.00686 PMID:29129177

Yohannes, A. M., & Alexopoulos, G. S. (2014). Depression and anxiety in patients with COPD. *European Respiratory Review : An Official Journal of the European Respiratory Society*, *23*(133), 345–349. doi:10.1183/09059180.00007813 PMID:25176970

Yohannes, A. M., Dryden, S., & Hanania, N. A. (2018). The Validity and Responsiveness of the Depression, Anxiety and Stress Scale (DASS-21) in Chronic Obstructive Pulmonary Disease. *Chest*. Advance online publication. doi:10.1016/j.chest.2018.12.010 PMID:30594559

Yu, T., Frei, A., ter Riet, G., & Puhan, M. A. (2018). Impact of Stressful Life Events on Patients with Chronic Obstructive Pulmonary Disease. *Respiration*, *95*(2), 73–79. doi:10.1159/000481714 PMID:29156451

Zappia, T., Peter, S., Hall, G., Vine, J., Martin, A., Munns, A., Shields, L., & Verheggenn, M. (2013). Home oxygen therapy for infants and young children with acute bronchiolitis and other lower respiratory tract infections: The HiTHOx program. *Issues in Comprehensive Pediatric Nursing*, *36*(4), 309–318. doi:10.3109/01460862.2013.834397 PMID:24083944

Zhu, N., Suarez-Lopez, J. R., Sidney, S., Sternfeld, B., Schreiner, P. J., Carnethon, M. R., Lewis, C., Crow, R. S., Bouchard, C., Haskell, W. L., & Jacobs, D. R. Jr. (2010). Longitudinal examination of age-predicted symptom-limited exercise maximum HR. *Medicine and Science in Sports and Exercise*, *42*(8), 1519–1527. doi:10.1249/MSS.0b013e3181cf8242 PMID:20639723

About the Contributors

David José Murteira Mendes, born in Évora (Portugal) in the 4th of July of 1966, achieved a PhD degree in Computer Science in Universidade de Évora (Portugal) in 2014. Previously he owns a MSc in Applied Artificial Intelligence also from the same University, a MBA from Universidad de Extremadura (Badajoz, Spain) a BSc in Computer Science from Universidade Nova de Lisboa (Portugal). He has developed a Software Engineer career from 1989 and developed mainly software for government organizations in particular for Hospitals intended both for management and clinical support. He acted as IT coordinator near the Mozambican Health Ministry after having designed the national Health Information System according to the governments memorandum "Health Strategic Program 2009/14". Currently as of 2018 he is R&D Manager for DECSIS, SA where he maintains the relations with academia regarding ICT applied to Healthy Ageing Environments. He has special interest in scuba diving being an active PADI instructor and underwater photographer.

* * *

Raquel Amorim is a nurse in the Hospital Center of Setúbal. Master of the Nursing Course, in the specialty of Rehabilitation Nursing. The research areas are the Elderly and the Aging, Rehabilitation Nursing and the Person in critical condition.

Carmen Cipriano-Crespo has a Degree in Social and Cultural Anthropology and Degree in Occupational Therapy. Doctor in Social and Cultural Anthropology in the UNED. She teaches at the Faculty of Occupational Therapy, Speech Therapy and Nursing in Talavera de la Reina, University of Castilla la Mancha (Spain). She has participated in research projects related to Narrative-Based Medicine, Gender Studies, Parenting Guidelines and Sleep Management in Families with children. He has published several articles and participated in national and international congresses.

David Conde-Caballero is a graduate in Nursing, Graduate in Podiatry, Graduate in Social and Cultural Anthropology. Doctor in Anthropology. Professor at the University of Extremadura (Spain), Faculty of Nursing and Occupational Therapy. He has worked on aspects related to food from the perspective of anthropology. In relation to care, he is the author of several publications that try to approach the power of narratives as first-order evidence in nursing care. Thus, Nursing Based on Narratives has been one of his objects of study, an approach from which he has been interested in pathologies such as HIV or Borderline Personality Disorders among many other situations.

Ana Costa is a nurse in the Hospital Center of Setúbal. Master of the Nursing Course, in the specialty of Rehabilitation Nursing. The research areas are the Elderly and the Aging, Rehabilitation Nursing and the Person in critical condition.

Patricia Domínguez Isabel Graduated in Nursing at the University of Castilla-La Mancha, Toledo. Author of scientific articles related to the history of nursing, gender and health. Member of the associated study HISAG-EP (History, Health, Gender, Spain-Portugal), which belongs to the structuring project UICISA: E (Research Unit, Coimbra).

Blanca Espina Jerez is graduated in Psychology, and specialist in Clinical Psychology. She is currently studying Nursing Degree at the University of Castilla La-Mancha (UCLM), Toledo, (Spain). She has published scientific papers in high impact journals and book chapters. At the same time, she has contributed to the scientific diffusion of her work in National and International Congresses, at university level and with general population. Blanca is part of the HISAG-EP Associated Study, belonging to the Structuring Project: History and Epistemology of Health and Disease of the UICISA-E Research Unit, University of Coimbra (Portugal). In 2016, she obtained a practical scholarship and contributed as a volunteer clinical psychology in Mexico City for three months. In 2018 she has received the recognition of The Social Council in the modality of "UCLM Student" for her excellent academic results.

Ana Patricia Miguel is a Registered Nurse since 2002. Until 2016 worked in A&E. Since 2017 in Gastroenterology Ward. Since 2015 work in pre-hospital emergency care.

M. Teresa Ortuño has a degree in Biological Sciences, Biochemistry specialty (University of Valencia, 1992); Health specialty in Clinical Pathology (BIR, 2003); PhD in Biological Sciences from the Universidad Complutense de Madrid (2004).

Post-specialized health-training contract "Río Hortega" (ISCiiiI) (2007-2010). Post-doctoral researcher at the Instituto de Investigaciones Biomédicas "Alberto Sols", Instituto de Investigación Sanitaria Hospital 12 de Octubre, and postdoctoral fellow at Dana Farber Cancer Institute (Boston, MA, USA). Principal Investigator of three health research projects and collaborating researcher in 10 research projects, of public financing and competitive regime. Evaluator of the Agencia Estatal de Investigación, the Fundación Progreso y Salud (Consejería de Salud de Andalucía), and the Institut National de la Santé et de la Recherche Médicale (Inserm, France). Associate Professor of the Faculty of Physiotherapy and Nursing of Toledo (UCLM, 2008-2018). Currently, Assistant Doctor Professor of the same Faculty since December 2018. Scientific publications indexed in JCR, and communications to National and International Congresses, related to Biochemistry, and Molecular and Cellular Biology.

Marlene Silvestre is a nurse in the medical service 3 in the University Hospital of the Algarve; Master student in Nursing at the Polytechnic Institute of Portalegre. Degree in Nursing at the University of Algarve's School of Health, since 2012.

Isabel Simões graduated as a Nurse in 1995. Education Science Bachelor in 2002; Specialist on Rehabilitation Nursing in 2006; Postgraduate in Health Services Management in 2017. Areas of Experience: Intensive Care, Vascular Surgery, Cardiology, Pneumology. Currently Chief Nurse of Pneumology Service at Hospital de Egas de Moniz in Lisbon.

João Vieira is an Adjunct Professor in the Polytechnic Institute of Beja, Department of Health. Master of Science in Nursing, in the specialty of Rehabilitation Nursing. Areas of interest in research are the Critically Ill Patient, Critical Care Nursing, Rehabilitation Nursing, Aging and the Elderly.

Index

I

L

M

N

O

P

Q

R

S

T

V

Purchase Print, E-Book, or Print + E-Book

IGI Global's reference books can now be purchased from three unique pricing formats:
Print Only, E-Book Only, or Print + E-Book.
Shipping fees may apply.

www.igi-global.com

Recommended Reference Books

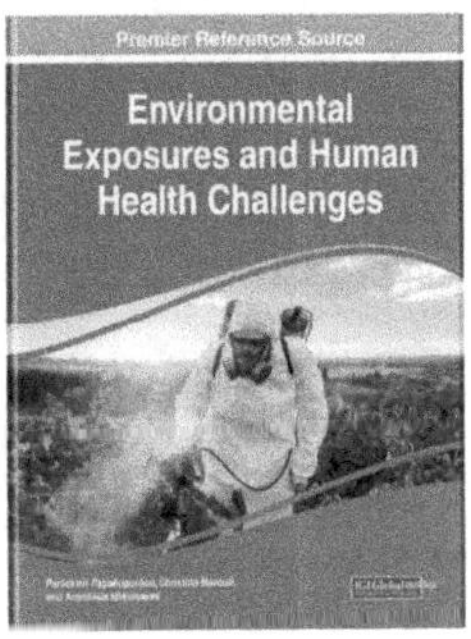

ISBN: 978-1-5225-7635-8
© 2019; 449 pp.
List Price: $255

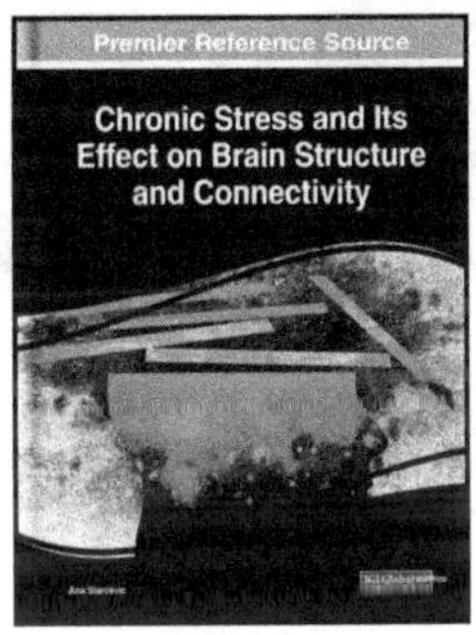

ISBN: 978-1-5225-7513-9
© 2019; 318 pp.
List Price: $225

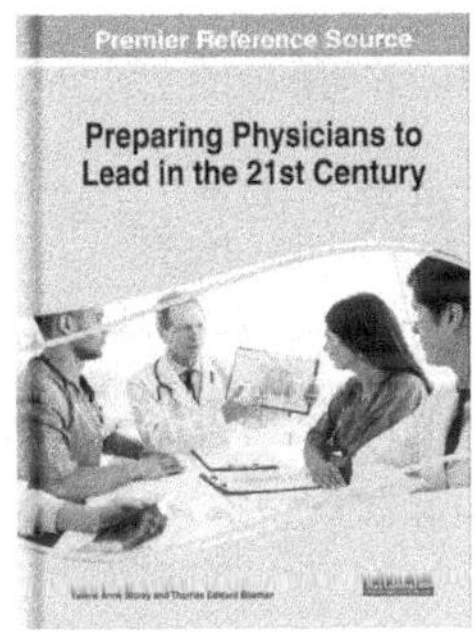

ISBN: 978-1-5225-7576-4
© 2019; 245 pp.
List Price: $245

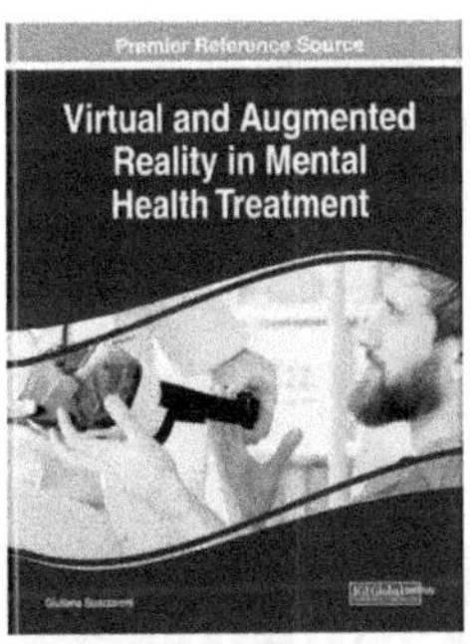

ISBN: 978-1-5225-7168-1
© 2019; 329 pp.
List Price: $265

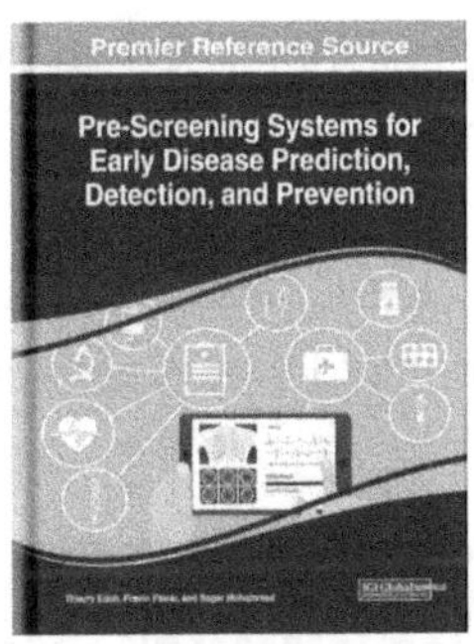

ISBN: 978-1-5225-7131-5
© 2019; 395 pp.
List Price: $245

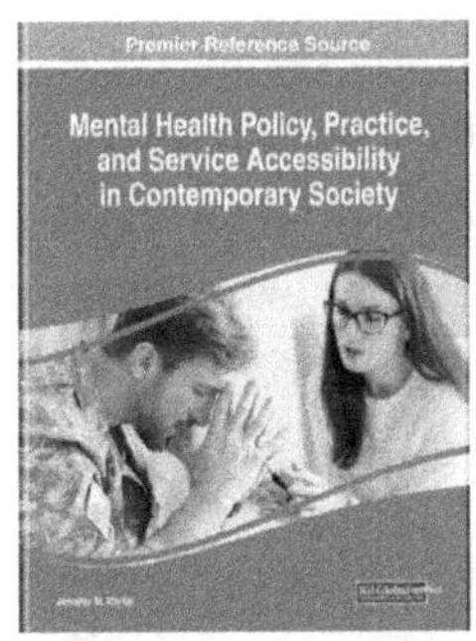

ISBN: 978-1-5225-7402-6
© 2019; 323 pp.
List Price: $245

Looking for free content, product updates, news, and special offers?
Join IGI Global's mailing list today and start enjoying exclusive perks sent only to IGI Global members.
Add your name to the list at **www.igi-global.com/newsletters.**

Publisher of Peer-Reviewed, Timely, and Innovative Academic Research

IGI Global
DISSEMINATOR OF KNOWLEDGE

www.igi-global.com Sign up at www.igi-global.com/newsletters facebook.com/igiglobal twitter.com/igiglobal

Ensure Quality Research is Introduced to the Academic Community

Become an IGI Global Reviewer for Authored Book Projects

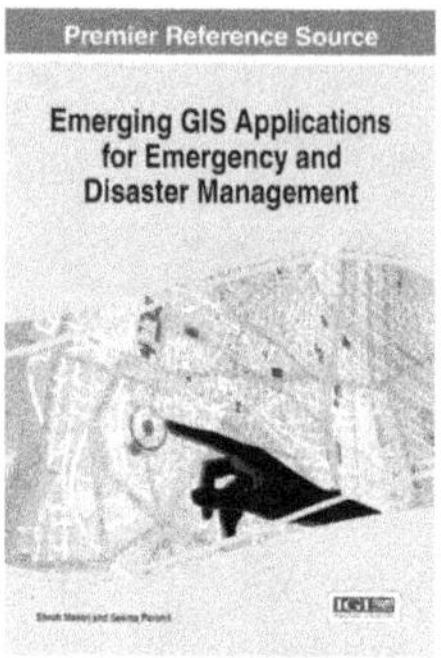

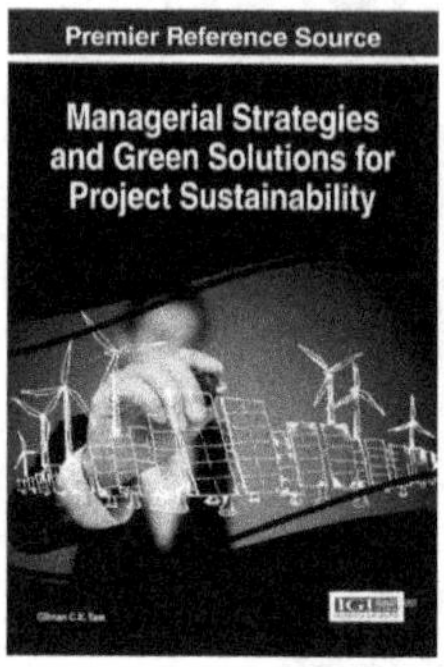

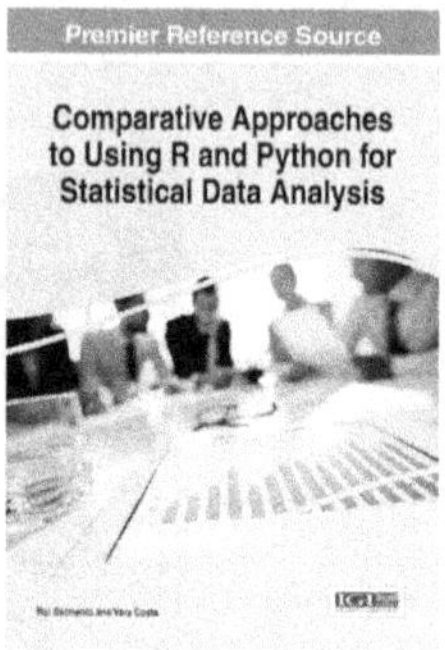

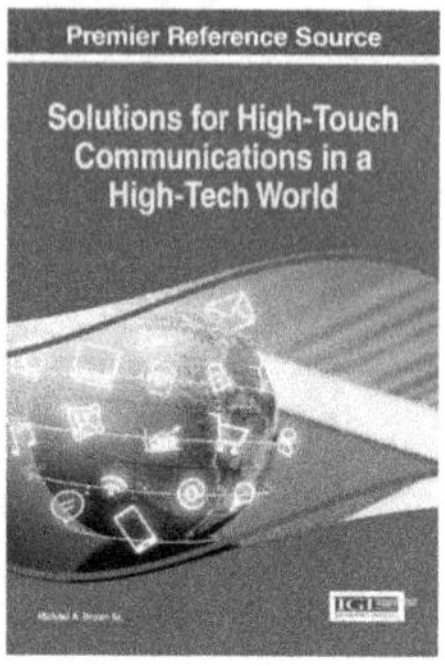

The overall success of an authored book project is dependent on quality and timely reviews.

In this competitive age of scholarly publishing, constructive and timely feedback significantly expedites the turnaround time of manuscripts from submission to acceptance, allowing the publication and discovery of forward-thinking research at a much more expeditious rate. Several IGI Global authored book projects are currently seeking highly-qualified experts in the field to fill vacancies on their respective editorial review boards:

Applications and Inquiries may be sent to:
development@igi-global.com

Applicants must have a doctorate (or an equivalent degree) as well as publishing and reviewing experience. Reviewers are asked to complete the open-ended evaluation questions with as much detail as possible in a timely, collegial, and constructive manner. All reviewers' tenures run for one-year terms on the editorial review boards and are expected to complete at least three reviews per term. Upon successful completion of this term, reviewers can be considered for an additional term.

If you have a colleague that may be interested in this opportunity, we encourage you to share this information with them.

IGI Global Proudly Partners With eContent Pro International

Receive a 25% Discount on all Editorial Services

Editorial Services

IGI Global expects all final manuscripts submitted for publication to be in their final form. This means they must be reviewed, revised, and professionally copy edited prior to their final submission. Not only does this support with accelerating the publication process, but it also ensures that the highest quality scholarly work can be disseminated.

English Language Copy Editing

Let eContent Pro International's expert copy editors perform edits on your manuscript to resolve spelling, punctuaion, grammar, syntax, flow, formatting issues and more.

Scientific and Scholarly Editing

Allow colleagues in your research area to examine the content of your manuscript and provide you with valuable feedback and suggestions before submission.

Figure, Table, Chart & Equation Conversions

Do you have poor quality figures? Do you need visual elements in your manuscript created or converted? A design expert can help!

Translation

Need your documjent translated into English? eContent Pro International's expert translators are fluent in English and more than 40 different languages.

Hear What Your Colleagues are Saying About Editorial Services Supported by IGI Global

"The service was very fast, very thorough, and very helpful in ensuring our chapter meets the criteria and requirements of the book's editors. I was quite impressed and happy with your service."

– Prof. Tom Brinthaupt,
Middle Tennessee State University, USA

"I found the work actually spectacular. The editing, formatting, and other checks were very thorough. The turnaround time was great as well. I will definitely use eContent Pro in the future."

– Nickanor Amwata, Lecturer,
University of Kurdistan Hawler, Iraq

"I was impressed that it was done timely, and wherever the content was not clear for the reader, the paper was improved with better readability for the audience."

– Prof. James Chilembwe,
Mzuzu University, Malawi

Email: customerservice@econtentpro.com **www.igi-global.com/editorial-service-partners**

IGI Global
DISSEMINATOR OF KNOWLEDGE
www.igi-global.com

Celebrating Over 30 Years of Scholarly Knowledge Creation & Dissemination

InfoSci®-Books

A Database of Over 5,300+ Reference Books Containing Over 100,000+ Chapters Focusing on Emerging Research

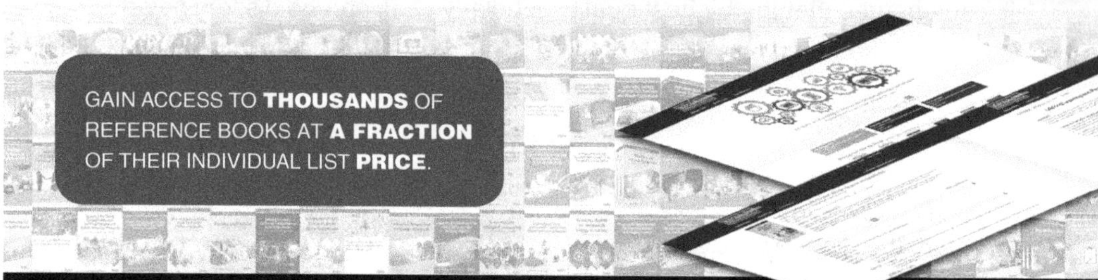

InfoSci®-Books Database

The **InfoSci®-Books** database is a collection of over 5,300+ IGI Global single and multi-volume reference books, handbooks of research, and encyclopedias, encompassing groundbreaking research from prominent experts worldwide that span over 350+ topics in 11 core subject areas including business, computer science, education, science and engineering, social sciences and more.

Open Access Fee Waiver (Offset Model) Initiative

For any library that invests in IGI Global's InfoSci-Journals and/ or InfoSci-Books databases, IGI Global will match the library's investment with a fund of equal value to go toward **subsidizing the OA article processing charges (APCs) for their students, faculty, and staff** at that institution when their work is submitted and accepted under OA into an IGI Global journal.*

INFOSCI® PLATFORM FEATURES

- No DRM
- No Set-Up or Maintenance Fees
- A Guarantee of No More Than a 5% Annual Increase
- Full-Text HTML and PDF Viewing Options
- Downloadable MARC Records
- Unlimited Simultaneous Access
- COUNTER 5 Compliant Reports
- Formatted Citations With Ability to Export to RefWorks and EasyBib
- No Embargo of Content (Research is Available Months in Advance of the Print Release)

**The fund will be offered on an annual basis and expire at the end of the subscription period. The fund would renew as the subscription is renewed for each year thereafter. The open access fees will be waived after the student, faculty, or staff's paper has been vetted and accepted into an IGI Global journal and the fund can only be used toward publishing OA in an IGI Global journal. Libraries in developing countries will have the match on their investment doubled.*

To Learn More or To Purchase This Database:
www.igi-global.com/infosci-books
eresources@igi-global.com • Toll Free: 1-866-342-6657 ext. 100 • Phone: 717-533-8845 x100

IGI Global
DISSEMINATOR OF KNOWLEDGE
www.igi-global.com

IGI Global
DISSEMINATOR OF KNOWLEDGE
www.igi-global.com

Publisher of Peer-Reviewed, Timely, and Innovative Academic Research Since 1988

IGI Global's Transformative Open Access (OA) Model: **How to Turn Your University Library's Database Acquisitions Into a Source of OA Funding**

In response to the OA movement and well in advance of Plan S, IGI Global, early last year, unveiled their OA Fee Waiver (Offset Model) Initiative.

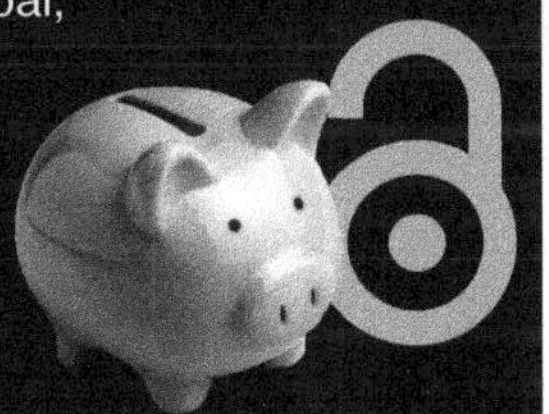

Under this initiative, librarians who invest in IGI Global's InfoSci-Books (5,300+ reference books) and/or InfoSci-Journals (185+ scholarly journals) databases will be able to subsidize their patron's OA article processing charges (APC) when their work is submitted and accepted (after the peer review process) into an IGI Global journal.*

How Does it Work?

1. When a library subscribes or perpetually purchases IGI Global's InfoSci-Databases including InfoSci-Books (5,300+ e-books), InfoSci-Journals (185+ e-journals), and/or their discipline/subject-focused subsets, IGI Global will match the library's investment with a fund of equal value to go toward subsidizing the OA article processing charges (APCs) for their patrons.

   Researchers: Be sure to recommend the InfoSci-Books and InfoSci-Journals to take advantage of this initiative.
2. When a student, faculty, or staff member submits a paper and it is accepted (following the peer review) into one of IGI Global's 185+ scholarly journals, the author will have the option to have their paper published under a traditional publishing model or as OA.
3. When the author chooses to have their paper published under OA, IGI Global will notify them of the OA Fee Waiver (Offset Model) Initiative. If the author decides they would like to take advantage of this initiative, IGI Global will deduct the US$ 1,500 APC from the created fund.
4. This fund will be offered on an annual basis and will renew as the subscription is renewed for each year thereafter. IGI Global will manage the fund and award the APC waivers unless the librarian has a preference as to how the funds should be managed.

Hear From the Experts on This Initiative:

"I'm very happy to have been able to make one of my recent research contributions, 'Visualizing the Social Media Conversations of a National Information Technology Professional Association' featured in the *International Journal of Human Capital and Information Technology Professionals*, freely available along with having access to the valuable resources found within IGI Global's InfoSci-Journals database."

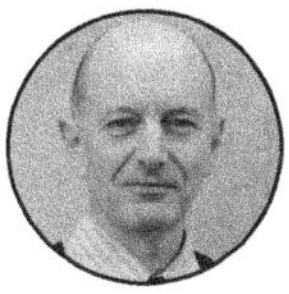

– **Prof. Stuart Palmer**,
Deakin University, Australia

For More Information, Visit: www.igi-global.com/publish/contributor-resources/open-access or contact IGI Global's Database Team at eresources@igi-global.com

www.ingramcontent.com/pod-product-compliance
Lightning Source LLC
LaVergne TN
LVHW081325300926
849161LV00008B/1878
* 9 7 8 1 7 9 9 8 3 5 3 1 8 *